P9-CAT-082

The Child with Multiple Birth Defects

OXFORD MONOGRAPHS ON MEDICAL GENETICS

General Editors
ARNO G. MOTULSKY   MARTIN BOBROW
PETER S. HARPER   CHARLES SCRIVER

Former Editors
J. A. FRASER ROBERTS   C. O. CARTER

OXFORD MONOGRAPHS ON MEDICAL GENETICS NO. 31

The Child with Multiple Birth Defects

SECOND EDITION

M. Michael Cohen, Jr.

Professor of Oral & Maxillofacial Pathology,
Pediatrics, Community Health & Epidemiology,
Health Services Administration,
Sociology & Social Anthropology
Dalhousie University
Halifax, Nova Scotia, Canada

New York   Oxford
OXFORD UNIVERSITY PRESS
1997

Oxford University Press

Oxford   New York
Athens   Auckland   Bangkok
Bogota   Bombay   Buenos Aires   Calcutta
Cape Town   Dar es Salaam   Delhi
Florence   Hong Kong   Istanbul   Karachi
Kuala Lumpur   Madras   Madrid   Melbourne
Mexico City   Nairobi   Paris   Singapore
Taipei   Tokyo   Toronto

and associated companies in
Berlin   Ibadan

Copyright © 1997 by Oxford University Press, Inc.

Published by Oxford University Press, Inc.,
198 Madison Avenue, New York, New York 10016

Oxford is a registered trademark of Oxford University Press

All rights reserved. No part of this publication may be reproduced,
stored in a retrieval system, or transmitted, in any form or by any means,
electronic, mechanical, photocopying, recording, or otherwise,
without the prior permission of Oxford University Press.

Library of Congress Cataloging-in-Publication Data
Cohen, M. Michael (Meyer Michael, Jr.), 1937–
The child with multiple birth defects /
M. Michael Cohen, Jr.—2nd ed.
p.   cm.   Includes bibliographical references and index.
ISBN 0-19-509926-5
1. Abnormalities, Human—Diagnosis.
2. Genetic disorders—Diagnosis.
3. Syndromes in children—Diagnosis.
I. Title.
[DNLM: 1. Abnormalities, Multiple.
QS 675 C678c 1997]   RB155.6.C64   1997
616'.043—dc20   DNLM/DLC   for Library of Congress   96-4650

1   3   5   7   9   8   6   4   2

Printed in the United States of America
on acid-free paper

To

Robert J. Gorlin
and
John M. Opitz

and to the memory of

David W. Smith
and
Josef Warkany

Foreword

I have often been asked by pediatric residents and tyro clinical geneticists, "How do you go about diagnosing syndromes?" Usually I have lamely told them that they should begin by examining as many atlases and texts on dysmorphology as they are able, but, in truth, this will only get them part way—and not very far at that.

My bias is that the really great diagnosticians are in a class by themselves, an order of magnitude better, seeming almost to intuit the answer to a clinical dilemma. Few achieve the clinical acumen of Michael Cohen. However, a *good* level of diagnostic excellence is easily achievable—with clinical experience and a great how-to book.

Before Mike Cohen's seminal text, there was no *vade mecum* that filled the bill. I view the book as a shibboleth to this field, which some have viewed as arcane. In the first two chapters, Dr. Cohen gives the reader the requisite vocabulary, which is so much a part of the field. He then discusses qualitative and quantitative approaches to dysmorphology. In single chapters, Dr. Cohen reviews and distills in a lively fashion an understanding of clinical genetics, teratogens, various syndrome classifications, and syndrome delineation. Two chapters really stand out as classic—ones that I secretly wish I had written myself—one on dysmorphic growth and development and another on psychosocial considerations. The material was "out there"—it just wasn't gathered together before this marvelous compendium was made. This text ranks high on my list of influential books.

Robert J. Gorlin
Regent's Professor Emeritus
University of Minnesota

Foreword to the First Edition

A syndrome is a disease picture composed of various signs and symptoms that "run together." The phenomenon of regular groupings of pathologic manifestations was known to Hippocrates and Galen, and their followers continued use of the concept, substituting "morbus" or "symptom complex" at times for the same idea. In 1957, Leiber and Olbrich published a *Dictionary of Clinical Syndromes* (Urban and Schwarzenberg, Munich) that not only listed thousands of then-known syndromes and their synonyms, definitions, components, and differential diagnoses with pertinent references but also analyzed the entities in regard to etiology, pathogenesis, nomenclature, and scientific value. One obvious justification for such a book was that the common medical dictionaries could not include all the established syndromes and their confusing names.

In recent years, this need has been further increased owing to the renewed interest of the medical profession in congenital disorders, particularly malformations, that have a marked tendency to multiple manifestations. A flood of observations of and publications on syndromes has pervaded the medical literature, and many volumes have appeared that aid practicing physicians in labeling their patients with congenital malformations. Such books, useful as they are for rapid diagnoses, represent a certain danger because the labels often are substitutes for understanding and analysis of the patients' anomalies, of the families' problems, and of the communities' burdens.

It is time to pause and review the abundance of publications, to classify and evaluate them, and to direct the flood into useful channels. The present volume has been written to do this. Dr. Michael Cohen has an encyclopedic knowledge of malformation syndromes and an analytical mind that enables him to discuss with clarity definitions, delineations, variabilities, heterogeneities, terminologies, and etiologies of syndromes. His efforts will benefit those who want to study syndromology in depth and those who want to write about various syndromes. No doubt this book will help to bring order into an area that has grown too fast and has become confusing to readers and contributors who did not grow up with the development of this field.

Josef Warkany, M.D., D.Sc.
Professor of Research Pediatrics
University of Cincinnati
Children's Hospital Research Foundation
Cincinnati, Ohio

Preface

The reason for writing the first edition of this book in 1982[1] was that medical genetics books of that era included very little about multiple congenital anomaly syndromes, and those that were mentioned—chromosomal syndromes and a few monogenic syndromes—received only cursory treatment. Sporadic syndromes, both common and uncommon, received no attention. More important, the process of syndrome delineation and its implications were never discussed at all. Opitz and Herrmann[5] characterized most medical curricula of that era:

Most schools continue to concentrate on teaching medical students primarily the manifestations of surgical lesions and of medical disease. A brief stay on pediatrics during medical school does not suffice to teach the student how to take a routine 3-generation pedigree, how to conduct a thorough physical examination including a dermatoglyphic study, or how to analyze a few aspects of pre- and postnatal growth and development. We know of few medical students who have learned to measure bones and to analyze their . . . [developmental] . . . characteristics from roentgenograms; far fewer have learned the use or need for anthropometric equipment; and virtually none can make an intelligent statement after inspection of the patient's teeth. Some of these skills are acquired by house-officers as they rotate through a genetics service. At the present time, though, few house-officers acquire the skill or experience required to practice good clinical genetics unless they take a fellowship in clinical genetics. . . .

This book was, and still is, an approach to the patient with multiple anomalies. It deals with the underpinnings of the field—the principles of syndromology. I have written it for students, residents, fellows, and anyone else who has an interest in syndromology. This book assumes some general understanding of the rudiments of both medicine and genetics. Topics such as embryology, advanced genetics, and specific clinical management receive no more than passing mention. These topics are covered in various textbooks. Nor is this book an encyclopedic treatise on specific syndromes. Many books cover that ground very well (see Table 11-2). The conceptual aspects of syndromology are emphasized here.

The field has advanced dramatically since the 1982 edition, necessitating fundamental changes. Thus, I have written a brand new book for Oxford University Press. The organization has changed since the last edition. Not only have new chapters been added, but all of the chapters have been placed in a more logical order. The book can be divided roughly into three general sections. In the first section, the building blocks for understanding syndromology are discussed in Chapters 1–7. In the second section, the formal aspects of syndromology proper are presented in Chapters 8–11. In the last section, topical subjects of importance in the field appear in Chapters 12–14.

The first two chapters detail the fundamental concepts and vocabulary used in dysmorphology. Chapter 1 discusses the nature of syndromes, associations, and sequences, and Chapter 2 explains the three basic types of major anomalies—malformations, deformations, and disruptions—and their interrelationships.

The next two chapters deal with minor anomalies and their diagnostic importance. Chapter 3 discusses minor anomalies in general, and Chapter 4 presents facial dysmorphology *per se* because so many minor anomalies occur in the facial region. Chapter 4 also illustrates the unusual types of major facial anomalies first brought to the world's attention by the French craniofacial surgeon Paul Tessier. Sophisticated craniofacial measurements are discussed at the end of Chapter 4, and a guide to physical measurements used in general dysmorphology is presented in Chapter 5. The etiologic aspects of syndromology are explained in Chapter 6 (genetics) and Chapter 7 (teratogens). The formal aspects of syndromology proper include syndrome classification (Chapter 8), the process of syndrome delineation (Chapter 9), and the heterogeneous nature of etiopathogenesis (Chapter 10), culminating in an approach to syndrome diagnosis (Chapter 11). Topical subjects appearing at the end of the book include dysmorphic growth and development (Chapter 12), mental deficiency (Chapter 13), and psychosocial aspects of dysmorphology (Chapter 14).

I have been interested in syndromology for a long time, and I have been lucky to have spent time learning the subject from Robert J. Gorlin, David W. Smith, John M. Opitz, and Josef Warkany. I have been influenced in different ways by each of these acknowledged masters.

I did a 5-year fellowship with my mentor Bob Gorlin in Minneapolis from 1966 to 1971. His work has been monumental. He was—and continues to be—the most seminal influence in my professional life. I have enjoyed helping him with two editions of *Syndromes of the Head and Neck*.[3,4]

During my years in Seattle as a Career Development Award Recipient from 1971 to 1981, I had frequent contact with Dave Smith and his fellows and collaborated with them on a number of projects and publications. Dave pioneered a new field, which he called *dysmorphology*, and he made many impressive and original contributions.

In 1976, in the middle of my Seattle career, I spent a year in Madison with John Opitz from whom I learned a lot. His many contributions to the field have been brilliant. I enjoy continued association with him and with the *American Journal of Medical Genetics*, first as a reviewer of numerous manuscripts and then as one of the Associate Editors of the Clinical Genetics Section.

Also during my time in Seattle, Joe Warkany spent summers there away from his home base of Cincinnati. He was a giant who drew on vast knowledge and experience, having begun the study of malformations during the 1940s when the subject was not popular. He left behind a staggering number of significant clinical and research publications.[2] In 1978, Joe and Ron Lemire asked me if I would join them in coauthoring a book entitled *Mental Retardation and Congenital Malformations of the Central Nervous System*.[6] During the following summer, Joe and I shared an office to work on his book.

In recent years, with annual trips to Bauru, Brazil, sponsored by Antonio Richieri-Costa, I have been shown patients with malformation syndromes that I had never seen before. I am grateful to him for showing me patients with so many newly recognized syndromes that have appeared in his recent publications.

I have asked Art Aylsworth (Chapel Hill) and Margot Van Allen (Vancouver) to read a draft of this text and offer critical comments. I am grateful to them for their help. In the final analysis, however, a book is an individual matter and I take full responsibility for what I have said.

Halifax, Nova Scotia   M. Michael Cohen, Jr.

REFERENCES

1. Cohen MM Jr: *The Child With Multiple Birth Defects.* New York: Raven Press, 1982.
2. Cohen MM Jr: Josef Warkany, 1902–1992: A personal remembrance. *J Craniofac Genet Dev Biol* 14:1–6, 1994.
3. Gorlin RJ, Pindborg JJ, Cohen MM Jr: *Syndromes of the Head and Neck.* Second Edition, New York: McGraw-Hill, 1976.
4. Gorlin RJ, Cohen MM Jr, Levin LS: *Syndromes of the Head and Neck.* Third Edition, New York: Oxford University Press, 1990.
5. Opitz JM, Herrmann J: The study of genetic diseases and malformations. *Birth Defects* 13(6):45–66, 1977.
6. Warkany J, Lemire RJ, Cohen MM Jr: *Mental Retardation and Congenital Malformations of the Central Nervous System.* Chicago: Yearbook Medical Publishers, 1981.

Acknowledgments

Many colleagues and friends have stimulated my thinking over the years. Foremost among these are Robert J. Gorlin (Minneapolis) and John M. Opitz (Helena). There are many others.

Pediatrics and/or Genetics: Arthur S. Aylsworth (Chapel Hill), Mason Barr, Jr. (Ann Arbor), Stan Blecher (Guelph), Robert J. Desnick (New York), Jaime L. Frías (Tampa), John M. Graham, Jr. (Los Angeles), Bryan D. Hall (Lexington), Ethylin Wang Jabs (Baltimore), Ronald J. Lemire (Seattle), Jules G. Leroy (Ghent), Mark S. Lubinsky (Milwaukee), Mark S. Ludman (Halifax), Maximilian Muenke (Philadelphia), Giovanni Neri (Rome), Antonio Richieri-Costa (Bauru), Robert J. Shprintzen (New York), Robert W. ten Bensel (Minneapolis), Margot I. Van Allen (Vancouver), Rosanna Weksberg (Toronto), and J. Philip Welch (Halifax).

Biochemistry: David E.C. Cole (Toronto).
Embryology: Jan E. Jirasek (Prague), Thomas H. Shepard (Seattle), and Kathleen K. Sulik (Chapel Hill).
Epidemiology: Irvin Emanuel (Seattle), J. David Erickson (Atlanta), Maria-Luisa Martínez-Frías (Madrid), Pierpaolo Mastroiacovo (Rome), and Godfrey Oakley (Atlanta).
Pathology: J. Bruce Beckwith (Loma Linda) and Enid Gilbert-Barness (Tampa).
Radiology: Leonard O. Langer, Jr. (Minneapolis) and Andrew K. Poznanski (Chicago).

I am grateful to the Audiovisual Department of the Faculty of Medicine at Dalhousie University for help and support. Jeff House, Senior Editor at Oxford University Press, has advised me about editorial matters and has been wonderful in expediting the second edition of this book. Finally, I wish to thank my administrator Ruth E. MacLean (Halifax) for her able executive skills. This book would not have been possible without her expertise.

Contents

The Child with Multiple Birth Defects

1

Syndromes, Associations, and Sequences

[The syndromologist has an] . . . encyclopedic memory . . . [and practices] . . . judicious use of idioglossia . . . [which] . . . confounds . . . [his or her] . . . colleagues. . . . [He or she is] . . . always able to spot dysmorphic features if they are—or should be—there. [The syndromologist] . . . measures everything (e.g., length of ear, nose, hand, penis) or distance between everything (e.g., inner canthi, nipples). . . . [He or she] . . . usually reaches a diagnosis or, if not, writes the patient up as a new syndrome.

From *Recognizable Patterns of Genetic Counsellors*, by Michael Partington.[31]

The epigraph is hilarious but largely accurate. Clearly, Michael Partington's unpublished compendium deserves to be published.

Syndromology is a broad and diverse endeavor spanning almost all areas of medicine. Approximately 1% of all newborns have multiple anomalies, or syndromes. Of these, about 40% can be diagnosed as having specific, recognized syndromes.[25] The other 60% have unknown entities that need to be further delineated. As an unknown syndrome becomes delineated, its phenotypic spectrum, its natural history, and its risk of recurrence become known, allowing for better patient care and family counseling. Although many syndromes are individually rare, in the aggregate they constitute a significant portion of medicine (Fig. 1-1).[5]

SYNDROME CONCEPTS

The word *syndrome* is derived from a Greek word that literally means *a running together*. The term has a long history of diverse usage. A similar fate has befallen

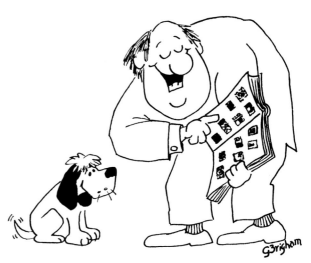

Figure 1-1. The syndromologist is sometimes mistaken for a collector of rare stamps. While some syndromes are individually rare, in the aggregate they make up a significant portion of medicine. From Cohen.[5]

many other words, such as *function, race,* and *intelligence.* The term *syndrome* has been applied to collections of signs, to groups of symptoms, and to mixed assortments of signs and symptoms. It has been attached to both specific and nonspecific entities. For some clinicians, the term refers to a group of manifestations when the cause is poorly understood, the term *disease* being reserved for disorders of known genesis. *Disease* usually connotes a progressive disorder or one in which deterioration occurs. In this context, the etiology may or may not be known. Thus, we speak of hand, foot, and mouth disease.[5] For some, such as Thomas Sydenham, syndrome and disease were equivalent concepts.[20]

Some use the term *syndrome* for multiple anomalies of genetic origin. The term has been applied to specific laboratory findings, such as high cerebrospinal fluid protein in the absence of cells—the diagnostic features of Guillain-Barré syndrome. It has even been used for apparently unconnected clinical findings, such as inability to recognize the fingers, left–right disorientation, agraphia, and acalculia—the features of Gerstmann syndrome; such findings have been observed with lesions of the parietal as well as with lesions of the frontal lobe. Occasionally, the term *syndrome* is applied to the more severe end of a teratogenic spectrum that grades into the normal range, such as fetal hydantoin syndrome.[5] Several papers[19,23,26] address various aspects of syndrome definition and meaning.

SYNDROME DEFINITION

Opitz[28] has distinguished causal or true syndromy from false syndromies, such as coincidental, associational, and symptomatic syndromies (Table 1-1). The International Working Group[1,34] recommended defining a syndrome as *a pattern of multiple anomalies thought to be pathogenetically related and not known to represent a single sequence or a polytopic field defect.**

*A polytopic field defect involves distantly located anatomic structures that are developmentally related. The term is more fully defined in Chapter 2 under the heading More Definitions.

Table 1-1. Some Concepts of Syndromy

Types of Syndromy	Characteristic Features	Examples*
True		
Causal	Etiologically defined disorder with pleiotropic effects	Trisomy 18 syndrome, Meckel syndrome
False		
Coincidental	Concurrence of more than one etiologically distinct disorder in the same patient	Trisomy 21 syndrome and neuro-fibromatosis in the same patient
Associational	Noncausal concurrence of several manifestations	
	Linkage or linkage-disequilibrium	Ankylosing spondylitis and HLA B27 allele
	Predispositional association	Autosomal recessive severe combined immunodeficiency and *Pneumocystis carinii* infection
Symptomatic	Etiologically nonspecific similar or identical sets of manifestations	Intrauterine growth retardation Nephrotic syndrome

Adapted from Opitz, 1979.[28]

SEQUENCE AND SYNDROME

A sequence, in turn, is defined as *a pattern of multiple anomalies derived from a single known or presumed prior anomaly or mechanical factors.* In a syndrome, the level of understanding of a pathogenetically related set of anomalies is usually lower than in a sequence in which the initiating event and the cascading of secondary events are frequently known. A syndrome may imply a unitary basis, e.g., Down syndrome; a sequence commonly has multiple causes, e.g., oligohydramnios sequence. Thus, syndromes and sequences differ from each other. Sequences are discussed further in Chapter 2.

ASSOCIATIONS

An association has been defined as *a nonrandom occurrence in two or more individuals of multiple anomalies not yet known to be a polytopic field defect,* sequence, or syndrome.*[1,34] With increasing knowledge, an association such as VACTERL or CHARGE (Table 1-2) may be broken apart into several sequences or syndromes. For example, the CHARGE association now includes some affected families with autosomal dominant inheritance and other affected families with autosomal recessive inheritance.[13]

Associations have been studied and discussed by Czeizel,[7] Khoury and his coworkers,[16-18] Evans and her coworkers,[9-12] Lubinsky,[21,21a,22] and Opitz.[26,27] If associations were completely broken down into sequences, polytopic field defects,[1] and/or syndromes, they should disappear in time. Although a number of entities have been identified in each association category, associations *per se* have *not* disappeared, and they do not show signs of disappearing. Thus, Opitz[26,27] suggested that associations may be better understood *biologically* than

Table 1-2. Four Associations

CHARGE[a]		VATER[b]		VACTERL[c]		MURCS[d]	
C	Coloboma	V	Vertebral anomalies	V	Vertebral defects	MU	Müllerian duct
H	Heart defect	A	Anal atresia	A	Anal atresia		aplasia
A	Atresia choanae	TE	TracheoEsophageal	C	Cardiovascular	R	Renal aplasia
R	Retarded growth and/or		fistula		anomalies	CS	Cervicothoracic
	CNS anomalies	R	Radial and Renal	TE	TracheoEsophageal		Somite dysplasia
G	Genital anomalies and/or		anomalies		fistula		
	hypogonadism			R	Radial and Renal		
E	Ear anomalies and/or				anomalies		
	deafness			L	Limb defects		

[a]Pagon et al.[30]

[b]Quan and Smith.[32]

[c]Khoury et al.[16] VACTERL is the expanded version of VATER.

[d]Duncan et al.[8]

statistically and offered the new definition of *patterns of multiple idiopathic anomalies of blastogenesis.* This is discussed further in Chapter 2.

NEW SYNDROMES

Syndromologists frequently postulate, discuss, and write about *new* syndromes, but they invariably mean *newly recognized* syndromes because the reported patients and their disorders existed before specific syndromologists encountered them. There are many legitimate newly recognized syndromes. Sometimes the condition is remarkably well described in the older literature. In some instances, the syndromologist who proposed the newly recognized syndrome is aware that the condition has been described previously. However, justification for new status is based on more definitive delineation of the condition.[5]

SYNDROME DESIGNATIONS

Several papers[3,14,15,35] have addressed the problems associated with syndrome designations. There are a bewildering variety of syndromes that must often be designated by some method other than by naming the condition after the basic defect. Because different systems of nomenclature are employed (Table 1-3), a single syndrome can be known by several terms, sometimes causing confusion (Figs. 1-2, 1-3). In general, a newly recognized syndrome can be denoted by (1) an eponym, (2) one or more striking features (Fig. 1-4), (3) an acronym, (4) a numeral, (5) a geographic term, or (6) some combination of the above. None of these systems of nomenclature is without fault. Each has advantages and disadvantages, and these have been discussed elsewhere.[3,14] In general, nomenclature usage evolves with time. Sometimes international working groups are very helpful in standardizing nomenclature in various subfields.

Mythical terms such as *elfin facies syndrome* and animal nomenclature such as *bird headed dwarf* are pejorative and should be discouraged. One commonly recognized principle in the field is never to use *apostrophe s* in eponymic designa-

Table 1-3. Syndrome Nomenclature

Basis of Nomenclature	Examples
Etiology	α-L-iduronidase deficiency, 47,XXY syndrome
Striking feature	Whistling face syndrome
Anatomic location	Nail-patella syndrome, tricho-rhino-phalangeal syndrome
Eponym	Peutz-Jeghers syndrome, Weaver syndrome
Acronym	LEOPARD syndrome[a]
Patient's name	Cowden syndrome, BBB/G syndrome[b]
Geographic location	Typus Amstelodamensis[c]
Numerical nomenclature	MPS IVA, type II achondrogenesis
Compound designations	Hurler syndrome (α-L-iduronidase deficiency), Taybi oto-palato-digital syndrome

Modified from Cohen.[3]

[a]Multiple Lentigines, Electrocardiographic conduction abnormalities, Ocular hypertelorism, Pulmonic stenosis, Atrial septal defect, Retardation of growth, and sensorineural Deafness.

[b]BBB/G syndrome is based on the initials of the original patient's surnames.

[c]Cornelia de Lange originally coined this geographic name for the syndrome that bears her name today.

tions.[6,35] Thus, we use *Apert syndrome*, not *Apert's syndrome*, because Apert neither had nor owned the syndrome he described. However, in my opinion, we should readily accept the use of the possessive case in *other* fields where it is common, for example, the use by pathologists of Burkitt's lymphoma or Paget's disease of the nipple.

POPULATION DEFINITION OF A SYNDROME

Not all abnormalities occur with the same frequency in a given syndrome. Some are common; others are rare. The term *phenotypic spectrum*[29] refers to the total number of abnormalities in a given syndrome and their respective frequencies in the syndrome population.

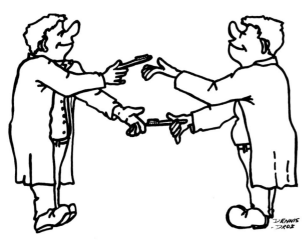

Figure 1-2. Academicians are more likely to share each other's toothbrush . . .

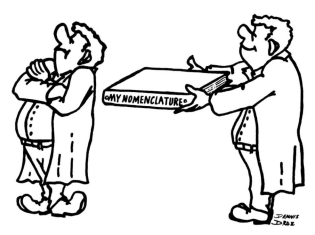

Figure 1-3. . . . than each other's nomenclature. From Cohen.[5]

It is sometimes asked if an occasionally observed abnormality is part of a syndrome. Since the pathogenesis of many syndromes is obscure, there is no direct way of knowing. However, by statistically defining the component abnormalities of a syndrome, it can be determined indirectly. Table 1-4 lists and Figure 1-5 illustrates the phenotypic spectrum of abnormalities (A, B . . . K) of a hypothetical syndrome together with their frequencies in the syndrome population and in a control population. If a given abnormality occurs with greater frequency in the syndrome population than as an isolated abnormality in the control population, it should be considered part of the syndrome. Thus, by comparing the frequencies in Table 1-4 and Figure 1-5, abnormalities A through H are obviously part of the syndrome. Even abnormality I (1% compared with 0.04%) should be considered part of the syndrome. This principle commits us to statements such as "cleft palate is part of Down syndrome" because it occurs with higher frequency than as an isolated defect in the control population.[4,5]

Abnormality J occurs with approximately the same frequencies in both syndrome and control populations (0.04% compared with 0.05%). Thus, it should not be considered part of the syndrome.[5]

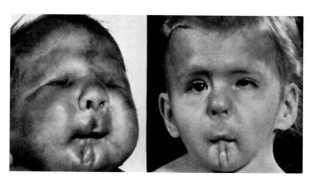

Figure 1-4. Whistling face syndrome. Nomenclature by striking feature. Left, from Rintala.[33] Right, courtesy of J. Külz, Rostock, Germany.

**Table 1-4. Statistical Definition
of a Hypothetical Syndrome**

Specific Abnormality	Frequency of Abnormality in Syndrome Population (% Values)	Frequency of Abnormality in Control Population (% Values)
A	100	1.00
B	90	0.15
C	65	0.35
D	52	0.09
E	43	0.75
F	36	0.17
G	11	0.06
H	3	0.12
L	1	0.04
J	0.04	0.05
K	0.00004	0.001

From Cohen.[5]

Note that abnormality K occurs with significantly lower frequency than as an isolated defect in the control population (0.00004% compared with 0.001%). Conspicuous absence of an abnormality should be considered part of the syndrome.[4,5] A suggested example has been osteogenesis imperfecta, which has been stated to be a cancer-resistant genotype.[24] Various malignant neoplasms have been said to occur at a lower rate in patients with this disorder than they do in normal first-degree relatives or in the general population, excluding osteosarcoma, which tends to occur with a slightly *increased* rate in osteogenesis imperfecta.

Thus far, we have discussed a control population without specifying its nature. If a syndrome is ascertained independently of its phenotype, which is possible with a chromosomal syndrome or mendelian disorder for which there is a laboratory test, an unbiased estimate of its phenotypic spectrum can be obtained. The ideal control population is one composed of unaffected first-degree relatives. However, it may not be practical to use first-degree relative populations. If the syndrome is rare, which is frequently the case, large syndrome and control populations may not be available. In such instances, it is difficult to establish low-frequency abnormalities as part of the syndrome with certainty, since large syndrome and control populations are required to do this.[4,5]

If ascertained independently of the phenotype, the syndrome can probably be compared directly with the frequencies of isolated abnormalities in the general population. One obvious advantage is that frequencies of various isolated abnormalities are readily available in the literature. Thus, a rough comparison can be made without extensive calculations. However, it should be recognized that the general population is not the same as a normal, first-degree relative population. Thus, the comparison should be made with caution, depending on the appropriateness of the general population utilized.[4,5]

Estimating the frequencies of various abnormalities from probands with a mendelian syndrome for which there is no known laboratory test truncates the syndrome toward the severe end of the phenotypic spectrum (Fig. 1-6). The

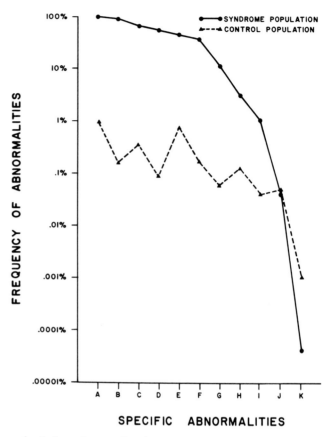

Figure 1-5. Statistical definition of a hypothetical syndrome. Graphic representation (logarithmic) of Table 1-3, comparing the frequencies of abnormalities in the syndrome population with the frequencies of the same abnormalities as isolated defects in a control population. Note that abnormalities A through I all occur with greater frequency in the syndrome population than in the control population. Therefore, they are all part of the syndrome. Since abnormality K occurs considerably less frequently in the syndrome population than in the control population, its absence should be considered part of the syndrome. Finally, since abnormality J occurs with approximately the same frequency in both syndrome and control populations, its occurrence in the syndrome is probably coincidental. From Cohen.[5]

ascertainment bias introduced by using probands probably cannot be balanced by including mildly affected patients born before the proband. Since there is a greater chance of ascertaining a family with several severely affected members than there is of ascertaining a single case, there is a bias in favor of severely affected patients. Adding the mildly affected cases that arise in all sibships to the study probably leads to a bimodal frequency distribution, reflecting the mild and severe ends of the phenotypic spectrum (Fig. 1-6). An unbiased estimate of the phenotypic spectrum of a mendelian syndrome for which there is no laboratory test can be obtained by including only those affected siblings born after the proband (Fig. 1-6). To avoid ascertainment bias, probands are excluded. The more families in the study, the greater the chance of balancing intra- and intersibship variabilities.[29]

In a recurrent-pattern syndrome,* there is an artificial homogeneity of cases

---

*A recurrent pattern syndrome can be informally defined here as a group of sporadically occurring patients who are thought to have the same syndrome. See Chapter 9 for formal definition.

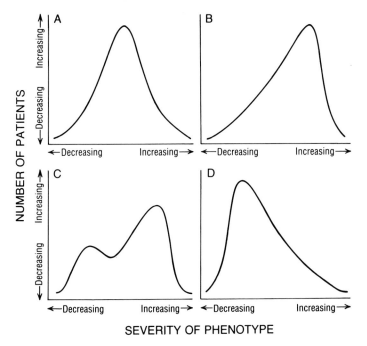

Figure 1-6. The phenotypic spectrum of a syndrome. A: The normal phenotypic spectrum that occurs when the syndrome population is ascertained independently of the phenotype, as is possible with a chromosomal syndrome or mendelian disorder with a laboratory test. This phenotypic spectrum also occurs when the ascertainment bias has been corrected in a mendelian syndrome by including only affected siblings born after the proband and excluding the proband. B: Syndrome population truncated toward the severe end of the phenotypic spectrum. Such artificial homogeneity occurs when a syndrome population is ascertained by phenotypic features as in a recurrent pattern syndrome. (See footnote on page 10.) C: Syndrome population with bimodal distribution emphasizing both severe and mild ends of the phenotypic spectrum. Such a distribution probably occurs in a mendelian syndrome population composed of probands plus previously unrecognized, mildly affected siblings who were born before the proband and actively searched for. D: Syndrome population truncated toward the mild end of the phenotypic spectrum. Such a distribution probably occurs in a mendelian syndrome population composed of previously unrecognized, mildly affected siblings who were born before the proband and actively searched for, the proband himself or herself being excluded in an attempt to correct ascertainment bias. From Cohen.[5]

that emphasizes the more severe aspects of the syndrome. The etiology is unknown, and the disorder cannot be ascertained independently of the phenotype. Nor can ascertainment bias be corrected for, as in a mendelian syndrome, because the affected individuals in the syndrome sample are unrelated. Thus, statistical definition of a syndrome is more complex in a recurrent-pattern syndrome.[4,5]

To determine the frequency with which a given abnormality probably occurs by chance in a recurrent-pattern syndrome, it is necessary to know the frequency of the syndrome in the general population and the frequency of the abnormality in question as an isolated trait in the general population. The probability that the abnormality occurs in the syndrome by chance is equal to the product of the two separate frequencies. Consider the recurrent-pattern syndrome shown in Table 1-5. For comparative purposes, the frequencies of abnormalities A through K in the syndrome population and the frequencies of abnormalities A through K as isolated traits in the general population are the same as those in Table 1-4. If a recurrent-pattern syndrome has a prevalence of 1 in 5,000 (2 ×

Table 1-5. Statistical Definition of a Recurrent-Pattern Syndrome[a]

Specific Abnormality	Frequency of Abnormality in General Population	Frequency of Abnormality in General Population × Frequency of Syndrome in General Population (2×10^{-4})	Frequency of Abnormality in Syndrome Population
A	10×10^{-3}	20×10^{-7}	1×10^{-0}
B	1.5×10^{-3}	3×10^{-7}	9×10^{-1}
C	3.5×10^{-3}	7×10^{-7}	6.5×10^{-1}
D	0.9×10^{-3}	1.8×10^{-7}	5.2×10^{-1}
E	7.5×10^{-3}	15×10^{-7}	4.3×10^{-1}
F	1.7×10^{-3}	3.4×10^{-7}	3.6×10^{-1}
G	0.6×10^{-3}	1.2×10^{-7}	1.1×10^{-1}
H	1.2×10^{-3}	2.4×10^{-7}	0.3×10^{-1}
I	0.4×10^{-3}	0.8×10^{-7}	0.1×10^{-1}
J	0.5×10^{-3}	1×10^{-7}	0.4×10^{-3}
K	0.1×10^{-4}	0.2×10^{-8}	0.4×10^{-6}

From Cohen.[5]

[a]Column 4 should be compard to column 3.

10^{-4}) in the general population, and an abnormality in question, say B, occurs as an isolated trait in 0.15% (1.5×10^{-3}) of the general population, then the probability that the abnormality occurs in the syndrome by chance is approximately 3×10^{-7}. The values for which various abnormalities occur in the syndrome population by chance are listed in column 3 of Table 1-5. By comparing these values to the actual frequencies with which abnormalities occur in the syndrome population (column 4), it should be noted that all abnormalities, including J and K, occur with higher frequencies in the syndrome population than expected on the basis of chance.[4,5]

There are many obstacles to determining the phenotypic spectrum for various syndromes at different stages of delineation. Thus, we should be wary of exact percentages given for various abnormalities in most syndrome review articles and textbooks. Percentages can be especially misleading in recurrent-pattern syndromes; they tend to be overestimates. Even in mendelian syndromes with or without laboratory definition, in chromosomal syndromes, or in teratogenic syndromes, no attempt is made to correct for ascertainment bias in the phenotypic frequencies given in most syndrome review articles.[4,5]

FORTUITOUS CONCURRENCE OF ANOMALIES

Two or more anomalies can concur fortuitously in the same individual. The anomalies are presumed to arise from different causes acting independently. The theoretical frequency with which this occurs can be calculated by summing the products of the frequencies of each possible combination of anomalies in the general population.[2] For example, if a total of only three anomalies existed hypothetically in the general population with frequencies of a, b, and c, respectively, then the frequencies of specific chance patterns in the population would be

$$f_1 = ab, \; f_2 = bc, \; f_3 = ac, \; \text{and} \; f_4 = abc$$

and the total frequency with which all chance patterns occur in the general population would be

$$\Sigma f = ab + bc + ac + abc$$

Most represent binary combinations of defects. Generally, the more anomalies there are, the rarer the occurrence. It should be carefully noted that, even though we can calculate the theoretical frequencies of chance concurrences in the general population, we cannot identify them individually as such. For example, in a patient with the binary combination of cleft palate and atrial septal defect, we cannot prove that the two anomalies have different causes. It is possible that they have the same cause.[2]

REFERENCES

1. Benirschke K, Cohen MM Jr, Hall JG, Lenz W, Lowry RB, Opitz JM, Pinsky L, Schwarzacher HG, Smith DW, Spranger J: Terms pertaining to morphogenesis and malformations. Birth Defects Meeting, June 8–11, 1980.
2. Cohen MM Jr: Interrelationships between common congenital malformations. *Lancet* 1:147, 1976.
3. Cohen MM Jr: Syndrome designations. *J Med Genet* 13:266–270, 1976.
4. Cohen MM Jr: Syndromology: An updated conceptual overview. 1. Syndrome concepts, designations, and population characteristics. *Int J Oral Maxillofac Surg* 18:216–222, 1989.
5. Cohen MM Jr: *The Child With Multiple Birth Defects*. First Edition. New York: Raven Press, 1982.
6. Coppes MJ, Beckwith B: Eponyms in medicine: Possessive or nonpossessive? *J Pediatr* 122:165, 1993.
7. Czeizel A: Schisis-association. *Am J Med Genet* 10:25–35, 1981.
8. Duncan PA, Shapiro LR, Stangel JJ, Klein RM, Adlonizio JC: The MURCS association: Müllerian duct aplasia, renal aplasia, and cervicothoracic somite dysplasia. *J Pediatr* 95:399–402, 1979.
9. Evans JA, Stranc LC, Kaplan P, Hunter AGW: VACTERL with hydrocephalus: Further delineation of the syndrome(s). *Am J Med Genet* 34:177–182, 1989.
10. Evans JA, Vitez M, Czeizel A: Congenital abnormalities associated with limb deficiency defects: A population study based on cases from the Hungarian Congenital Malformation Registry (1975–1984). *Am J Med Genet* 49:52–66, 1994.
11. Evans JA, Vitez M, Czeizel A: On the biological nature of associations: Evidence from a study of radial ray deficiencies and associated malformation. In Opitz JM (ed): *Blastogenesis—Normal and Abnormal*. Wiley-Liss for the March of Dimes— Birth Defects Foundation. BD:OAS, 1993.
12. Evans JA, Vitez M, Czeizel A: Patterns of acrorenal malformation associations. *Am J Med Genet* 44:413–419, 1992.
13. Gorlin RJ, Cohen MM Jr, Levin LS: *Syndromes of the Head and Neck*. Third edition. New York: Oxford University Press, 1990.
14. Herrmann J, Opitz JM: Naming and nomenclature of syndromes. *Birth Defects* 10(7):69–86, 1974.
15. Jablonski S: Syndrome: Le mot de jour. *Am J Med Genet* 39:342–346, 1991.

16. Khoury MJ, Cordero JF, Greenberg R, James LM, Erickson JD: A population study of the VACTERL association: Evidence for its etiologic heterogeneity. *Pediatrics* 71:815–820, 1983.

17. Khoury MJ, Cordero JG, Mulinare J, Opitz JM: Selected midline defect associations: A population study. *Pediatrics* 84:266–272, 1989.

18. Khoury MJ, James LM, Erickson JD: On the measurement and interpretation of birth defect associations in epidemiologic studies. *Am J Med Genet* 37:229–236, 1990.

19. Khoury MJ, Moore CA, Evans JA: On the use of the term "syndrome" in clinical genetics and birth defects epidemiology. *Am J Med Genet* 49:26–28, 1994.

20. Kogoj F: Symptomenkomplexe, Syndrome und Semisyndrome. *Wien Med Wochenschr* 106:787–789, 1956.

21. Lubinsky M: Current concepts. VATER and other associations: Historical perspectives and modern interpretations. *Am J Med Genet Suppl* 2:9–16, 1986.

21a. Lubinsky M: Epidemiologies of blastogenic defects: Genetic associations and inherited anomalies rare in mendelian syndromes. *Am J Med Genet* (in press).

22. Lubinsky MS: Properties of associations: Identity, nature, and clinical criteria, with a commentary on why CHARGE and Goldenhar are not associations. *Am J Med Genet* 49:21–25, 1994.

23. Lubinsky MS: The syndrome as finding or as cause: Suggested terminology. *Am J Med Genet* 20:727–728, 1985.

24. Lynch HT, Lemon HM, Krush AJ: A note on "cancer-susceptible" and "cancer-resistant" genotypes. *Nebr State Med J* 51:209–211, 1966.

25. Marden PM, Smith DW, McDonald MJ: Congenital anomalies in the newborn infant, including minor variations. *J Pediatr* 64:358–371, 1964.

26. Opitz JM: Associations and syndromes: Terminology in clinical genetics and birth defects epidemiology: Comments on Khoury, Moore, and Evans. *Am J Med Genet* 49:14–20, 1994.

27. Opitz JM: Blastogenesis and the "primary field" in human development. *Birth Defects* 29(1):3–37, 1993.

28. Opitz JM: Terminological and epistemological considerations of human malformations. In Harris H. and Hirschhorn K (eds): *Advances in Human Genetics.* New York: Plenum, 1979, pp. 71–107.

29. Opitz JM, Herrmann J, Dieker H: The study of malformation syndromes in man. *Birth Defects* 5(2):1–10, 1969.

30. Pagon RA, Graham JM Jr, Zonana J, Yong S: Coloboma, congenital heart disease, and choanal atresia with multiple anomalies: CHARGE association. *J Pediatr* 99:223–227, 1981.

31. Partington MW: *Recognizable Patterns of Genetic Counsellors* (with apologies to D.W.S.). Unpublished compendium, 1977.

32. Quan L, Smith DW: The VATER association. *J Pediatr* 82:104–107, 1973.

33. Rintala AE: Freeman-Sheldon's syndrome: Cranio-carpo-tarsal dystrophy. *Acta Paediatr Scand* 57:553–556, 1968.

34. Spranger J, Benirschke K, Hall JG, Lenz W, Lowry RB, Opitz JM, Pinsky L, Schwarzacher HG, Smith DW: Errors of morphogenesis: Concepts and terms. Recommendations of an International Working Group. *J Pediatr* 100:160–165, 1982.

35. Warkany J: Syndromes. *Am J Dis Child* 121:365–370, 1971.

2

Malformations, Deformations, and Disruptions

Anomalies can be divided into malformations, deformations, and disruptions (Fig. 2-1). Syndactyly is a malformation that results from an intrinsically abnormal developmental process occurring during the embryonic period. Clubfoot is a deformation that can result from mechanical compression during the fetal period. Digital amputation in association with an aberrant tissue band represents disruption of an otherwise intrinsically normal developmental process. Several other examples of malformations, deformations, and disruptions are given in Table 2-1 and shown in Figure 2-2. Most anomalies observed at birth can be sorted into one of the three basic categories, and *there are practical reasons for doing so because the clinical implications of each category are different.* These differences are further explored in this chapter.

DEFINITIONS*

The following definitions have been recommended by the International Working Group.[3,79]

Malformation: A morphologic defect of an organ, part of an organ, or a larger region of the body resulting from an intrinsically abnormal developmental process

---

Association is discussed in Chapter 1, and a new working definition by Opitz[62] is presented later in this chapter under More Definitions.

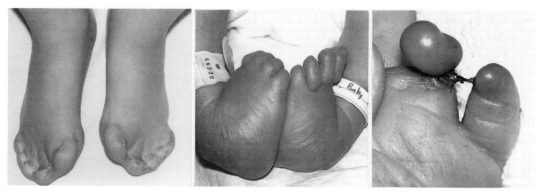

Figure 2-1. Three basic types of anomalies affecting limbs. Left: Syndactyly, a malformation. Center: Clubfoot, a deformation. Right: Digital amputation in association with amniotic band. From Cohen.[12]

Deformation: An abnormal form or position of a part of the body caused by nondisruptive mechanical forces

Disruption: A morphologic defect of an organ, part of an organ, or a larger region of the body resulting from a breakdown of, or an interference with, an originally normal developmental process

Sequence: A pattern of multiple anomalies derived from a single known or presumed prior anomaly or mechanical factor

Syndrome: A pattern of multiple anomalies thought to be pathogenetically related and not known to represent a sequence or a polytopic field defect.*

Other terms will be introduced later in this chapter, under Some Other Definitions and Some Further Definitions.

MALFORMATIONS

Approximately 2%–3% of all newborns have significant malformations. A classification of malformations with examples is presented in Table 2-2. There are three general classes of malformations: incomplete morphogenesis, redundant morphogenesis, and aberrant morphogenesis. The most common class is incomplete morphogenesis in which a developmental arrest occurs, as in renal agenesis. If the ureteric bud fails to contact the metanephric blastema or if the blastema fails to respond to it, the kidney does not form. Some of the other subtypes of incomplete morphogenesis with examples are listed in Table 2-2. Redundant morphogenesis is much less common. In this class of malformations, the redundant structure passes through the same stage of morphogenesis at the same time as its normal counterpart.

A good example is an ear tag in the presence of an otherwise normal ear. Such a tag may be interpreted as a supernumerary auricular hillock. Aberrant morphogenesis is rare and has no counterpart in normal morphogenesis. A mediastinal thyroid gland serves as an example because it is never found in this location at any stage of normal morphogenesis. Because the classification of

*The term *polytopic field defect* involves distantly located anatomic structures that are developmentally related. It is fully defined later in this chapter, under More Definitions.

Table 2-1. Basic Types of Anomalies

Types of Anomalies	Process	Examples
Malformation	Intrinsically abnormal developmental process	Cleft lip, polydactyly
Deformation	Mechanical compression	Clubfoot, plagiocephaly
Disruption	Breakdown of otherwise normal developmental process	Amniotic band amputation, porencephaly

malformations presented in Table 2-2 is not at all inclusive and because nothing is implied about mechanisms, it is a classification of convenience rather than of scientific merit. The subject of malformations is discussed extensively by Warkany.[93]

Malformations can be relatively simple or complex. The later the defect is initiated, the simpler the malformation. Malformations initiated early during organogenesis tend to have more far-reaching consequences (Table 2-3). A malformation sequence has already been defined as multiple defects derived from a single known or presumed structural defect. The primary defect sets off a chain of secondary and tertiary events, resulting in what appear to be multiple anomalies. Some malformation sequences are shown in Figure 2-3.

In holoprosencephaly, the first malformation sequence, the embryonic forebrain fails to cleave sagittally into cerebral hemispheres, transversely into telencephalon and diencephalon, and horizontally into olfactory and optic bulbs. Holoprosencephaly varies in its degree of severity. At the mild end of the spectrum is simple absence of the olfactory tracts and bulbs. Holoprosencephaly is associated with facial dysmorphism (Fig. 2-4), which also varies from mild to

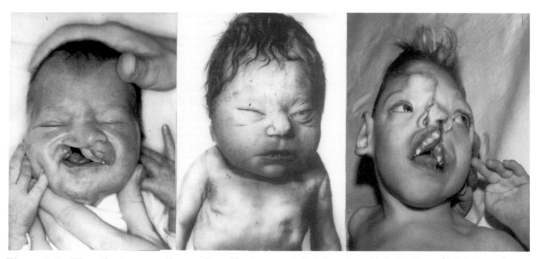

Figure 2-2. Three basic types of anomalies affecting craniofacial regions. Left: Unilateral cleft lip-palate, a malformation. It occurs twice as commonly on the left side. Center: Potter deformities with compressed appearance secondary to oligohydramnios, which causes intrauterine compression. A deformation. Right: Bizarre asymmetric clefting of nose, lip, and palate together with asymmetric anteriorly placed encephaloceles, the result of amniotic bands during intrauterine life. A disruptive process. Center, from Smith.[78a] Right, From Cohen.[12]

Table 2-2. Abnormal Morphogenesis Resulting in Malformations

Types of Abnormal Morphogenesis	Examples of Malformations	Relative Frequency as a Class
Incomplete morphogenesis		Common
Lack of development	Absent nostril, renal agenesis	
Hypoplasia	Microcephaly, micrognathia	
Incomplete closure	Cleft palate, iris coloboma	
Incomplete separation	Syndactyly	
Incomplete septation	Ventricular septal defect	
Incomplete migration	Exstrophy of the cloaca	
Incomplete rotation	Malrotated gut	
Incomplete resolution of early form	Choanal atresia, Meckel diverticulum	
Persistence of early location	Low-set ears, undescended testes	
Redundant morphogenesis	Supernumerary ear tag, polydactyly	Uncommon
Aberrant morphogenesis	Mediastinal thyroid gland, paratesticular spleen	Rare

severe expression. A single eye or closely set eyes, proboscis formation, single nostril nose, flattened nose, and median cleft lip may be observed variably or in combination. All malformations encountered trace their origin developmentally to a single primary defect in morphogenesis thought to be an abnormality in the prechordal mesoderm.[10,11]

Table 2-3. Timing of Selected Malformations

Malformation	Defect in	Cause Prior to
Holoprosencephaly	Prechordal mesoderm	23 Days
Sirenomelia	Caudal axis	23 Days
Anencephaly	Anterior neuropore	26 Days
Meningomyelocele	Posterior neuropore	28 Days
Transposition of the great vessels	Direction of development of bulbous cordis septum	36 Days
Radial aplasia	Development of radius	38 Days
Cleft lip	Development of primary palate	6 Weeks
Ventricular septal defect	Closure of ventricular septum	6 Weeks
Diaphragmatic hernia	Closure of pleuropotential canal	6 Weeks
Syndactyly	Programmed cell death between digits	6 Weeks
Duodenal atresia	Recanalization of duodenum	7–8 Weeks
Omphalocele	Intestinal loop return to abdominal cavity	10 Weeks
Bicornuate uterus	Fusion of lower portion of müllerian ducts	10 Weeks
Cleft palate	Development of secondary palate	10 Weeks
Hypospadias	Fusion of urethral folds	12 Weeks
Cryptorchidism	Descent of testes	7–9 Months

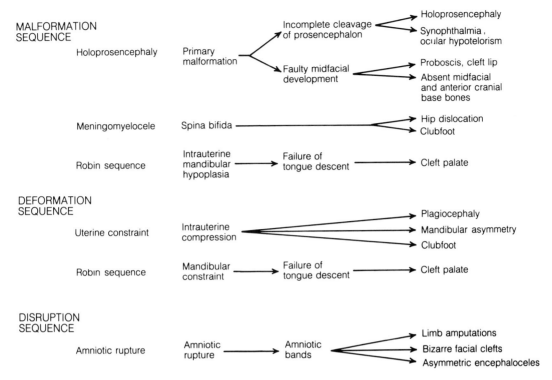

Figure 2-3. Schematic representation of several malformation, deformation, and disruption sequences. From Cohen.[12]

The second malformation sequence is meningomyelocele in which spina bifida, a malformation, leads to congenital hip dislocation and clubfoot, two deformations. The relationship between malformations and deformations is considered further in another section of this chapter.

Finally, the Robin sequence can be considered a malformation sequence in some instances, such as the partial trisomy 11q syndrome. With the dysmorphic development and growth deficiency that accompanies most chromosomal syndromes, the initiating event in Robin sequence in this syndrome may be intrinsic mandibular hypoplasia.[12]

Malformations can be minimally or maximally expressed. For example, bifid uvula is a minimal expression of cleft palate. More complex malformations also can be minimally or maximally expressed, as exemplified in holoprosencephaly and its attendant facial dysmorphism (Fig. 2-4). Two holoprosencephalic faces at opposite ends of the phenotypic spectrum but within the same family are shown in Figure 2-5.

A syndrome has been defined as a pattern of multiple anomalies thought to be pathogenetically related and not representing a sequence. In a syndrome, the level of understanding of a pathogenetically related set of anomalies is usually lower than in a sequence in which the initiating event and the cascading of secondary events are frequently known. A syndrome commonly, but not always, implies a unitary etiology, e.g., del(4p) syndrome; a sequence commonly has multiple causes, e.g., oligohydramnios sequence.

A true malformation syndrome is characterized by embryonic pleiotropy in which a pattern of developmentally unrelated malformation sequences occurs;

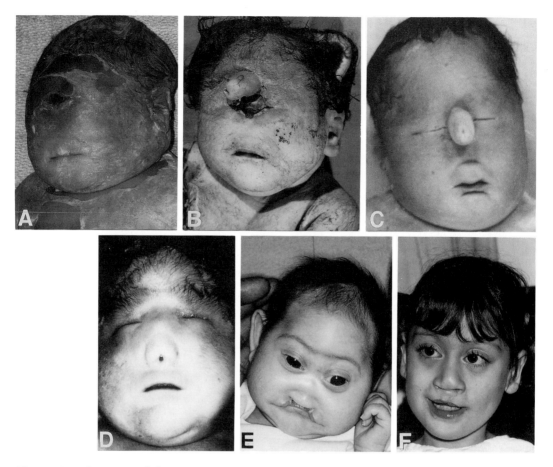

Figure 2-4. Spectrum of dysmorphic faces associated with variable degrees of holoprosencephaly. A: Cyclopia without proboscis formation. Note single central eye. B: Cyclopia with proboscis. C: Ethmocephaly. D: Cebocephaly. Ocular hypotelorism with single-nostril nose. E: Median cleft lip, flat nose, and ocular hypotelorism. F: Ocular hypotelorism and surgically repaired cleft lip. A–D, F, from Cohen et al.[13] E, from DeMyer and Zeman.[15] Montage from Cohen.[12]

that is, the malformations that make up the syndrome occur in embryonically noncontiguous areas. They are not related to one another at the descriptive embryonic level; at a more basic level, the malformations have—or are presumed to have—a common cause and are thus pathogenetically related. The difference between a malformation sequence and a malformation syndrome is diagrammed in Figure 2-6. When holoprosencephaly occurs alone, it is a malformation sequence, but, when it occurs with multiple noncontiguous anomalies in trisomy 13 syndrome (Fig. 2-7) or with multiple noncontiguous anomalies in the autosomal recessively inherited Meckel syndrome, it is a malformation syndrome composed of several malformation sequences.[12]

Each syndrome of known etiology has a syndrome-specific frequency with which a given malformation occurs in the syndrome population. Furthermore, for some types of malformations, each syndrome of known etiology has a syndrome-specific range of anatomic variation. Both syndrome-specific frequencies and anatomic ranges of variation, with holoprosencephaly as an example, are shown in Table 2-4.

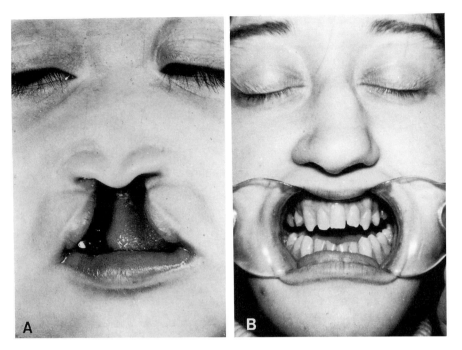

Figure 2-5. A: Holoprosencephaly with median cleft lip, flat nose, and ocular hypotelorism. From Patel et al.[74] B: Mother of infant shown in A. She has microform of same malformation sequence. Note single maxillary central incisor and mild ocular hypotelorism. Courtesy of R.B. Lowry, Calgary, Alberta, Canada.

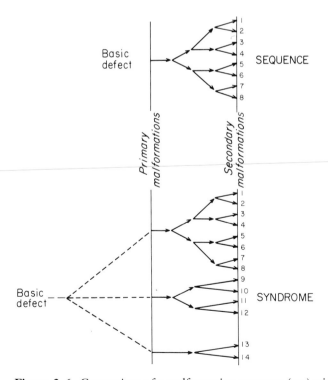

Figure 2-6. Comparison of a malformation sequence (top) with a true malformation syndrome (bottom). Isolated holoprosencephaly is an example of a malformation sequence. The combination of holoprosencephaly, ventricular septal defect, and polydactyly, caused by trisomy 13, is a malformation syndrome. From Cohen.[12]

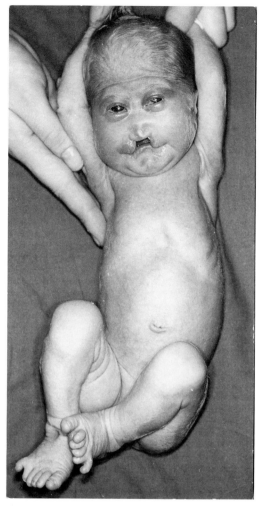

Figure 2-7. Trisomy 13 syndrome. Ocular hypotelorism, median cleft lip, polydactyly. The patient also had a ventricular septal defect. From Conen et al.[13a]

DEFORMATIONS

Approximately 1%–2% of all newborns have deformations. Some important deformities include clubfoot, hip dislocation, and postural scoliosis. Other congenital deformations are listed in Table 2-5 and are discussed extensively elsewhere by Dunn,[17–26] Graham,[31–36] and others.[5–9,38,52,57–60,73,75,76,81] Two craniofacial deformations are pictured in Figures 2-8 and 2-9. Deformations arise most frequently during late fetal life. Since the most common cause is intrauterine molding by mechanical forces, the musculoskeletal system is usually affected. The most important factor contributing to deformations is lack of fetal movement, whatever the cause. Deformations may result from mechanical, malformational, or functional causes, and these predisposing factors are listed in Table 2-6.

Table 2-4. Some Syndrome-Specific Frequencies and Syndrome-Specific Ranges of Holoprosencephaly

Condition	Estimated Frequency of Holoprosencephaly Within Diagnostic Category (%)	Range of Holoprosencephalic Facial Appearances Within Diagnostic Category
Autosomal recessive holoprosencephaly	100	Wide range: Cyclopia to median or lateral cleft lip
Trisomy 13 syndrome	70	Wide range: Cyclopia to median or lateral cleft lip
Autosomal recessive campomelic dysplasia	18	Narrow range: Absent olfactory tracts and bulbs and nondiagnostic face for holoprosencephaly
Deletion 13q syndrome	10	Narrow range: Ocular hypertelorism, iris coloboma, minor facial dysmorphism
Deletion 18p syndrome	10	Wide range: Cyclopia to median or lateral cleft lip
Infants of diabetic mothers	1–2	Wide range: Cyclopia to median or lateral cleft lip

From Cohen.[10]

Mechanical Causes

Mechanical causes of deformations are most common. Correlating various pregnancy factors to be statistically associated with the occurrence of congenital deformations (Fig. 2-10), Dunn[19,21] postulated how such factors might be interrelated (Fig. 2-11). First pregnancies tend to be associated with unstretched uterine and abdominal muscles. This can result in uteroplacental insufficiency, which, in turn, can lead to oligohydramnios. Breech presentation is common since the uterus is too compressed to allow the fetus to rotate into the cephalic position (Figs. 2-12, 2-13). Uterine restraints on fetal movement allow mild but persistent extrinsic forces to deform the fetus. For the first days after birth, infants with deformities usually can be folded into their atypical prenatal postures (Figs. 2-8, 2-14). Radiographically, the close correspondence between the abnormal posture of the fetus before delivery and the posture of the infant after birth has been observed repeatedly. Such posture has been termed the *position of comfort* by Chapple and Davidson.[6]

If various postural deformities have a mechanical origin, more than one deformation might be expected to occur in some patients. In a study of approximately 4,500 newborns, Dunn[20,21] indicated that one-third of all newborns with deformations had two or more deformities (Fig. 2-15). A deformation sequence can be specified as multiple deformations derived from a single known or presumed mechanical factor or prior structural defect.[45] Figure 2-3 shows two deformation sequences. In the first example, intrauterine compressive forces have led to three deformations (plagiocephaly, mandibular asymmetry, and clubfoot) in the same patient. In the second example, micrognathia, caused by intrauterine constraint, had led to failure of the tongue to descend, resulting in cleft palate. Thus, Robin sequence can be considered on a *malformational* or *deformational* basis, depending on whether the initiating event causing intra-

Table 2-5. Congenital Deformations^a

Craniofacial	Pectus excavatum
Vertex birth molding	Postural scoliosis
Craniotabes	Thoracic cage constraint-induced lung hypoplasia
Deformational dolichocephaly	Limbs
Deformational plagiocephaly	Dislocated radial head
Torticollis-induced plagiocephaly	Constraint-induced radial palsy
Constraint-induced craniosynostosis	Hip dislocation
Potter facies	Genu recurvatum
Compression-induced facial palsy	Tibial torsion
Nasal deformation	Sciatic nerve compression palsy
Auricular deformation	Potter limbs
Micrognathia	Arthrogryposis
Mandibular asymmetry	Talipes calcaneovalgus
Torticollis	Talipes equinovarus
Trunk	Metatarsus adductus
Pectus carinatum	Deformed toes

^aThis table contains some normally occurring deformations, e.g., vertex birth molding and tibial torsion. Some, such as dolichocephaly, micrognathia, clubfoot, Potter facies, and scoliosis, can occur on a malformational or on a deformational basis.

uterine micrognathia is mandibular hypoplasia or extrinsic mechanical forces acting on the mandible.[12]

Malformational Causes

In Dunn's study of newborns,[18] 7.6% of all malformations were associated with deformations. When this relationship occurred, the malformations primarily involved the central nervous system and the urinary tract, and, most frequently, the deformations were secondary to the malformations. Both central nervous system and urinary tract malformations cause deformations by interfering with

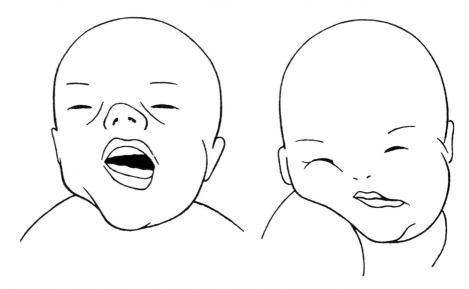

Figure 2-8. Mandibular deformation resulting from sharply lateroflexed position of the head *in utero* with the shoulder pressed against the mandible for a long period of time. Courtesy of Mead Johnson and Co.

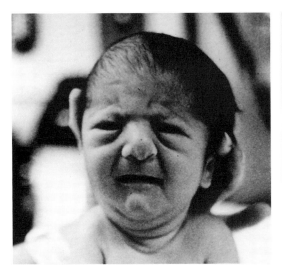 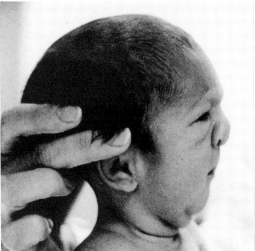

Figure 2-9. Compression of the face, particularly the nose, from prolonged transverse presentation with the head retroflexed and the face compressed against the lateral wall of the uterus. From Graham.[33]

fetal movements. Figure 2-3 gives an example of a malformation sequence that results in two deformations. Spina bifida, a malformation, leads to congenital hip dislocation and clubfoot since the malformations may produce partial paralysis of the legs. The resultant muscular imbalance is an intrinsic deforming force that limits the fetus's ability to kick and hence to change its position, thus altering the direction along which extrinsic deforming forces may be acting. Hip dysplasia, hip dislocation, and clubfoot may be explained on this basis, as may the hypoplastic lower limbs, a growth disturbance caused by deficient innervation.

An adequate quantity of amniotic fluid protects the fetus from extrinsic forces. Some amniotic fluid crosses the amnion as a transudate, but most is produced by fetal urine. Any malformation of the urinary tract that significantly

Table 2-6. Predisposing Factors in Deformations[a]

Mechanical	Malformed fetus
Unstretched uterine and abdominal musculature	Large fetus
(associated with first pregnancies)	Large head
Small maternal size	Malformational
Small pelvis	Spina bifida
Small uterus	Other central nervous system malformations
Unicornuate uterus	Bilateral renal agenesis
Bicornuate uterus	Severe hypoplastic kidneys
Uterine leiomyomas	Severe polycystic kidneys
Unusual implantation site	Urethral atresia
Amniotic tear with chronic leakage	Functional
Oligohydramnios (various causes)	Neurological disturbances
Unusual fetal position (breech, transverse lie,	Muscular disturbances
face, brow)	Connective tissue defects
Early pelvic engagement of fetal head	
Twin fetuses	

[a]Some factors can act alone, some act in concert, and some categories overlap.

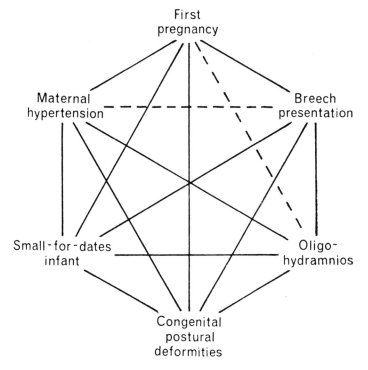

Figure 2-10. Each unbroken line represents a statistically significant association. Interrupted lines represent probable but unproved associations. From Dunn.[19]

reduces the output of fetal urine results in lack of amnionic fluid, thus also producing the deformities of Potter sequence (Figs. 2-16, 2-17).[81] Malformations such as bilateral renal agenesis, severe hypoplastic kidneys, severe polycystic kidneys, and urethral atresia can cause primary oligohydramnios and its consequences. Obstruction of the penile urethra may lead not only to oli-

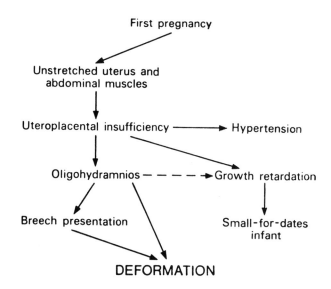

Figure 2-11. Diagram illustrating sequence of events leading to intrauterine deformation. From Dunn.[19]

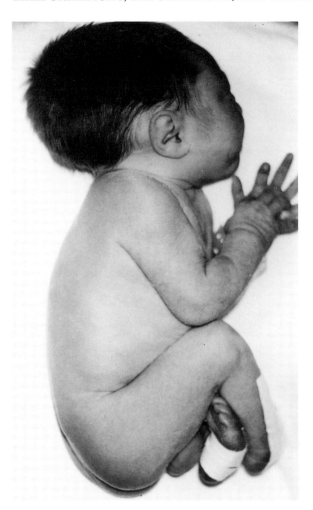

Figure 2-12. One-third of all deformations occur in infants with breech presentations. Prolonged breech presentation resulting in elongated head with prominent occipital shelf. Talipes equinovarus treated by taping. From Graham.[33]

gohydramnios but also to urethral obstruction sequence, more commonly known as *prune belly syndrome* (Fig. 2-18).[72] A severe caudal axis malformation sequence such as sirenomelia, in which kidneys and genitalia are both missing, also produces oligohydramnios and the deformed face and hands of the Potter sequence (Figs. 2-16B, 2-17C).

Functional Causes

Functional causes of deformation include various forms of congenital hypotonia and neuromuscular types of arthrogryposis. Congenital hypotonia may be accompanied by micrognathia, microglossia, prominent lateral palatine ridges, abnormal flexion creases, pes planovalgus, and other deformities. The arthrogryposes are characterized by congenital immobility of the limbs and fixation of the joints in certain positions (Figs. 2-19 to 2-22).[16,39]

In the fetal akinesia sequence, chronic lack of movement leads to multiple

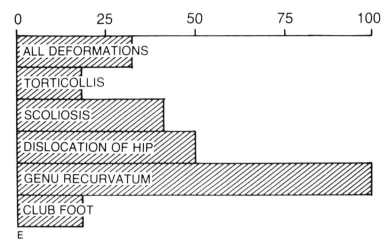

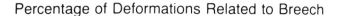

Figure 2-13. Percentage of breech presentations associated with particular deformations from study of 6,000 newborn infants. From Dunn.[17]

joint contractures, micrognathia, polyhydramnios, pulmonary hypoplasia, fetal growth retardation, and short umbilical cord (Figs. 2-23, 2-24). This deformation sequence is etiologically heterogeneous and can result from various neuropathies and myopathies acting during late gestation.[61]

DISRUPTIONS

The frequency of disruptions in newborn infants is unknown, but the range may be between 1% and 2%. Historically, the work of Torpin[83] is significant because

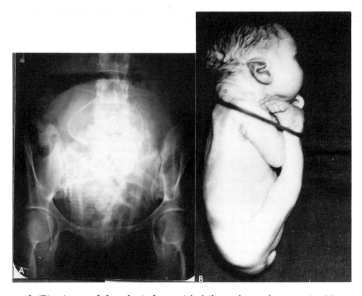

Figure 2-14. Prenatal (A) and postnatal (B) views of female infant with bilateral renal agenesis. Note oligohydramnios and compressed appearance with breech presentation and extended legs. Deformities include dolichocephaly, Potter facies, and congenital hip dislocation. From Dunn.[20]

CONGENITAL POSTURAL DEFORMITIES	Facial deformities	Plagiocephaly	Mandibular asymmetry	Sternomastoid torticollis	Scoliosis—postural	Congenital dislocation of the hip	Talipes
Facial deformities		S	S*	S	S*	S*	S*
Plagiocephaly	S		S*	S*	S*	S*	N
Mandibular asymmetry	S*	S*		S*	N	S*	S*
Sternomastoid torticollis	S	S*	S*		S*	N	S*
Scoliosis—postural	S*	S*	N	S*		S*	S
Congenital dislocation of the hip	S*	S*	S*	N	S*		S*
Talipes	S*	N	S*	S*	S	S*	

Abbreviations: N: not significant; S: $P < 0.05$; S*: $P < 0.001$

Figure 2-15. Statistically significant associations between various congenital postural deformities, showing tendency of deformations to cluster in the same patient. Approximately one-third of all newborns with deformations have multiple deformations. From Dunn.[19]

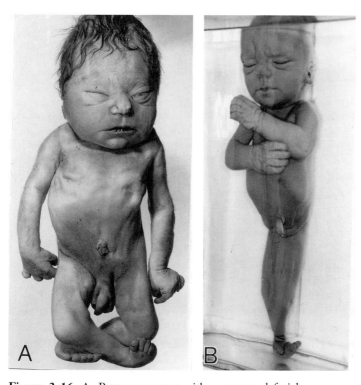

Figure 2-16. A: Potter sequence with compressed facial appearance and limb positioning deformities. From Smith.[78a] B: Sirenomelia, a severe caudal axis malformation sequence in which kidneys and genitalia are missing. Note Potter facies and upper limb deformities. Courtesy of the Warren Anatomical Museum, Harvard University.

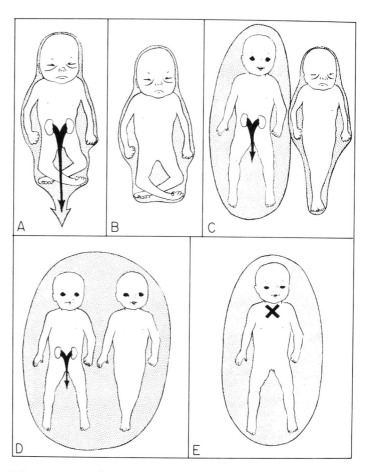

Figure 2-17. Oligohydramnios has different causes and, except under unusual circumstances, leads to facial and limb deformities of Potter sequence. Normally, small amounts of amniotic fluid cross amnion as a transudate, but most amniotic fluid results from fetal urination. A: Amniotic tear with chronic leakage of fluid leading to oligohydramnios, Potter facies, and limb positioning defects. Both kidneys are present, and urination is normal. B: Bilateral renal agenesis. C: Monozygotic twins with separate amnions. Fetus on left has kidneys, and enough fetal urine is contributed to amniotic fluid to protect fetus from deformities of Potter sequence. Fetus on right has sirenomelia in which both kidneys and genitalia are absent. Since there is no urinary contribution to amniotic fluid, compression results in facial and upper limb deformities of Potter sequence. D: Monozygotic twins sharing common amniotic sac. Note that although fetus on right has sirenomelia, Potter deformities are not present because fetus on left provides enough urine in amniotic fluid to protect co-twin from deformities of Potter sequence. E: Fetus has bilateral renal agenesis and therefore does not contribute fetal urine to amniotic fluid. Potter sequence is based on a neurologic swallowing deficit because amniotic fluid crossing amnion remains external to fetus, protecting it from extrinsic, deforming forces. From Cohen.[12]

he recognized the consequences of amniotic rupture. The most important studies of disruption are those of Van Allen[84–87] and Van Allen and associates.[89–91] Many others have also made contributions.[1,2,37,40,41–43,45,48,56,58,61,77,78]

Disruptions have a number of causes, including vascular factors, anoxia, infections, radiation, teratogens, amniotic entanglement, mechanical factors, and dysplastic* lesions. Both the type and the severity of a vascular disruption depend on gestational timing, location, degree of tissue damage, and the pres-

*See discussion of dysplasia in the last section of this chapter, Other Definitions.

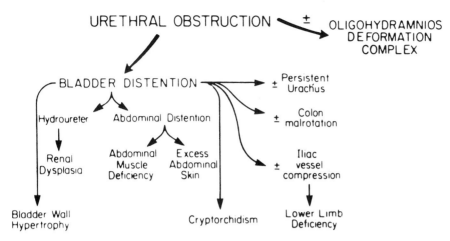

Figure 2-18. Urethral obstruction sequence. From Pagon et al.[72]

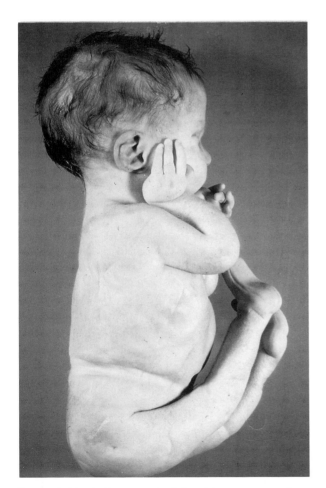

Figure 2-19. Arthrogrypotic deformities on a central nervous system basis. Courtesy of J.B. Beckwith, Loma Linda, California.

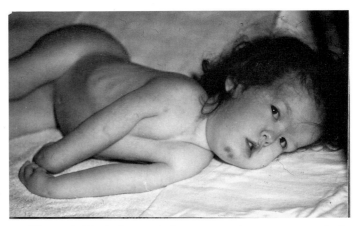

Figure 2-20. Arthrogryposis on a central nervous system basis.

ence or absence of secondary adhesions between adjacent structures. The resultant anomalies are distinctive in appearance because of tissue loss, aberrant differentiation of contiguous tissues, and incomplete development. Distortions that occur during the fetal period tend to be less severe than those during the embryonic period because vascular disruptions are usually confined to a more limited area from an occluded blood vessel or vessels or from vascular insufficiency limited to within areas of watershed blood supply (Table 2-7).[84,85]

Some anomalies, resulting from embryonic disruption, can closely mimic primary malformations. For example, early amnion disruption sequence can

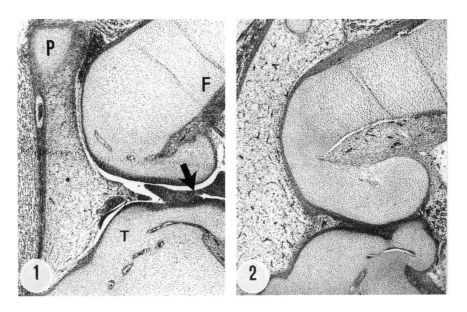

Figure 2-21. Experimental paralysis in chick embryos produced by neuromuscular blocking agents results in joint fixation. Limb movement is essential for joint cavity formation. (1) Normal knee joint, sagittal section. Note joint cavity forming. Arrow indicates cruciate ligament. F, femur; T, tibia; P, patella. (2) Chick embryo paralyzed by neuromuscular blocking agent. Note absence of joint cavitation and cruciate ligament. From Drachman and Sokoloff.[16]

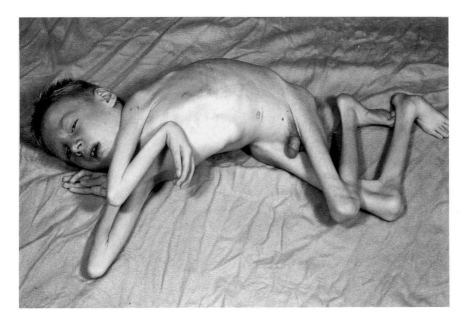

Figure 2-22. Amyotonia congenita with abnormal limb positioning.

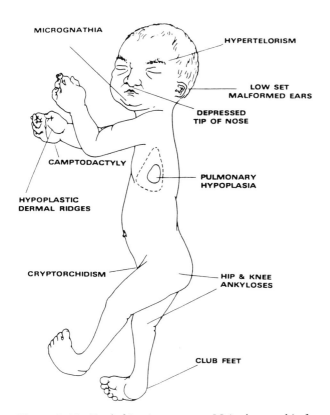

MICROGNATHIA

HYPERTELORISM

LOW SET
MALFORMED EARS

DEPRESSED
TIP OF NOSE

CAMPTODACTYLY

PULMONARY
HYPOPLASIA

HYPOPLASTIC
DERMAL RIDGES

CRYPTORCHIDISM

HIP & KNEE
ANKYLOSES

CLUB FEET

Figure 2-23. Fetal akinesia sequence. Main dysmorphic features. Adapted from Pena and Shokeir.[75]

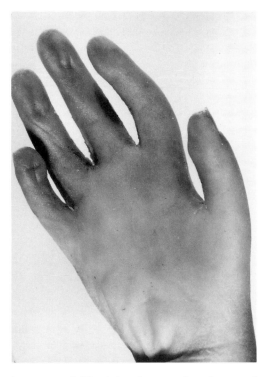

Figure 2-24. Fetal akinesia sequence. Pena-Shokeir syndrome, type I. Hand showing complete absence of palmar and digital creases. From Punnett et al.[76]

produce anencephaly, orofacial clefting, or limb reduction defects. Therefore caution should be exercised in the interpretation of such anomalies; *they may be malformations or disruptions, and diagnosis of a disruption should not be made unless the patient has other features consistent with a disruptive etiology.*[84,85] For example, anencephaly in the presence of amniotic bands or orofacial clefting with ampu-

Table 2-7. Mechanisms of Vascular Disruption in the Embryo and Fetus

Mechanism	Resultant Structural Anomalies
Disruption of embryonic capillary plexus	Early amnion disruption sequence, limb–body wall complex, limb reduction anomalies, oromandibular–limb hypogenesis
Persistence of embryonic vessels	Structural anomalies of the limbs, e.g., radial aplasia, tibial aplasia, clubfoot, fibular aplasia
Premature ablation of embryonic vessels	Subclavian artery supply disruption sequence (Poland sequence, Moebius sequence, Klippel-Feil sequence), horseshoe kidney, gastroschisis
Failure of maturation of vessels	Capillary hemangiomas, arteriovenous fistulas, Berry aneurysms
Occlusion (external compression) of vessels	Anomalies associated with leiomyomas, tubal pregnancies, and bicornate uterus
Occlusion (emboli thrombosis) of vessels	See Table 2-8 for twin anomalies, comparable anomalies in singletons
Altered hemodynamics	Anomalies associated with maternal cocaine use

Adapted from Van Allen.[84]

tations and ring constrictions would be interpreted as a disruption. In some limb anomalies with unusual vascular patterns, it is not always clear whether the vascular pattern is a cause or an effect. For example, it has been postulated that in sirenomelia the pathogenesis may be based on the presence of a single large artery arising high in the abdominal cavity. This *steal vessel* assumes the function of the umbilical arteries and diverts nutrients from the caudal end of the embryo. Arteries below the steal vessel are underdeveloped, the dependent caudal tissues also being underdeveloped.[80] However, others (M. Barr, Jr., personal communication, 1992) attribute the unusual vascular pattern to be a secondary effect of the sirenomelic malformation.

Monozygotic twins have a 50% higher frequency of anomalies than singletons. Many such anomalies are disruptions and may be caused by arterial-to-venous anastomoses between the twins because the placenta is shared. Causes of vascular disruption include (1) placental emboli resulting in the death of one twin, together with anomalies of the other twin due to showers of emboli followed by infarction; (2) thromboplastin from a dead co-twin causing anomalies in the surviving twin from disseminated intravascular coagulation; (3) transient hypo- or hypertension from altered fetal dynamics; or (4) hypo- or hyperperfusion from disparate placental blood flow, resulting in altered growth and anomalies.[84,85] Anomalies reported in twins, following the *in utero* demise of co-twins, and anomalies occurring in discordant twins are summarized in Table 2-8. Central nervous system anomalies followed by gastrointestinal and urogenital anomalies occur most frequently.

Some examples of perfused twins following twin reversed arterial perfusion (TRAP) sequence are shown in Figure 2-25. In this disruption sequence, artery-to-artery anastomosis results in a pump twin and a perfused twin. The pump

Table 2-8. Some Structural Anomalies Reported in Twins That Have Been Attributed to Vascular Disruption

Central nervous system	Toe reduction
Parietal, occipital infarcts	Gangrene, arterial thrombosis
Cerebellar infarcts	Craniofacial
Porencephaly	Orofacial clefts
Hydranencephaly	Hemifacial microsomia (some cases)
Hydrocephalus	Lung
Multicystic encephalomalacia	Arterial thrombi
Microcephaly	Pulmonary infarcts
Transverse myelia	Urogenital
Gastrointestinal	Renal cortical infarction
Hepatic infarct	Renal medullary infarction
Subhepatic cyst	Unilateral renal atresia
Splenic infarct	Horseshoe kidney
Gallbladder atresia	Splenogonadal fusion
Small bowel atresia	Bilateral anorchia
Colonic atresia	Miscellaneous
Appendiceal atresia	Cutis aplasia
Gastroschisis	Oromandibular–limb hypogenesis
Limbs	Poland disruption sequence
Transverse limb reduction	Limb–body wall complex
Constriction bands	Amnion disruption sequence
Distal syndactyly	Twin reversed arterial perfusion sequence
Digital amputations and rings	

Adapted from Van Allen.[84]

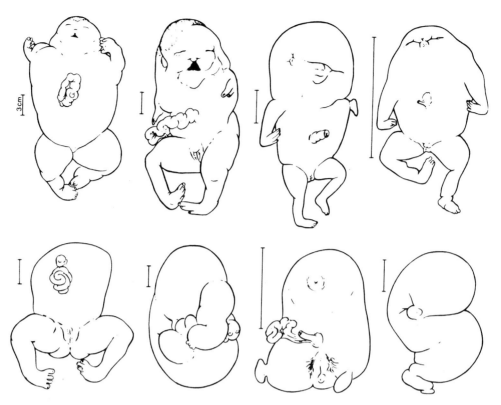

Figure 2-25. Some examples of twin reversed arterial profusion (TRAP) sequence. Note graded loss of normal form with relative sparing of lower portion of body. From Van Allen et al.[91]

twin develops volume overload, increased cardiac work, and congestive heart failure, resulting in intrauterine growth retardation, intrauterine death or prematurity, or edema, ascites, or frank fetal hydrops. The perfused twin, with reversed circulation and blood deficient in oxygen and nutrients, develops disruption of existing structures, incomplete morphogenesis, and malformations of the developing tissues.[91]

Amnion rupture sequence is associated with a wide spectrum of anomalies. The findings depend on the severity of the disruptive insult and the time during the embryonic or fetal period that such an event takes place. Amnion rupture sequence can result, variably, in anencephaly with amniotic bands, craniofacial clefts, orofacial clefting, encephaloceles, extrathoracic heart, omphalocele, limb–body wall deficiency, limb reduction defects, amputations, ring constrictions, and distal syndactyly. Anecdotal case reports have suggested a number of etiologies, including abdominal trauma, chorioamnionitis, IUD removal, maternal oophorectomy, ingestion of bisulfan (an antimitotic drug for the treatment of chronic myelogenous leukemia that can result in thrombocytopenia as a complication), amniocentesis, and chorionic villus sampling.[84,85] Factors involved in limb–body wall disruption are shown in Figure 2-26 and illustrated in Figures 2-27 and 2-28. A case with craniofacial involvement and digital amputations is shown in Figures 2-29 and 2-30.

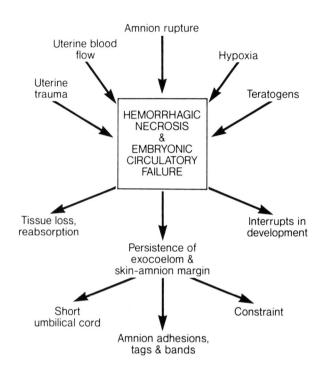

LIMB BODY WALL COMPLEX
disruption of embryonic vasculature

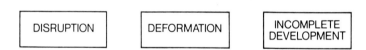

Figure 2-26. Diagram of factors in limb–body wall complex. From Van Allen et al.[86]

COMPARISON OF MALFORMATIONS, DEFORMATIONS, AND DISRUPTIONS

Table 2-9 summarizes a general comparison of malformations, deformations, and disruptions. Table 2-10 lists times of onset of various types of anomalies.

Malformations tend to arise during the embryonic period at the time of organogenesis. Deformations, on the other hand, tend to arise during the fetal period and are alterations in the shape of previously normal parts. Thus, deformations tend to affect intact regions. A clubfoot is not an organ defect but a regional defect, since the limbs have already formed. With simple clubfoot, for example, five digits and a proper number of phalanges and metatarsals are present. Disruptions can arise during the embryonic or the fetal period and affect areas.

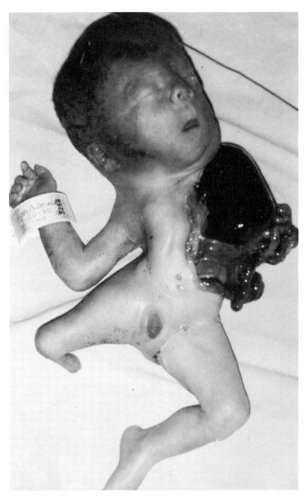

Figure 2-27. Limb–body wall complex showing disruptions and deformations. Thoracoabdominal wall deficiency, absent left arm, hypoplastic right leg, severe scoliosis, deformed ears, and retroflexion of the neck. From Miller et al.[58]

Although the distinction between malformations and deformations based on the embryonic and fetal periods is useful, rigid adherence to these time periods can be misleading. Some malformations such as cleft soft palate and some instances of hypospadias arise during the fetal period, and still others may be defined as a delay or error in perinatal transition as in patent ductus arteriosus (Table 2-10). It is not always correct to speak of a malformation as necessarily being caused *at* the specific time that it arose during development. Technically, the only statement that can be made about cause in relation to embryonic timing is that something happened *before* the latest point in time at which a given malformation might arise. The cause of the malformation might have occurred at that time, *but it might have occurred earlier.* This principle is illustrated by any monogenic malformation syndrome. For example, suppose a patient with Meckel syndrome (Fig. 2-31) has encephalocele, polycystic kidneys, polydactyly, ventricular septal defect, and cleft palate. The embryonic timing of each of these malformations is different. This is true for many malformation syndromes. The only statement that can be made about cause is that something

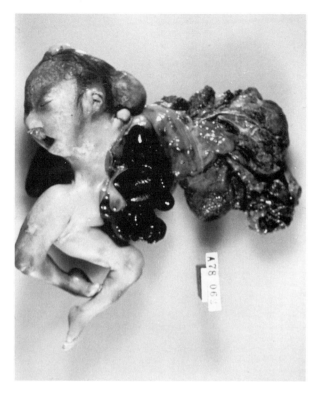

Figure 2-28. Limb–body wall complex. Stillborn (29 weeks) with left thoracoabdominal wall deficiency, severe scoliosis, encephalocele, cleft lip, and short umbilical cord. From Miller et al.[58]

must have happened before the earliest induced malformation. In the case of Meckel syndrome, the earliest malformation occurred at 4 weeks of development, but because the syndrome has autosomal recessive inheritance, the abnormality was present earlier than 4 weeks of development, specifically, at the zygotic stage of development. Two mutant genes in the homozygous state were present at that time.[12]

It has been stated that deformations arise most commonly during the fetal period. The fetus is especially prone to deformation because of its skeletal plasticity and rapid rate of growth in a potentially constraining intrauterine environment. That rapid growth can be a factor in prenatal deformations is easily realized because a fetus of 28 weeks doubles its body weight in 6 weeks. In contrast, during postnatal growth, a 5-year-old boy requires 6 years to double his body weight. Deformations, however, can arise during the postnatal period, as in cases of progressive scoliosis, for example, or in patients with severe cerebral palsy who develop craniofacial deformity, scoliosis, and contractures. Torticollis of long standing can result in asymmetry. Postnatal deformities also may be induced deliberately, as in the cultural practice of Chinese foot binding in young girls and in the practice of splinting the head between boards during infancy to form a pointed skull (Fig. 2-32). The same principles are used by orthopedic surgeons who correct deformities by postural means. Deformations are distinctly uncommon during the embryonic period, but may occur, as in those cases of Robin sequence arising from early severe mandibular constraint. Timing of anomalies is least exact with disruptions. As indicated, some struc-

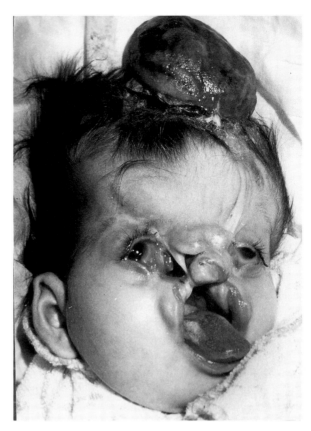

Figure 2-29. Amnion rupture sequence. Absent membrane bones of skull with protrusion of cranial contents. Bilateral facial clefts extending through premaxilla, lips, lateral nose, medial orbits, and skull. Note tissue band traversing forehead. From Granick et al.[37]

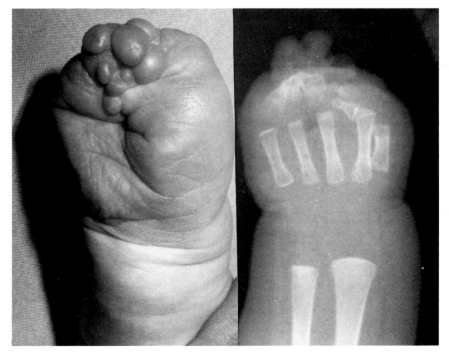

Figure 2-30. Amnion rupture sequence. From case shown in Figure 2-29. Note severe digital amputations. From Granick et al.[37]

Table 2-9. General Comparison of Malformations, Deformations, and Disruptions

Features	Malformations	Deformations	Disruptions
Time of occurrence	Embryonic	Fetal	Embryonic/fetal
Level of disturbance	Organ	Region	Area
Perinatal mortality	+	−	+
Clinial variability of any given anomaly	Moderate	Mild	Extreme
Multiple causes of any given anomaly	Very frequent	Less common	Less common
Spontaneous correction	−	+	−
Correction by posture	−	+	−
Correction by surgery	+	−/+	+
Relative recurrence rate	Higher	Lower	Extremely low
Approximate frequency in newborns	2%–3%	1%–2%	1%–2%

tural anomalies such as anencephaly or orofacial clefting can be either malformations or disruptions, so that interpretation must be cautious. For anencephaly to be considered a malformation, it must arise before closure of the anterior neuropore at 26 days of development. However, the same anomaly can arise *after* closure of the anterior neuropore by damage to the cranial tissues by a disruptive process.

Some degree of perinatal mortality is listed in every statistical survey of malformations because of the high frequency of central nervous system and cardiovascular anomalies. Disruptions that are induced during the embryonic period can also be devastating and incompatible with life. In contrast, simple amputations and constrictions of digits that may occur during the fetal period

Table 2-10. Time of Onset of Various Types of Anomalies

Time of Onset	Susceptibility	Examples
Malformations		
Embryonic	Common	Anencephaly, cleft lip, syndactyly
Fetal	Less common	Posterior cleft palate, hypospadias
Perinatal	Uncommon	Patent ductus arteriosus, cryptorchidism
Deformations		
Embryonic	Low	Robin sequence arising from early mandibular constraint
Fetal	High	Clubfoot, congenital hip dislocation, congenital postural scoliosis
Postnatal	Medium	Postnatal developing scoliosis, deformities resulting from severe cerebral palsy
Disruptions		
Embryonic	Common	Limb–body wall complex
Fetal	Less common	Amputation and ring constriction of digits

Patient with the Meckel Syndrome

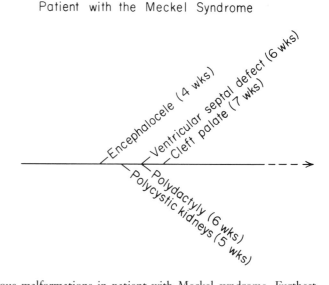

Figure 2-31. Embryonic timing for various malformations in patient with Meckel syndrome. Furthest horizontal point at left indicates zygote formation. Arrow points in direction of birth. From Cohen.[12]

are obviously compatible with life. The perinatal mortality tends to be extremely low in surveys of deformations.

Clinical variability is most extensive in disruptions. Among vascular disruptions, each one is practically unique. For example, compare the different phenotypes found in the TRAP sequence shown in Figure 2-25. With disruptions produced by some teratogens such as alcohol or hydantoin there is usually less variability. Malformations are moderately variable in how they are expressed (e.g., cleft lip-palate, omphalocele, hypospadias), and deformations tend to be mildly variable in comparison to malformations.

Malformations are the most causally heterogeneous of the three types of anomalies. For example, holoprosencephaly is a component part of more than 60 syndromes. Craniosynostosis is present in about 90 syndromes, and cleft lip-

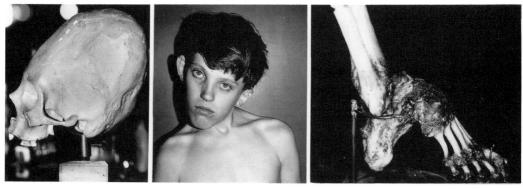

Figure 2-32. Postnatal deformation. Left: Cultural head molding. Courtesy of Vrolik Museum, Amsterdam. Center: Torticollis of long standing, resulting in asymmetry. Note eyes not on same level. From Cohen.[12] Right: Chinese foot binding with resultant deformity. Courtesy of the Warren Anatomical Museum, Harvard University.

palate is a feature in over 300 syndromes (see Chapter 9, Tables 9-3 through 9-5). Deformations and disruptions can be causally heterogeneous, but less so than malformations. In deformations like contractures, causes include constraint or some intrinsic neuromuscular or connective tissue problem. Probably the fetal akinesia sequence is the most causally heterogeneous of deformations; the phenotype can arise from oligohydramnios or from various abnormalities of myoneural dysfunction. Hydranencephaly, a disruption, has been associated with hemorrhagic states such as Factor XIII deficiency, death of a monozygotic co-twin, toxoplasmosis, herpes simplex, and maternal hypoxemia.[85]

Malformations and disruptions that are compatible with life can only be corrected by surgical means. In contrast, spontaneous correction or correction by posturing is possible with many deformations. Dunn[19] noted that 90% of deformations correct spontaneously after birth. That self-correction commonly occurs is not surprising because, following birth, the infant is no longer subject to intrauterine constraining forces. Tibial torsion present in newborns, for example, undergoes spontaneous correction in most cases. For various types of deformations, the degree to which self-correction is possible depends on how long during fetal life the constraining forces were acting and on the severity of the deformation (Fig. 2-33). Postural correction is feasible in many cases of scoliosis, congenital hip dislocation, and clubfoot. Obviously, for severe deformations surgery may be required. Spontaneous correction of malformations is rare, except for small atrial and ventricular septal defects, and correction by posturing is not possible.

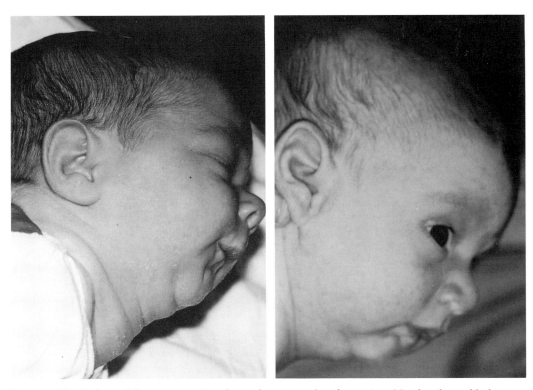

Figure 2-33. Prolonged face presentation during last 2 months of gestation. Nasal and mandibular compression shows partial self-resolution by 6 weeks of age. From Graham.[33]

The relative recurrence rate* row in Table 2-9 refers to each type of anomaly *as a whole class.* For example, each specific isolated malformation usually occurs as a sporadic event, but in a few instances mendelian inheritance may be present. When all malformations are considered together, their rate of recurrence is higher because each malformation has a minority of recurrent cases, which drives up the overall rate. In contrast, deformations have a lower recurrence rate. Some, such as clubfoot, have a multifactorial recurrence rate; others may have a negligible recurrence rate. For disruptions, the rate of recurrence is extremely low. Although disruptions are almost always sporadic events, an occasional recurrence is reported.[54]

Some approximate frequencies of various anomalies are listed in Table 2-9. Kalter and Warkany[47] have noted that from numerous surveys over a 30 year period, a 3% frequency has emerged for malformations in newborn infants. However, most surveys have not separated deformations and disruptions from malformations, hence the frequency estimate of 2%–3% in Table 2-9. Birth prevalence will also vary depending on the type of survey and on the ascertainment technique used (e.g., birth certificates vs. hospital discharge diagnoses).[28] Specific malformations occur with different rates in different populations. For example, cleft lip with or without cleft palate is much more common in the white population than in the black population, whereas with polydactyly the reverse is the case.[29] The frequency of malformations is higher in miscarried fetuses and stillborn infants, as is the frequency of chromosomal abnormalities. The frequency also increases as infancy progresses because some malformations (e.g., occult cardiovascular defects) are not diagnosed during the neonatal period.[88] Deformations at birth have an estimated frequency of 1%–2%, the most important surveys being closer to the top end of the range.[19] The frequency of disruptions in newborn infants is unknown,[85] an estimate of 1%–2% being suggested in Table 2-9. Of fetuses identified as having anomalies by ultrasound, approximately 9.2% result from vascular disruption.[85] According to Luebke et al.,[56] about 3.6% of *stillborns* have structural anomalies attributed to vascular disruption.

INTERRELATIONSHIPS BETWEEN MALFORMATIONS, DEFORMATIONS, AND DISRUPTIONS

Although distinctions between malformations, deformations, and disruptions are useful for clinical purposes, the three classes of anomalies are interrelated and may overlap in some instances (Fig. 2-34). It has been observed that malformations can result in deformations, as with the deformational sequelae of meningomyelocele. It has also been stated that some anomalies, such as Robin sequence, may be malformational or deformational, depending on the initiating factor. Plagiocephaly may occur on a malformational basis by unilateral coronal synostosis or by the rarely occurring lambdoid synostosis,[9] or it may occur on a deformational basis (Fig. 2-35). However, deformational constraint, particularly if prolonged, can also result in craniosynostosis in some cases as well (Fig. 2-36).[8]

Sometimes the same mechanism can result in different classes of anomalies. For example, intrauterine compression during the fetal period can result in

---

*With malformations, deformations, and disruptions, we speak of *empiric recurrence rates*, which are commonly interpreted as *true risks* when in fact they are not.

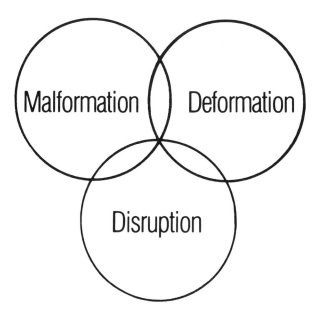

Figure 2-34. Venn diagram showing interrelationships between malformations, deformations, and disruptions. From Cohen.[12]

deformations, but, when severe compression is present earlier during the embryonic period, disruptions can be produced. Cases of limb–body wall complex (Figs. 2-27 and 2-28) have both disruptive and deformational components.[58] In this condition, amnion rupture sequence can lead to two types of disruptions: (1) compression-related defects such as limb deficiency, body wall deficiency, and neural tube defects; and (2) band- or adhesion-related defects such as craniofacial clefts. Deformations resulting from compression may include severe scoliosis, retroflexion of the neck, and ear deformities. Some cases of urethral obstruction sequence (Fig. 2-18) are associated with lower limb deficiency, which may possibly result from vascular compromise of the iliofemoral

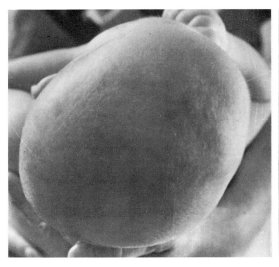
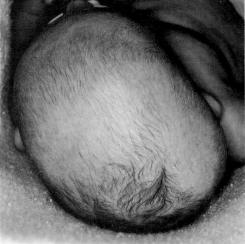

Figure 2-35. Deformational plagiocephaly. Left: Mild degree. From Cohen.[12] Right: Severe degree. Persistent head turn to left is caused by cervical and thoracic vertebral anomalies. From Graham.[33]

CATEGORIES OF PLAGIOCEPHALY

TYPE   ETIOLOGY

Nonsynostotic plagiocephaly

Coronal plagiocephaly   Constraint-related

Lambdoid plagiocephaly   Other etiologies

Figure 2-36. Categories of plagiocephaly and their causes. Other etiologies include genetic causes and unknown causes. From Cohen.[8]

vessels by the distended bladder.[72,85] The expanded Goldenhar spectrum with severe secondary disruption[56] is shown in Figure 2-37 and diagrammed in Figure 2-38. Figure 2-39 shows a schematic representation of amnion rupture sequence in which all three kinds of anomalies—malformations, deformations, and disruptions—are produced.[40,44] Frank malformations may include classic cleft lip, classic cleft palate, choanal atresia, proboscis formation, and omphalocele. Oligohydramnios may result in intrauterine crowding and tethering of fetal parts, producing deformations such as clubfoot. Finally, aberrant tissue bands may produce disruptions such as craniofacial cleavages, which do not conform to the normal planes of embryonic facial closure.

MORE DEFINITIONS[3,62–71,79]

Developmental fields: Units of the embryo in which the development of complex structures is determined and controlled in a spatially coordinated, temporally synchronous, and epimorphically hierarchical manner

Monotopic field: Developmental field involving closely contiguous anatomic structures

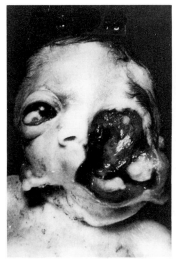
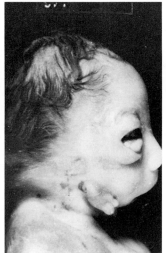
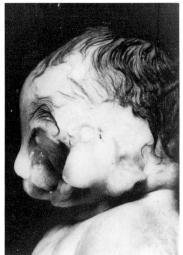

Figure 2-37. Bizarre case of expanded Goldenhar spectrum with secondary disruptions. From Luebke et al.[56]

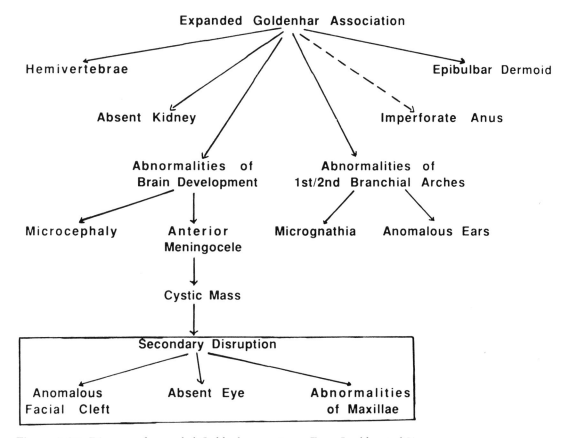

Figure 2-38. Diagram of expanded Goldenhar spectrum. From Luebke et al.[56]

Polytopic field: Developmental field that involves more distantly located anatomic structures but that depends on the nature of the inductive or developmental relationship

Developmental field defect: Dysmorphogenetically reactive unit, i.e., a set of embryonic primordia that react identically to different dysmorphogenetic causes. Can be monotopic or polytopic

Midline: Refers to the embryo, during early blastogenesis, reacting as a pluripotential single unit, or primary field. Defects of blastogenesis are confined to the midline*

Association: Nonrandom occurrence in two or more individuals of multiple, idiopathic anomalies of blastogenesis†

DEVELOPMENTAL FIELD DEFECTS‡

Although Opitz has stated repeatedly that the concept of developmental fields has had a long history in biology, his own contributions have been extremely

---

*The midline has been said to be developmentally weak as a consequence of determinative field properties.[55]

†Opitz[66] proposed this new working definition of an association. Compare with the earlier definition of the International Working Group given in Chapter 1.

‡Although the developmental field concept has become more popular in recent years,[64] its utility has been questioned by some.[30,46]

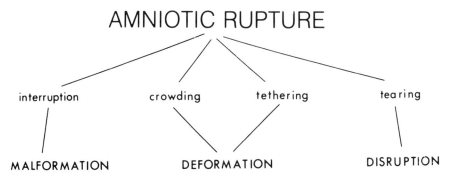

Figure 2-39. Schematic representation of various mechanisms of injury with amnion rupture. From Higginbottom et al.[40]

important as well as numerous.[62-71] In the definition of developmental field (*vide supra*), three terms require further explanation. First, *spatial coordination* refers to the processes whereby components of a complex structure assume their proper location and orientation with respect to each other by a combination of morphogenetic movement, growth, and inductive interactions.[67] Second, *temporal synchronization* refers to the proper timing of contiguous morphogenetic events to ensure normal development. Finally, *epimorphically hierarchical* refers to progression from the less complex to the more highly differentiated stage of embryonic development.

The developmental field concept has two main implications: (1) etiologic heterogeneity and (2) a possible explanation for the occurrence of "association" in the same patient.

In a developmental field defect, the embryonic field reacts identically to different causes.[65,67] For example, holoprosencephaly is a monotopic field defect that can be caused by trisomy 13, an autosomal gene mapped to 7p16, or the diabetic state of a pregnant woman.[10,11] Some genetic disorders such as Kallmann syndrome have absence of the olfactory tracts and bulbs only, without ever having severe holoprosencephaly. Such a restrictive malformation may represent a field-within-a-field or nested field.[82] Acrofacial dysostosis, the combination of mandibulofacial dysostosis and limb defects, constitutes a polytopic developmental field defect. Nager acrofacial dysostosis, for example, may be heterogeneous, occurring as an autosomal recessive or autosomal dominant trait or with complex chromosome abnormalities.[69,71] Thus, monotopic and polytopic developmental field defects refer to clinical outcomes, not to initial morphogenetic relationships. Furthermore, polytopic field defects should be distinguished from sequences.[70]

Midline anomalies are particularly common.[67,68] They include defects with a midline origin as well as symmetric structures influenced by midline primordia or morphogenetic events at the midline.[14,68] It has been shown in a number of studies that midline defects tend to be statistically associated with other midline defects.[15,49-51] Clinical/epidemiologic assessment of the primary midline developmental field and analysis of normal body symmetry and asymmetry have been carried out by Martínez-Frías et al.[56a,56b]

Opitz,[62,63] noting that the accepted definition of association[3,79] was statistical rather than biological, observed that ideally any given association should be broken apart into one or more sequences, syndromes, or field defects. However, even though some entities have split from associations, associations still remain

Table 2-11. Contrast Between Blastogenetic and Organogenetic Anomalies

Feature	Blastogenesis	Organogenesis
Timing	Karyogamy to end of gastrulation (stage 12, days 27–28)	Stage 13 (day 28) to end of eighth week (stage 22, days 55–56)
Field	Primary field	Secondary fields
Severity	Tend to be more severe	Tend to be less severe
Complexity	Tend to be more complex	Tend to be less complex
Extent	Tend to be multisystem, polytopic	Tend to be localized, monotopic
Lethality	More common	Less common
Monozygotic twinning	More common	Less common or not a factor
Sex differences	Tend to be less apparent	Tend to be more apparent
Midline	Confined to midline	Not confined to midline
Multiple anomalies: associative vs. syndromic	Usually associative	More likely syndromic

Adapted from Opitz.[62]

and have not disappeared, suggesting a biological definition for associations: *patterns of multiple anomalies of blastogenesis.* Opitz[62] made use of his concept of associations in contrasting blastogenetic with organogenetic anomalies (Table 2-11) (see also Lubinsky.[53a])

OTHER DEFINITIONS

Because definitions are given in Chapters 1 and 2, the following two definitions are discussed at the end of this chapter even though they are not directly related to the major topics.

The International Working Group[3,79] defined *dysplasia* as

An abnormal organization of cells into tissue(s) and its morphologic result(s). In other words: a dysplasia is the process (and the consequences) of dyshistogenesis.

I prefer the term *dyshistogenesis.* Some problems of dyshistogenesis are shown in Figure 2-40. The term *dysplasia* has been used loosely. For example, in pathology dysplasia is applied to cervical and oral epithelial lesions, but not to neoplasms of mesodermal origin.* In dysmorphology, dysplasia has been used for very different types of disorders such as frontonasal dysplasia, *dysplastic* ear, renal dysplasia, cleidocranial dysplasia, and septo-optic dysplasia. Even the use of the term in pathology, where it is most common, has been questioned.[53]

Warburg and Møller[92] have defined *dystrophy* as

The process and consequences of hereditary progressive affections of specific cells in one or more tissues that initially show a normal function.

They note that the term *abiotrophy* has previously been applied but is no longer used. They also note that *degeneration* is an equivocal term applied to both hereditary and acquired conditions. Warburg and Møller[92] further observe that

---

*Fibrous dysplasia cannot be properly classified as a neoplasm.

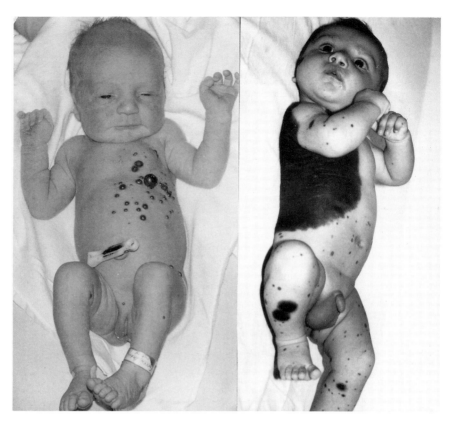

Figure 2-40. Examples of dyshistogenesis. Left: Multiple hemangiomas. Right: Huge nevus and smaller multiple nevi.

dyshistogenetic tissues present with abnormal structure and function at birth in contrast to dystrophies, which are genetically programmed for later onset.

REFERENCES

1. Baker CJ, Rudolph AJ: Congenital ring constrictions and intrauterine amputations. *Am J Dis Child* 121:393–400, 1971.
2. Bavinck JN, Weaver DD: Subclavian artery supply disruption sequence: Hypothesis of a vascular etiology for Poland, Klippel-Feil, and Möbius anomalies. *Am J Med Genet* 23:903–918, 1986.
3. Benirschke K, Cohen MM Jr, Hall JG, Lenz W, Lowry RB, Opitz JM, Pinsky L, Schwarzacher HG, Smith DW, Spranger J: Terms pertaining to morphogenesis and malformations. March of Dimes Birth Defects Meeting, June 8–11, 1980.
4. Brown FE, Colen LB, Addante RR, Graham JM Jr: Correction of congenital auricular deformities by splinting in the neonatal period. *Pediatrics* 78:406–411, 1986.
5. Browne D: Congenital deformities of mechanical origin. *Proc R Soc Med* 29:1409–1431, 1936.
6. Chapple CC, Davidson DT: A study of the relationship between fetal position and certain congenital deformities. *J Pediatr* 18:483–493, 1941.
7. Clarren SK: Plagiocephaly and torticollis: Etiology, natural history, and helmet treatment. *J Pediatr* 98:92–95, 1981.

8. Cohen MM Jr: Discussion: Frontal plagiocephaly: Synostotic, compensational, or deformational. *Plast Reconstr Surg* 89:32–33, 1992.

9. Cohen MM Jr: Letter to the Editor: Lambdoid synostosis is an overdiagnosed condition. *Am J Med Genet* 61:98–99, 1996.

10. Cohen MM Jr: Perspectives on holoprosencephaly: Part I. Epidemiology, genetics, and syndromology. *Teratology* 40:211–235, 1989.

11. Cohen MM Jr: Perspectives on holoprosencephaly. Part III. Spectra, distinctions, continuities, and discontinuities. *Am J Med Genet* 34:271–288, 1989.

12. Cohen MM Jr: *The Child With Multiple Birth Defects.* New York: Raven Press, 1982.

13. Cohen MM Jr, Jirasek JE, Guzman RT, Gorlin RJ, Peterson MQ: Holoprosencephaly and facial dysmorphia: Nosology, etiology and pathogenesis. *Birth Defects* 7(7):125–135, 1971.

13a. Conen PE, Erkman B, Metaxotou C: The "D" syndrome. *Am J Dis Child* 111:236–247, 1966.

14. Czeizel A: Schisis association. *Am J Med Genet* 10:25–35, 1981.

15. DeMyer WE, Zeman W: Alobar holoprosencephaly (arhinencephaly) with median cleft lip and palate: Clinical, electroencephalographic and nosologic considerations. *Confin Neurol* 23:1–36, 1963.

16. Drachman DB, Sokoloff L: The role of movement in embryonic joint development. *Dev Biol* 14:401–420, 1966.

17. Dunn PM: Breech delivery: Perinatal morbidity and mortality. 5th European Congress of Perinatal Medicine, Uppsala, Sweden, p 54, 1976.

18. Dunn PM: Congenital dislocation of the hip (CHD): Necropsy studies at birth. *Proc R Soc Med* 62:1035–1037, 1969.

19. Dunn PM: Congenital postural deformities. *Br Med Bull* 32:71–76, 1976.

20. Dunn PM: Congenital postural deformities: Perinatal associations. *Proc R Soc Med* 65:735–738, 1972.

21. Dunn PM: Congenital postural deformities: Further perinatal associations. *Proc R Soc Med* 67:1174–1178, 1974.

22. Dunn PM: Congenital sternomastoid torticollis: An intrauterine postural deformity. *Arch Dis Child* 49:824–825, 1974.

23. Dunn PM: Growth retardation of infants with congenital postural deformities. *Acta Med Auxol* 7:63–68, 1975.

24. Dunn PM: Maternal and fetal aetiological factors. 5th European Congress of Perinatal Medicine, Uppsala, Sweden, p 76, 1976.

25. Dunn PM: Maternal and fetal aetiological factors in breech deliveries. Symposium II, Fifth European Congress of Perinatal Medicine, Sweden, pp 77–81, 1976.

26. Dunn PM: Perinatal observations on the etiology of congenital dislocation of the hip. *Clin Orthop* 11:11–22, 1976.

27. Durkin-Stamm MV, Gilbert EF, Ganick DJ, Opitz JM: An unusual dysplasia-malformation-cancer syndrome in two patients. *Am J Med Genet* 1:279–289, 1978.

28. Edmonds LD, Layde PM, James LM et al: Congenital malformations surveillance: Two American systems. *Int J Epidemiol* 10:247–252, 1981.

29. Erickson JD: Racial variations in the incidence of congenital malformations. *Ann Hum Genet* 39:315–320, 1976.

30. Fraser FC: The origins, natural history and fate of the developmental field defect. *Proc Greenwood Genet Center* 8:152, 1989.

31. Graham JM Jr: Alterations in head shape as a consequence of fetal head constraint. *Semin Perinatol* 7:257–269, 1983.

32. Graham JM Jr: Causes of limb reduction defects: The contribution of fetal constraint and/or vascular disruption. *Clin Perinatol* 13:575–591, 1986.

33. Graham JM Jr: *Smith's Recognizable Patterns of Human Deformation.* Second edition. Philadelphia: WB Saunders, 1988.

34. Graham JM Jr, deSaxe M, Smith DW: Sagittal craniostenosis: Fetal head constraint as one possible cause. *J Pediatr* 95:747, 1979.

35. Graham JM Jr, Higginbottom MC, Smith DW: Preaxial polydactyly of the foot

associated with early amnion rupture: Evidence for mechanical teratogenesis? *J Pediatr* 98:943–945, 1981.

36. Graham JM Jr, Miller ME, Stephan MJ, Smith DW: Limb reduction anomalies and early in utero limb compression. *J Pediatr* 96:1052–1056, 1980.

37. Granick MS, Ramasastry S, Vries J, Cohen MM Jr: Severe amniotic band syndrome occurring with unrelated syndactyly. *Plast Reconstr Surg* 80:829–832, 1987.

38. Haberkern CM, Smith DW, Jones KL: The "breech head" and its relevance. *Am J Dis Child* 133:154–156, 1979.

39. Herrmann J, Opitz JM: Naming and nomenclature of syndromes. *Birth Defects* 10(7):69–86, 1974.

40. Higginbottom MC, Jones KL, Hall BD, Smith DW: The amniotic band disruption complex: Timing of amniotic rupture and variable spectra of consequent defects. *J Pediatr* 95:544–549, 1979.

41. Hoyme HE, Higginbottom MC, Jones KL: The vascular pathogenesis of gastroschisis: Intrauterine interruption of the omphalomesenteric artery. *J Pediatr* 98:228–231, 1981.

42. Hoyme HE, Higginbottom MC, Jones KL: Vascular etiology of disruptive structural defects in monozygotic twins. *Pediatrics* 67:288–291, 1981.

43. Hoyme HE, Jones KL, Van Allen MI: Vascular pathogenesis of transverse limb reduction defects. *J Pediatr* 101:839–843, 1982.

44. Hunter AGW, Carpenter BF: Implications of malformations not due to amniotic bands in the amniotic band sequence. *Am J Med Genet* 24:691–700, 1986.

45. Jones KL, Smith DW, Hall BD, Hall JG, Ebbin AJ, Massoud H, Golbus MS: A pattern of craniofacial and limb defects secondary to aberrant tissue bands. *J Pediatr* 83:90–95, 1974.

46. Kallen B: *Epidemiology of Human Reproduction.* Boca Raton, FL: CRC Press, 1988, pp 31–35.

47. Kalter H, Warkany J: Congenital malformations: Etiologic factors and their role in prevention. *N Engl J Med* 308:424–431, 1983.

48. Kennedy LA, Persaud TVN: Pathogenesis of developmental defects induced in the rat by amniotic sac puncture. *Acta Anat* 97:23–35, 1977.

49. Khoury MJ, Cordero JF, Rasmussen S: Invited editorial comment: Ectopia cordis, midline defects and chromosome abnormalities: An epidemiologic perspective. *Am J Med Genet* 30:811–817, 1988.

50. Khoury MJ, Cordero JF, Mulinare J, Opitz JM: Selected midline defect associations: A population study. *Pediatrics* 84:266, 1989.

51. Khoury MJ, James LM, Erickson JD: On the measurement and interpretation of birth defect associations in epidemiologic studies. *Am J Med Genet* 37:229–236, 1990.

52. Koskinen-Moffett LK, Moffett BC Jr, Graham JM Jr: Cranial synostosis and intrauterine compression: A developmental study of human sutures. In Dixon AD and Sarnat BG (eds): *Factors and Mechanisms Influencing Bone Growth.* New York: Alan R. Liss, 1982, pp 365–378.

53. Koss LG: Dysplasia. A real concept or a misnomer? *Obstet Gynecol* 51:374–379, 1978.

53a. Lubinsky M: Epidemiologies of blastogenic defects: Genetic associations and inherited anomalies in rare mendelian syndromes. *Am J Med Genet* (in press).

54. Lubinsky M, Sujansky E, Sanger W, Salyards P, Severn C: Familial amniotic bands. *Am J Med Genet* 14:81–88, 1983.

55. Lubinsky MS: Midline developmental "weakness" as a consequence of determinative field properties. *Am J Med Genet Suppl* 3:23–28, 1987.

56. Luebke HJ, Reiser CA, Pauli RM: Fetal disruptions: Assessment of frequency, heterogeneity, and embryologic mechanisms in a population referred to a community-based stillbirth assessment program. *Am J Med Genet* 36:56–72, 1990.

56a. Martínez-Frías ML: Primary midline developmental field. I. Clinical and epidemiological characteristics. *Am J Med Genet* 56:374–381, 1995.

56b. Martínez-Frías ML, Urioste M, Bermejo E, Rodríguez-Pinilla E, Valentín F, Paisán L, Martínez S, Egüés J, Gómez F, Aparicio P, Cucalón F, Arroyo A, Meipp C, Vázquez S, Rodríguez JI, Rosa A, García J, Jiménez N, Moro C: Primary midline developmental field. II. Clinical/epidemiological analysis of alteration of laterality (normal body symmetry and asymmetry). *Am J Med Genet* 56:382–388, 1995.

57. Miller ME, Dunn PM, Smith DW: Uterine malformations and fetal deformation. *J Pediatr* 94:387–390, 1979.

58. Miller ME, Graham JM Jr, Higginbottom MC, Smith DW: Compression-related defects from early amnion rupture: Evidence for mechanical teratogenesis. *J Pediatr* 98:292–297, 1981.

59. Miller ME, Higginbottom MC, Smith DW: Short umbilical cords: Its origin and relevance. *Pediatrics* 67:618–621, 1981.

60. Miller ME, Jones MC, Smith DW: Tension: The basis of umbilical cord growth. *J Pediatr* 101:844, 1982.

61. Moessinger AC: Fetal akinesia sequence: An animal model. *Pediatrics* 72:857–863, 1983.

62. Opitz JM: Blastogenesis and the "primary field" in human development. *Birth Defects* 29(1):3–37, 1993.

63. Opitz JM: Editorial: Associations and syndromes: Terminology in clinical genetics and birth defects epidemiology: Comments on Khoury, Moore, and Evans. *Am J Med Genet* 49:14–20, 1994.

64. Opitz JM: Editorial comment: Developmental field theory and observations— Accidental progress? *Am J Med Genet Suppl* 2:1–8, 1986.

65. Opitz JM: Editorial comment: The developmental field concept. *Am J Med Genet* 21:1–11, 1985.

66. Opitz JM: *The Developmental Field Concept.* New York: Alan R. Liss, 1986.

67. Opitz JM: The developmental field concept in clinical genetics. *J Pediatr* 101:805–809, 1982.

68. Opitz JM, Gilbert EF: Editorial comment: CNS anomalies and the midline as a "developmental field." *Am J Med Genet* 12:443–455, 1982.

69. Opitz JM, Gilbert SF: Editorial comment: Developmental field theory and the molecular analysis of morphogenesis: A comment on Dr. Slavkin's observations. *Am J Med Genet* 47:687–688, 1993.

70. Opitz JM, Lewin SO: The developmental field concept in pediatric pathology— Especially with respect to fibular a/hypoplasia and the DiGeorge anomaly. *Birth Defects* 23(1):277–292, 1987.

71. Opitz JM, Mollica F, Sorge G, Milana G, Cimino G: Acrofacial dysostoses: Review and report of a previously undescribed condition: The autosomal or X-linked dominant Catania form of acrofacial dysostosis. *Am J Med Genet* 47:660–678, 1993.

72. Pagon R, Smith DW, Shephard TH: Urethral obstruction malformation complex: A cause of abdominal muscle deficiency and the "prune belly." *J Pediatr* 96:900–906, 1979.

73. Palacios J, Rodriguez JI: Extrinsic fetal akinesia and skeletal development. A study in oligohydramnios sequence. *Teratology* 42:1–5, 1990.

74. Patel H, Dolman CL, Byrne MA: Holoprosencephaly with median cleft lip. *Am J Dis Child* 124:217–225, 1972.

75. Pena SDJ, Shokeir MHK: Syndrome of camptodactyly, multiple ankyloses, facial anomalies, and pulmonary hypoplasia: A lethal condition. *J Pediatr* 85:373–375, 1974.

76. Punnett HH, Kistenmacher ML, Valdes-Dapena M, Ellison RT: Syndrome of ankylosis, facial anomalies, and pulmonary hypoplasia. *J Pediatr* 85:375–377, 1974.

77. Robinson LK, Hoyme HE, Edwards DK, Jones KL: Vascular pathogenesis of unilateral craniofacial defects. *J Pediatr* 111:236–239, 1987.

78. Russell LJ, Weaver DD, Bull MJ, Weinbaum M: In utero brain destruction resulting

in collapse of the fetal skull, microcephaly, scalp rugae, and neurologic impairment: The fetal brain disruption sequence. *Am J Med Genet* 17:509–521, 1964.

78a. Smith DW: *Recognizable Patterns of Human Malformation*. Third Edition. Philadelphia: WB Saunders, 1982.

79. Spranger JW, Benirschke K, Hall JG, Lenz W, Lowry RB, Opitz JM, Pinsky L, Schwarzacher HG, Smith DW: Errors of morphogenesis: Concepts and terms. *J Pediatr* 100:160–165, 1982.

80. Stevenson RE, Jones KL, Phelan MC, Jones MC, Barr M Jr, Clericuzio C, Harley RA, Benirschke K: Vascular steal: The pathogenetic mechanism producing sirenomelia and associated defects of the viscera and soft tissues. *Pediatrics* 78:451–457, 1986.

81. Thomas IT, Smith DW: Oligohydramnios, cause of the non-renal features of Potter's syndrome, including pulmonary hypoplasia. *J Pediatr* 84:811–814, 1974.

82. Toriello HV: Letter to the Editor: The arhinencephaly field defect. *Am J Med Genet Suppl* 2:73–76, 1986.

83. Torpin R: *Fetal Malformations Caused by Amnion Rupture During Gestation*. Springfield, IL: Charles C. Thomas, 1968.

84. Van Allen MI: Structural anomalies resulting from vascular disruption. *Pediatr Clin North Am* 39:255–277, 1992.

85. Van Allen MI: Structural anomalies from vascular disruption. In Gilbert-Barness E (ed.): *Potter's Pathology of the Fetus and Infant*. W.B. Saunders, in press.

86. Van Allen MI, Curry C, Gallagher L: Limb–body wall complex: I. Pathogenesis. *Am J Med Genet* 28:529–548, 1987.

87. Van Allen MI, Curry C, Walden CE, Gallagher L, Patten RM: Limb–body wall complex: II. Limb and spine defects. *Am J Med Genet* 28:549–565, 1987.

88. Van Allen MI, Hall JG: Congenital anomalies. In Bennett JC, Plum F (eds) *Cecil Textbook of Medicine*, 20th edition. W.B. Saunders, Philadelphia. Chapt. 27, pp 157–159,1996.

89. Van Allen MI, Myhre S: Ectopia cordis thoracalis with craniofacial defects resulting from early amnion rupture. *Teratology* 32:19–24, 1985.

90. Van Allen MI, Siegel-Bartelt J, Dixon J, Zuker RM, Clarke HM, Toi A: Constriction bands and limb reduction defects in two newborns with fetal ultrasound evidence for vascular disruption. *Am J Med Genet* 44:598–604, 1992.

91. Van Allen MI, Smith DW, Shepard TH: Twin reversed arterial perfusion (TRAP) sequence: A study of 14 twin pregnancies with acardius. *Semin Perinatol* 7:285–293, 1983.

92. Warburg M, Møller HU: Dystrophy: A revised definition. *J Med Genet* 26:769–771, 1989.

93. Warkany J: *Congenital Malformations: Notes and Comments*. Chicago: Year Book Medical Publishers, 1971.

3

Minor Anomalies

Minor anomalies have been discussed extensively in the pediatric and genetic literature.[8a,14,19,23,27,32,32a,35] Among the terms used have been *minor congenital anomalies, mild errors of morphogenesis,*[27] and *informative morphogenetic variants.*[35] Opitz[32,32a] suggested that minor anomalies represent either defects of organogenesis, arising during embryogenesis and termed *mild malformations,* or defects of phenogenesis, arising during fetal or early postnatal life and representing quantitative differences between individuals. In his most recent review of minor anomalies, Merlob[27] used the subtitle, "One of the most controversial subjects in dysmorphology." The subject is also extremely complex. The most exhaustive review is that of Frías and Carey.[8a] In this chapter, the clinical utility is discussed, and some of the problems raised by various studies of minor anomalies are then reviewed.

CLINICAL UTILITY

A distinction can be made between major and minor anomalies. Major anomalies such as omphalocele, tetralogy of Fallot, and cleft lip are of obvious surgical, medical, or cosmetic importance. Minor anomalies are not of serious surgical or medical significance, although in some instances they may be of cosmetic concern, as with prominent epicanthic folds. Rarely, they may cause complications, as in an infected branchial cleft fistula. A representative but by no means exhaustive list of minor anomalies is presented in Table 3-1, and some selected anomalies are shown in Figure 3-1.

Minor anomalies have different causes. They may be malformations (e.g., an ear tag), deformations (e.g., altered mechanical forces deforming the external ear), disruptions (e.g., short terminal phalanges in the fetal hydantoin syndrome), or dysplasias (e.g., pigmented nevus).

Table 3-1. Minor Anomalies

Head	Neck
Aberrant scalp hair patterning	Mild webbed neck
Flat occiput	Branchial cleft fistula
Bony occipital spur	Hands
Third frontanel	Rudimentary polydactyly
Eyes	Duplication of thumbnail
Epicanthic folds	Single palmar crease
Epicanthus inversus	Unusual dermatoglyphics
Upward slanting palpebral fissures	Clinodactyly (5)
Downward slanting palpebral fissures	Short fingers (4, 5)
Short palpebral fissures	Feet
Dystopia canthorum	Syndactyly (2–3)
Minor hypertelorism	Gap between toes (1–2)
Minor hypotelorism	Short great toe
Minor ptosis	Recessed toes (4, 5)
Coloboma	Thickened nails
Ears	Prominent calcaneus
Primitive shape	Skin
Lack of helical fold	Hemangioma (other than face or neck)
Asymmetric size	Pigmented nevi
Posterior angulation	Mongoloid spot (whites)
Small ears	Depigmented spot
Protuberant ears	Unusual placement of nipples
Absent tragus	Accessory nipples
Double lobule	Café-au-lait spot
Auricular tag	Body
Auricular pit	Diastasis recti
Narrow external auditory meatus	Umbilical hernia
Nose	Minor hypospadias
Small nares	Deep sacral dimple
Notched alas	Skeletal
Oral regions	Cubitus valgus
Borderline small mandible	Prominent sternum
Incomplete form of cleft lip	Depressed sternum
Bifid uvula	Shieldlike chest
Aberrant frenula	Genua valga
Enamel hypoplasia	Genua vara
Malformed teeth	Genu recurvatum

Adapted from Marden et al.[19]

Many studies and discussions of minor anomalies have been published.[2,5,6,10–15,19,22–28,32,35,42,46] Some have been specialized papers[16,17,20,33,34,41,43–45] and topics have included single umbilical artery,[3,4,7] supernumerary nipples,[21,30,31,47] and dermatoglyphics,[36,38,39] among others. Internal minor anomalies have been discussed by Willis.[49] Although an association between minor anomalies and neurological or behavioral problems has been suggested in several studies,[8,9,29,37,40,48] assessment of minor anomalies in early life has not been found to be a practical screening device for predicting later aberrant behavior.[18] Accardo et al.[1] found that minor anomalies were not related to hyperactivity or attention deficits in a referred population.

Because minor anomalies may serve as indicators of altered morphogenesis and may sometimes imply more serious structural defects, they may be valuable diagnostic clues for specific patterns of malformation. Many malformation syn-

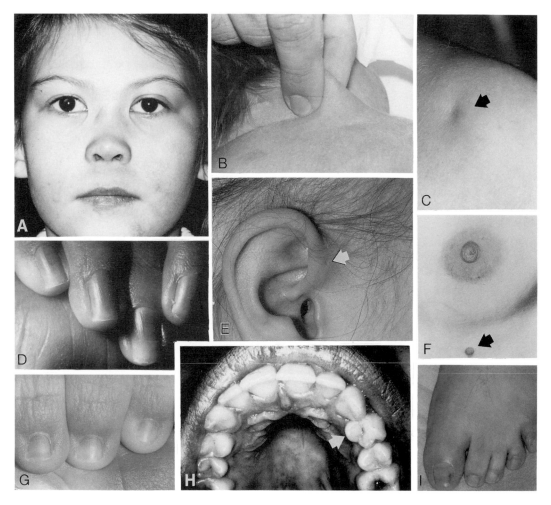

Figure 3-1. Selected minor anomalies. A: Epicanthic folds. B: Loose skin on posterior neck. C: Acromial dimple. D: Hyperconvex fingernails. E: Ear pit. F: Supernumerary nipple. G: Small deeply set nails. H: Accessory cusp on tooth. I: Partial soft tissue syndactyly.

dromes have characteristic facial appearances, and minor anomalies constitute most of the diagnostic features (see Chapter 4).

A landmark study of minor anomalies was carried out by Marden et al.[19] in 1964. The occurrence of single minor anomalies is common in the general population, existing in approximately 15% of all newborns. The occurrence of two is less common, and the presence of three or more minor anomalies is distinctly unusual, occurring in approximately 1% of all newborns. Of great interest, however, is the occurrence of a major malformation in association with 90% of all newborns with three or more minor anomalies.[19]

The implication is clear: Any newborn with three or more minor anomalies should be carefully evaluated for possible hidden major malformations such as cardiac, renal, or vertebral defects. Before ascribing significance to any minor anomaly, it should be ascertained whether the anomaly is present in any other member of the family. The significance of continuous or discontinuous minor anomalies in families is discussed further in the section on variant additive patterns in Chapter 6.

Minor anomalies occur with high frequency in many malformation syndromes. For example, in Down syndrome, 79% of all malformations detectable by clinical examination are minor anomalies; in trisomy 18 syndrome, 38%; in trisomy 13, 50%; and in Turner syndrome, 73%.[42] They also noted that 42% of patients with idiopathic mental retardation have three or more malformations of which 80% are minor; thus, the presence of minor anomalies may be considered an aid in the prognosis of mental deficiency. The significance of minor anomalies is summarized in Table 3-2.

REVIEW OF PROBLEMS

A major source on the complex problems surrounding the topic of minor anomalies is Pinsky,[35] who noted that single minor anomalies commonly have minor impact. For example, most cases of preauricular pits and tags are of no significance to the family[20] instead of being a marker of more extensive pleiotropic effects of the type observed in the branchio-oto-renal syndrome or in familial oculo-auriculo-vertebral syndrome. Occasional single minor anomalies do have major impact. For example, single umbilical artery[3,4,7] or supernumerary nipples[21,30,31,47] indicates that the patient should be evaluated to rule out urinary tract anomalies.

The topic of single umbilical artery and supernumerary nipples, however, is complex. Some infants with either of these have associated multiple malformations, and, often, syndrome diagnosis *per se* suggests careful assessment for renal anomalies. Other studies of single umbilical artery and supernumerary nipples have shown no increase in associated anomalies. Because there may be selection bias for multiple malformations in some studies, it has been suggested that when either single umbilical artery or supernumerary nipples occurs in an otherwise normal infant, no renal evaluation is necessary. The topic is particularly well discussed by Frías and Carey.[8a]

Analysis of multiple minor anomalies can sometimes be very useful. Rex and Preus[39] showed that 95% of patients with Down syndrome can be diagnosed with 99.9% confidence by using a diagnostic index based on the combination of hallucal patterning, second finger patterning, height of the palmar axial triradius, Brushfield spots, ear length, internipple distance as a ratio of chest circumference, wide gap between the second and third toes, and excess skin on the back of the neck.

The frequency of various minor anomalies found in any study depends on the age or age range of the population studied. Some minor anomalies are not necessarily present at birth. Café-au-lait spots may be of prenatal origin but

Table 3-2. Significance of Minor Anomalies

Fact	Implication
In newborns with three or more minor anomalies, 90% have major anomaly	Search for occult major anomaly
Minor anomalies present in many multiple congenital anomaly syndromes	Aid in diagnosis
42% of idiopathic mental retardation cases have three or more anomalies of which 80% are minor anomalies	Aid in prognosis

might not appear until some time after birth. High-arched palate is diagnosed much more frequently in children than in newborn infants. Mild epicanthic folds may regress with growth of the nasal bridge.

Studies of minor anomalies may also differ according to racial background. Sacral dimples are more common in whites, whereas prominent heels are more common in blacks. Holmes[10] found marked differences in the incidences of several anomalies in black and white infants.

The frequencies of specific minor anomalies in any given population vary. Mildly bifid tongue and ectopic anus are very uncommon. On the other hand, Brushfield spots and mild epicanthic folds are so common that they should be considered normal variants rather than minor anomalies.

Finally, studies may define a larger or a smaller number of minor anomalies, and this obviously affects the incidence of minor anomalies in populations. Holmes[10] found a higher incidence of one, two, or three or more minor anomalies than reported by Marden et al.[19] Since Holmes noted presence or absence of over 75 specific minor anomalies, he concluded that the higher incidence occurred because he identified a larger number of specific anomalies.

REFERENCES

1. Accardo PJ, Tomazic T, Morrow J, Haake C, Whitman BY: Minor malformations, hyperactivity, and learning disabilities. *Am J Dis Child* 145:1184–1187, 1991.
2. Alper J, Holmes LB, Mihm MC: Birthmarks with serious medical significance: Nevo-cellular nevi, sebaceous nevi, and multiple café-au-lait spots. *J Pediatr* 95:696–700, 1979.
3. Bourke WG, Clarke TA, Mathews TG, O'Halpin D, Donoghue VB: Isolated single umbilical artery—The case for routine renal screening. *Arch Dis Child* 68:600–601, 1993.
4. Bryan EM, Kohler HG: The missing umbilical artery. I. Prospective study based on a maternity unit. *Arch Dis Child* 49:844–852, 1974.
5. Carey JC: Invited editorial comment: Study of minor anomalies in childhood malignancy. *Eur J Pediatr* 144:250–251, 1985.
6. Crichton JU, Dunn HG, McBurney AK, Robertson A-M, Tredger E: Minor congenital defects in children of low birth weight. *J Pediatr* 80:830–832, 1972.
7. Csécsei K, Kovács T, Hinchliffe A, Papp Z: Incidence and associations of single umbilical artery in prenatally diagnosed malformed, midtrimester fetuses: A review of 62 cases. *Am J Med Genet* 43:524–530, 1992.
8. David TJ, Osborne CM: Scalp hair patterns in mental subnormality. *Med Genet* 13:123–126, 1976.
8a. Frías JL, Carey JC: Mild errors of morphogenesis. *Adv Pediatr* 43 (in press).
9. Gaily E, Granstrom M-L, Hiilesmaa V, Bardy A: Minor anomalies in offspring of epileptic mothers. *J Pediatr* 112:520–529, 1988.
10. Holmes LB: Racial differences in minor anomalies and normal physical variants in newborn infants. Teratology Society Abstract. Fourteenth Annual Meeting, Vancouver, British Columbia, 1974.
11. Holmes LB: *The Malformed Newborn: Practical Perspectives.* Boston: Massachusetts Development Disabilities Council, 1976.
12. Holmes LB: Minor anomalies in newborn infants. *Am J Hum Genet* 34:94A, 1982.
13. Holmes LB, Kleiner BC, Leppig KA, Cann CI, Munoz A, Polk BF: Predictive value of minor anomalies: II. Use of cohort studies to identify teratogens. *Teratology* 36:291–297, 1987.
14. Hook EB, Marden PM, Reiss NP, Smith DW: Some aspects of the epidemiology of human minor birth defects and morphological variants in a completely ascertained newborn population (Madison study). *Teratology* 13:47–56, 1976.

15. Hoyme HE: Minor malformations. Significant or insignificant? *Am J Dis Child* 141:947, 1987.

16. Jacobs AH, Walton RG: The incidence of birthmarks in the neonate. *Pediatrics* 58:218–222, 1976.

17. Kraus BS, Jordan RE, Nery EB, Kaplan S: Abnormalities of dental morphology in mentally retarded individuals: A preliminary report. *Am J Ment Defic* 71:828–839, 1967.

18. LaVeck B, Hammond MA, LaVeck GD: Minor congenital anomalies and behavior in different home environments. *J Pediatr* 96:940–993, 1980.

19. Marden PM, Smith DW, McDonald MJ: Congenital anomalies in the newborn infant, including minor variations. *J Pediatr* 64:358–371, 1964.

20. Meggyessy V, Mehes K: Preauricular pits in Hungary: Epidemiologic and clinical observations. *J Craniofac Genet Dev Biol* 2:215–218, 1982.

21. Meggyessy V, Mehes K: Association of supernumerary nipples with renal anomalies. *J Pediatr* 111:412–413, 1987.

22. Meggyessy V, Révhelyi M, Méhes K: Minor malformations in mental retardation of various etiology. *Acta Paediatr Acad Sci Hung* 21:175–180, 1980.

23. Méhes K: *Minor Malformations in the Neonate.* Budapest: Akadémiai Kiado, 1983.

24. Méhes K: Minor malformations in the neonate: Utility in screening infants at risk of hidden major defects. In Marois M (ed): *Prevention of Physical and Mental Congenital Defects, Part C: Basic and Medical Science, Education, and Future Strategies.* New York: Alan R. Liss, pp 45, 1984.

25. Méhes K, Kozsztolányi G: Morphologic variants in parents of children with malformation syndromes: Are they indicators of somatic mosaicism? *Clin Genet* 38:114–116, 1990.

26. Méhes K, Signer E, Pluss JH, Muller JH, Stalder G: Increased prevalence of minor anomalies in childhood malignancy. *Eur J Pediatr* 144:243–249, 1985.

27. Merlob P: Mild errors of morphogenesis: One of the most controversial subjects in dysmorphology. *Issues Rev Teratol* 7:57–102, 1994.

27a. Merlob P, Aitkin I: Time trends (1980–1987) of ten selected informative morphogenetic variants in a newborn population. *Clin Genet* 38:33–37, 1990.

28. Merlob P, Papier CM, Klingberg MA, Reisner SH: Incidence of congenital malformations in the newborn, particularly minor abnormalities. In Marois M (ed): *Prevention of Physical and Mental Congenital Defects, Part C: Basic and Medical Sciences, Education, and Future Strategies.* New York: Alan R. Liss, pp 51–55, 1984.

29. Miller G: Minor congenital anomalies and ataxic cerebral palsy. *Arch Dis Child* 64:557–562, 1989.

30. Mimouni F: Association of supernumerary nipples and renal anomalies. Letter to the Editor. *Am J Dis Child* 142:591, 1988.

31. Mimouni F, Merlob P, Reisner SH: Occurrence of supernumerary nipples in newborns. *Am J Dis Child* 137:952–953, 1983.

32. Opitz JM: Invited editorial comment: Study of minor anomalies in childhood malignancy. *Eur J Pediatr* 144:252–254, 1985.

32a. Opitz JM: Pathogenetic analysis of certain developmental and genetic ectodermal defects. *Birth Defects* 24(2):75–102, 1988.

33. Pape KE, Pickering D: Asymmetric crying facies: An index of other congenital anomalies. *J Pediatr* 81:21–30, 1972.

34. Perlman M, Reisner SH: Asymmetric crying facies and congenital anomalies. *Arch Dis Child* 48:627–629, 1973.

35. Pinsky L: Informative morphogenetic variants. Minor congenital anomalies revisited. In H. Kalter (ed): *Issues in Dermatology.* Vol 3. New York: Plenum Press, 1985, pp 135–170.

36. Preus M, Fraser FC: Dermatoglyphics and syndromes. *Am J Dis Child* 124:933–943, 1972.

37. Quinn PQ, Rapoport JL: Minor physical anomalies and neurologic status in hyperactive boy. *Pediatrics* 53:742–746, 1974.

38. Reed TE, Borgaonkar DS, Coneally PM, Yu P, Nance WE, Christian JC: Dermatoglyphic nomogram for the diagnosis of Down's syndrome. *J Pediatr* 77:1024–1032, 1970.
39. Rex AP, Preus M: A diagnostic index for Down syndrome. *J Pediatr* 100:903–906, 1982.
40. Rosenberg JB, Weller GM: Minor physical anomalies and academic performance in young school age children. *Dev Med Child Neurol* 15:131–135, 1973.
41. Smith DW: Commentary: Redundant skin folds in the infant—Their origin and relevance. *J Pediatr* 95:1021–1022, 1979.
42. Smith DW, Bostian KE: Congenital anomalies associated with idiopathic mental retardation. *J Pediatr* 65:189–196, 1964.
43. Smith DW, Cohen MM Jr: Widow's peak scalp hair anomaly and its relation to ocular hypertelorism. *Lancet* 2:1127–1128, 1973.
44. Smith DW, Gong BT: Scalp hair patterning as a clue to early fetal brain development. *J Pediatr* 83:374–380, 1973.
45. Smith DW, Takashima H: Protruding auricle: A neuromuscular sign. *Lancet* 1:747–749, 1978.
46. Tirosh E, Jaffe M, Dar H: The clinical significance of multiple hair whorls and their association with unusual dermatoglyphics and dysmorphic features in mentally retarded Israeli children. *Eur J Pediatr* 146:568–570, 1987.
47. Varsano IB, Jaben L, Garty B-Z, Mukamed MM, Grünebaum M: Urinary tract abnormalities in children with supernumerary nipples. *Pediatrics* 73:103–105, 1984.
48. Waldrop MF, Bell RQ, McLaughlin B, Halverson CF: Newborn minor physical anomalies predict short attention span, peer aggression, and impulsivity at age 3. *Science* 199:563–565, 1978.
49. Willis RA: *The Borderland of Embryology and Pathology.* Second edition. London: Butterworths, 1962.

4

Facial Dysmorphology

Many malformation syndromes have distinctive facial appearances, and, because minor anomalies affecting the head and neck are particularly common, they frequently account for many of the diagnostic features. The diagnoses of Down syndrome, de Lange syndrome, Williams syndrome, and Weaver syndrome are evident by the facial features alone (Fig. 4-1). In Figure 4-2, a girl with Down syndrome, treated by minor plastic surgical procedures,[28] can no longer be recognized facially as having Down syndrome.

FACIAL GESTALT AND SYNDROME DIAGNOSIS

Because some dysmorphic features defy measurement and even convincing verbal description, photographic documentation is important in syndromology; phenotypic features can change with time. In some conditions, such as de Lange syndrome, the phenotypic features, especially of the face, are usually constant enough at any age to impart the correct diagnostic impression, and the striking resemblance of affected individuals transcends the racial background of the patients.[29] Occasionally, mild expression may render clinical diagnosis difficult, particularly at birth. In a few instances, the characteristic phenotype of de Lange syndrome evolves with time (Fig. 4-3).[47] The facial features of Williams syndrome become more distinctive from infancy to childhood.[43] The Down syndrome face, so distinctive during infancy, is not recognizable during fetal life except in late gestation. In other conditions, such as the cri-du-chat syndrome, the phenotypic features tend to become less distinct with time.[7] Finally, some dysmorphic faces are so distinctive and unique (Fig. 4-4) that no other phenotype needs to be considered in the differential diagnosis.

The longitudinal study of facial changes over time in various syndromes was pioneered by Allanson and her coworkers.[1-6,30] At one time, heterogeneity was

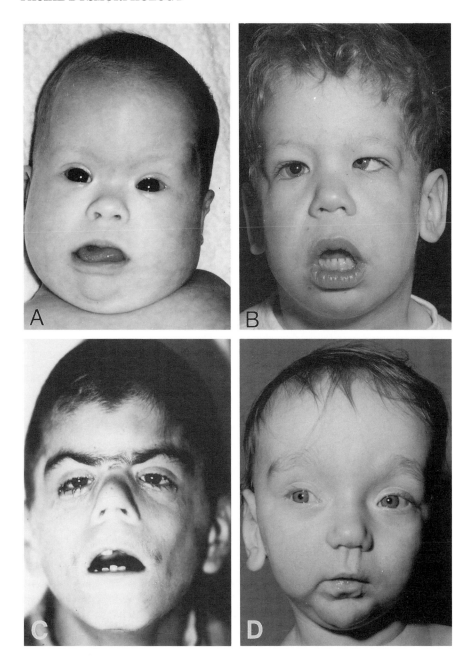

Figure 4-1. Four faces with minor anomalies. A: Down syndrome. Upslanting palpebral fissures, epi-canthic folds, low nasal bridge, small nose, protruding tongue. B: Williams syndrome. Strabismus, flat midface, anteverted nostrils, long philtrum, thick lips. (Courtesy of J.M. Opitz, Helena, MT). C: de Lange syndrome. Confluent eyebrows, long curly eyelashes, anteverted nostrils, long philtrum. D: Weaver syndrome. Broad forehead, ocular hypertelorism, long philtrum, micrognathia. From Cohen.[17]

suspected in Noonan syndrome. However, the facial phenotype changes with age (Fig. 4-5), suggesting a homogeneous syndrome. In the newborn, features include ocular hypertelorism, downslanting palpebral fissures, deeply grooved philtrum with high, wide peaks of the vermilion border, highly arched palate, micrognathia, low-set and posteriorly angulated ears with thick helices, and

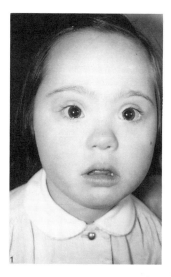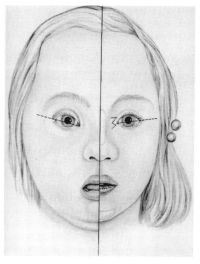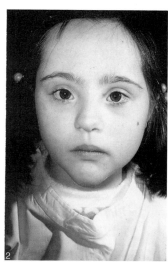

Figure 4-2. Left: Five-year-old girl with typical facial features of Down syndrome. Center: Plastic surgical procedures included elimination of epicanthic folds, correction of upslanting palpebral fissures, elevation of nasal dorsum and glabella, wedge excision for macroglossia, advancement genioplasty, and removal of fatty tissue under chin. All procedures carried out in a single operation. Right: Same girl postsurgically at 9 years of age. Note absence of Down syndrome facial features. From Höhler.[29]

excessive nuchal skin with low posterior hairline. During infancy, the head is relatively large with a turricephalic configuration. Ocular hypertelorism, prominent eyes, and thick hooded eyelids are characteristic. The nasal bridge is low, and the nose has a wide base with a bulbous tip. During childhood, the face may appear coarse or myopathic. The facial contour becomes more triangular with age. During adolescence and young adulthood, the eyes are less prominent, and the nose has a thin, high bridge and a wide base. The neck appears longer with accentuated webbing or prominent trapezius. In older adults, the nasolabial folds are prominent, the anterior hairline is high, and the skin appears wrinkled and transparent. Features present regardless of age include blue-green irides, halo iris, arched eyebrows, and low-set, posteriorly angulated ears with thick helices.[3,8] The hair may be wispy during infancy and curly or woolly in older children and adolescence. Malocclusion occurs in approximately one-third of the cases.[3]

Changes in Rubinstein-Taybi syndrome are illustrated in Figure 4-6. A hamartomatous condition like Proteus syndrome, which may develop facial changes in some instances,[18] is shown in Figure 4-7. Studies of facial alterations with time in a number of syndromes are listed in Table 4-1.

UNUSUAL CRANIOFACIAL ANOMALIES AND THE TESSIER CLASSIFICATION

Tessier[59] described an anatomic and descriptive classificatory system in which the various types of bony and soft tissue defects, which he called *clefts*, are situated along definite axes with numbers assigned to the sites of clefting, depending on their relationships to the sagittal midline (Fig. 4-8). Clefting may involve bone and/or soft tissue but rarely to the same extent. From the sagittal

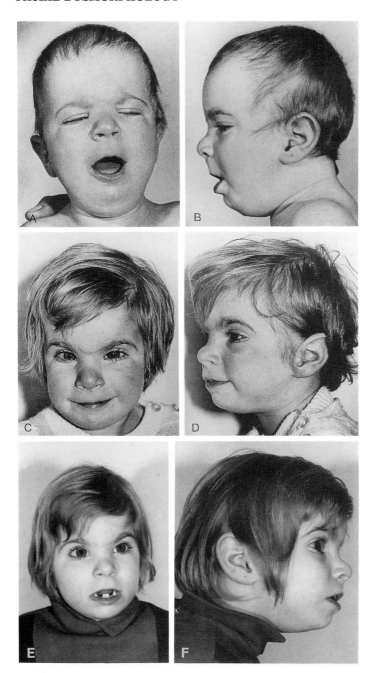

Figure 4-3. Photographic documentation showing evolution of the de Lange phenotype. A,B: Patient at 8 months of age. Microcephaly, downslanting palpebral fissures, right epicanthic fold, convergent strabismus, small nose with anteverted nostrils, and slight posterior angulation of the ears. C,D: Patient at 21 months of age with de Lange phenotype evident. From Passarge et al.[47] E,F: Patient at 3 years of age. Courtesy of E. Passarge, Hamburg, Germany.

midline to the infraorbital foramen, abnormalities of soft tissue predominate. From the infraorbital foramen to the temporal bone, however, osseous defects are more severe than those of soft tissue, a notable exception being the ear. Clefts through the orbit use the lower eyelid as an equator. Cleft numbered lines may be either northbound (cranial) or southbound (facial). Cranial num-

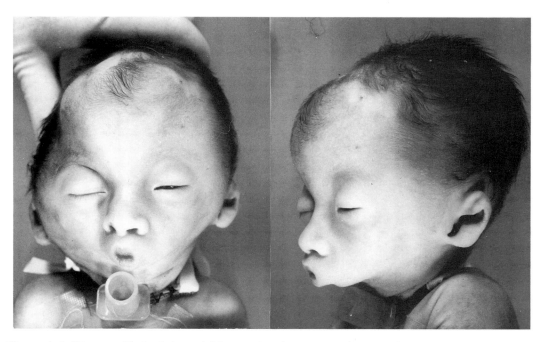

Figure 4-4. Hypomandibular faciocranial dysostosis, a distinctive and unique phenotype. From Ludman et al.[36]

bered lines have facial numbered counterparts, yet these numbers are different to avoid the implication that they necessarily have the same etiopathogenesis. Thus, the Tessier classification permits description of both the location and the extent of unusual facial clefts.

In some instances, overlying soft tissue defects predict the possibility of underlying bony clefts. Elsewhere I have referred to such features (e.g., colobomatous notching of the upper or lower eyelids or the nostrils or interruption of the eyelashes or the eyebrows) as *Tessier signs*.[15] Also included in this category are hairline indicators that may point to the cleft (Fig. 4-9).[42] Several osseous types of clefts are illustrated in Figure 4-10, and clinical examples are shown in Figures 4-11 to 4-15. It is not uncommon for several different Tessier clefts to occur in the same patient.

The causes of most Tessier clefts are unknown. The overwhelming majority occur sporadically. An exception is mandibulofacial dysostosis (Fig. 4-12), which is autosomal dominantly inherited. Many Tessier clefts are malformations that can be explained by faulty embryogenesis. However, others represent disruptions, particularly those associated with amniotic bands.

MEASUREMENT, CRANIOFACIAL EVALUATION, AND THE DYSMORPHIC FACE

Objective measurements often belie subjective clinical impression. Illusory hypertelorism may be created by a flat or low nasal bridge, epicanthic folds, dystopia canthorum, exotropia, or widely spaced eyes.[19] Patients with Down syndrome are commonly described as having highly arched palates. However, a metric study[55] has shown that palatal height tends to be in the normal range and

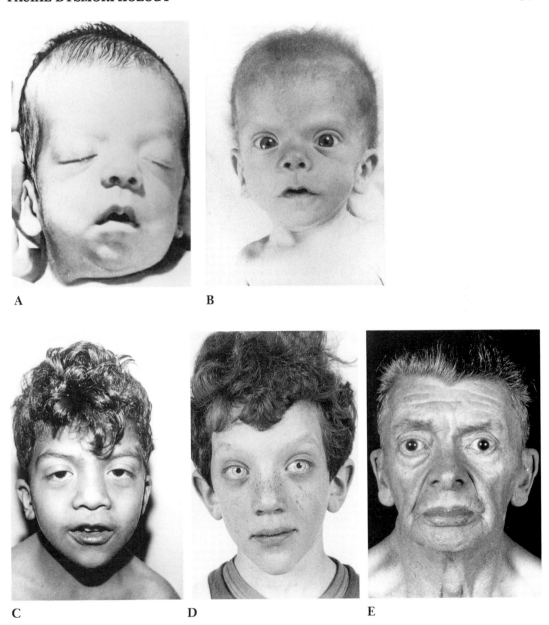

A   B

C   D   E

Figure 4-5. Noonan syndrome. From Allanson et al.[3] A: Facial appearance in newborn. Courtesy of M. Preus, Montreal. B: Facial appearance during infancy. Courtesy of H. Hughes, Cardiff, Wales. C: Face of 4-year-old boy. Courtesy of M. Preus, Montreal. D: Face of 12-year-old boy. Courtesy of H. Hughes, Cardiff, Wales. E: Face of older adult. Courtesy of J. Hall and D. Witt, Vancouver.

is not markedly high. On the other hand, palatal width in Down syndrome tends to be more narrow than in normal controls, resulting in the illusion of highly arched palate (Fig. 4-16). Some features such as epicanthic folds cannot be precisely measured but can be graded as being mild, moderate, or severe. Other features such as Brushfield spots are of the presence–absence type.

In evaluating the dysmorphic face, it is usually the more practical and efficient but less accurate measures that are used. Soft tissue measurements take precedence over radiographic ones, and the use of simple rather than sophisticated techniques is the rule. Although many elegant techniques and studies are avail-

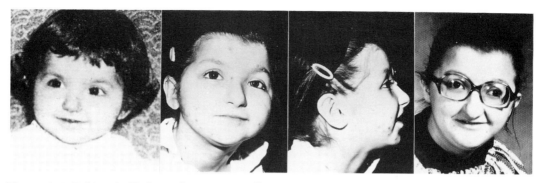

Figure 4-6. Rubinstein-Taybi syndrome. From Allanson.[1] Series of photographs during infancy, at age 7 years, and in adulthood. Courtesy of M. Partington, Australia.

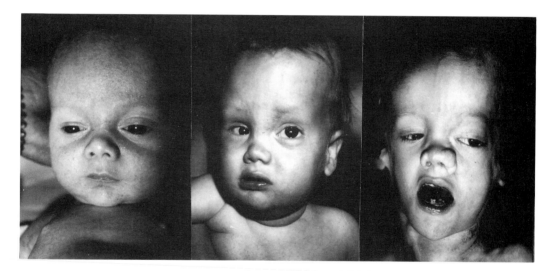

Figure 4-7. Proteus syndrome. Evolution of facial dysmorphism. Left: Age 1 month. Center: Age 5 months. Right: Age 5½ years. Note connective tissue nevus on left side of nose. From Cohen.[18]

Table 4-1. Studies of Facial Alterations in Various Syndromes

Syndrome	Reference
Beckwith-Wiedemann syndrome	Hunter and Allanson[30]
Cri-du-chat syndrome	Breg et al.[7]
de Lange syndrome	Passarge et al.[47] Allanson and Ireland[5]
Down syndrome	Allanson et al.[6]
Noonan syndrome	Allanson et al.[3]
Rubinstein-Taybi syndrome	Allanson,[1] Allanson and Hennekam[4]
Sotos syndrome	Allanson and Cole[2]
Williams syndrome	Morris et al.[43] (see Fig. 4-1)

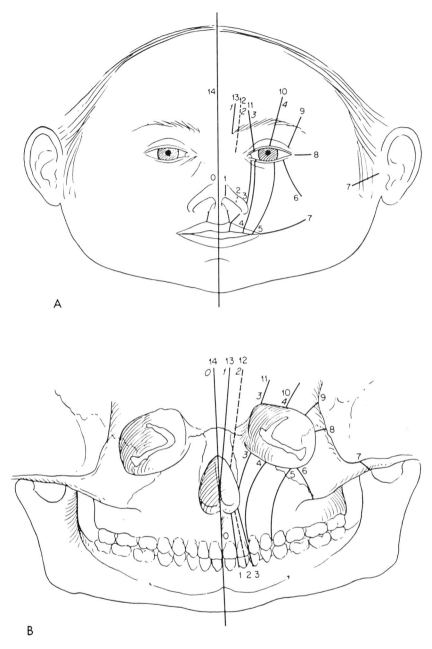

Figure 4-8. Tessier craniofacial clefting system. A: Soft tissue clefts. B: Bony clefts. Dotted lines represent uncertain localization or uncertain clefting. Note that northbound cranial line has a different number than its counterpart southbound facial line. Thus, system is descriptive and anatomic and avoids etiologic and/or pathogenetic speculation. For example, the cause of a No. 10 cleft may possibly be different than the cause of a No. 4 cleft. From Tessier.[59]

able, they may be too technical, expensive, and time consuming to be used routinely in the overall work-up of the patient with multiple anomalies. On the other hand, elaborate techniques such as cephalometrics are very useful for specific clinical purposes such as treatment planning for craniofacial surgery and evaluation of long-term results. Roentgencephalometry can also be used for

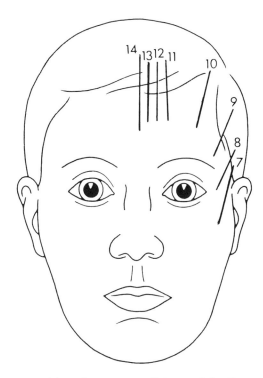

Figure 4-9. Diagram of hairline indicators that are superior and lateral extensions of Tessier clefts. From Moore et al.[42]

research purposes to study both normal and abnormal growth and development of the craniofacial complex.[11,12,32,33,49,50]

Decisions must be made about which measurements are to be taken on various patients, and, as already indicated, this depends partly on the particular patient being evaluated and partly on the clinical purpose or purposes for which the patient is examined. For example, simple measurements of the inner and outer canthal distances suffice for the general dysmorphology examination. On the other hand, careful radiographic measurements of the interorbital distance are necessary for the patient undergoing subtotal ethmoidectomy for the correction of ocular hypertelorism. Finally, a canthal index from a frontal photograph of any size provides an indication of the degree of ocular hypertelorism in a case of consultation by correspondence.[19]

Facial Anthropometry

Direct anthropometric measurement is an efficient and noninvasive way of describing craniofacial morphology (Fig. 4-17). A major advantage is its technical simplicity. Anthropometry can be used to evaluate patients, to plan facial surgery, to quantify features of malformation syndromes, and to compare differences between populations. Methodological and analytical aspects have been well reviewed by Ward.[62] Many standardized craniofacial variables are available.[21–23,31,40,52,53,56,63] Anthropometric measurements for dysmorphic conditions have been provided by several authors.[21,22,41,46,58]

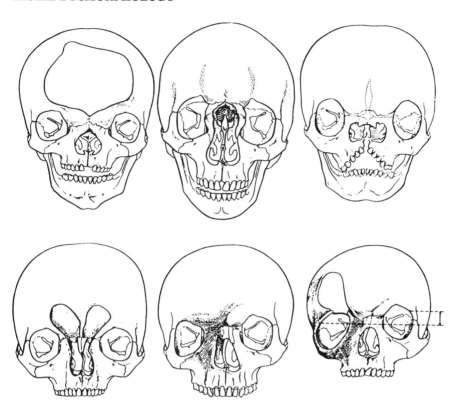

Figure 4-10. Upper left: Cleft No. 14. Median craniofacial dysraphism involving encephalocele, hypertelorism, bifid nose, and diastema between maxillary central incisors. Upper middle: Cleft No. 14. Median frontonasal encephalocele and dystopia canthorum. Note sparing of upper cranial region and tooth bearing part of maxilla. Upper right: Cleft Nos. 0, 14. Median craniofacial dysraphism with encephalocele or calcification of falx cerebri or both, duplication of crista galli, hypertelorism, bifid nose, absence of vomer, and keel-shaped maxillary dental arch. Lower left: Bilateral cleft No. 13. Bilateral paramedian encephaloceles and hypertelorism. This case was associated with colobomatous notching of both nostrils. Lower middle: Cleft Nos. 2, 12. Unilateral involvement affecting facial component more severely than cranial component. Cleft is either through frontal process of maxilla or between maxilla and nasal bone. Note unilateral hypertelorism. Patient had cleft through medial part of right nostril. Lower right: Cleft No. 10. Unilateral large defect of frontal bone involving supraorbital rim and orbital roof with encephalocele, unilateral hypertelorism, and dystopia with lateral rotation of affected orbit. From Tessier.[59]

Stengel-Rutkowski et al.[58] presented a photoanthropometric method that permits objective definition of facial structures from frontal and lateral photographs. Because each measurement is a ratio of one linear distance to another in the same photograph, measurements are comparable in photographs of different sizes and in photographs taken at different distances from the subject. The method can be applied to cases from the literature in which suitable photographs are available. Stengel-Rutkowski et al.[58] studied 18 parameters in 100 normal children and compared the results with those of 25 chromosomal patients and 75 nonchromosomal patients. Values below the 3rd and above the 97th centiles were considered abnormal. Frequently observed dysmorphism involved prominence of the chin, inner canthal distance, interalar distance, and ear width. Photo anthropometric techniques have also been applied to human teratogenic conditions.[6a,9]

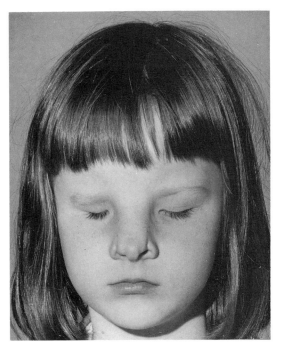 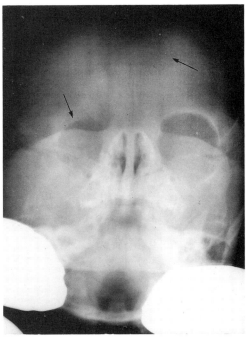

Figure 4-11. Unilateral microphthalmia, ocular hypertelorism, and bilateral notching of nostrils. Midline cranium bifidum defect (Tessier No. 14 cleft) on radiograph but not evident clinically. Note difference in size of orbits. From Sedano et al.[54]

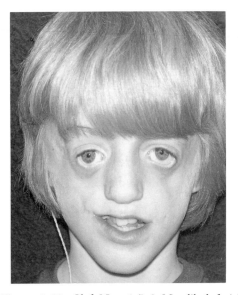 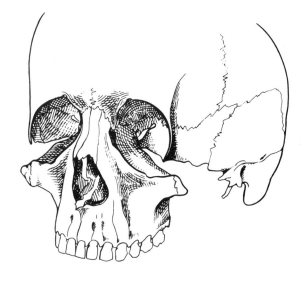

Figure 4-12. Cleft Nos. 6, 7, 8. Mandibulofacial dysostosis. Left: Clinical appearance showing downslanting palpebral fissures and malar deficiency. Note abnormal shape of lower eyelids, which often have missing lashes medially. From Cohen.[17] Right: Bony clefting of ovoid-shaped orbits with absence of zygomatic arches. From Tessier.[59]

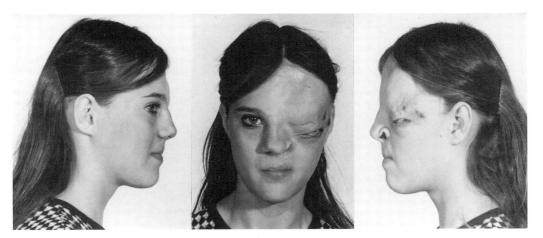

Figure 4-13. Lateral and downward displacement of left eye. Note interruption of eyebrow on affected side and repaired cleft lip. Tessier No. 10 cleft resulted in prolapse of brain into orbit and downward and lateral displacement of eyeglobe. Patient CCFA No. 1240, Age 14-7. Courtesy of S. Pruzansky, Chicago, Illinois. From Cohen.[14]

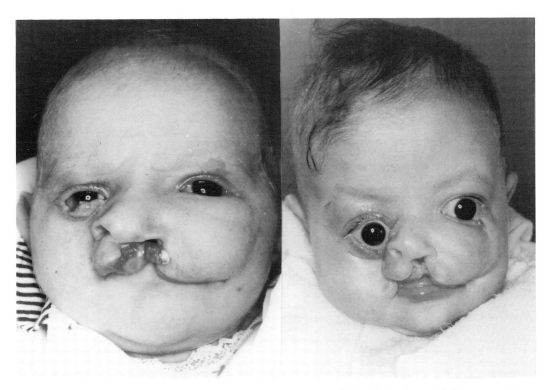

Figure 4-14. Multiple clefts. Left: Cleft lip with Tessier No. 7 cleft on left side and cleft Nos. 5 and 6 on right. Right: Cleft lip-palate with Tessier No. 6 cleft on left side and No. 4 cleft on right. Courtesy of A. Richieri-Costa, Bauru, Brazil. From Cohen.[14]

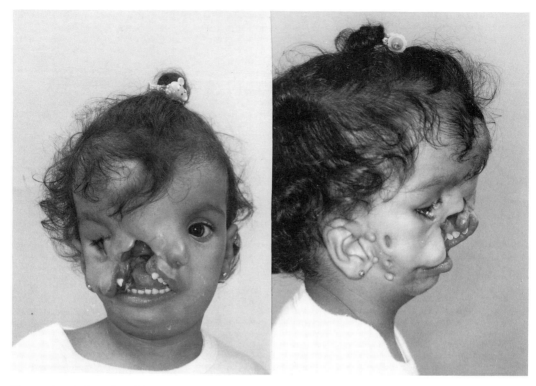

Figure 4-15. Complex clefting. Hairline indicator points to cleft area. CT scan showed anterior cranium bifidum occultum and gap in sphenoid bone. Note ear tags. Courtesy of A. Richieri-Costa, Bauru, Brazil.

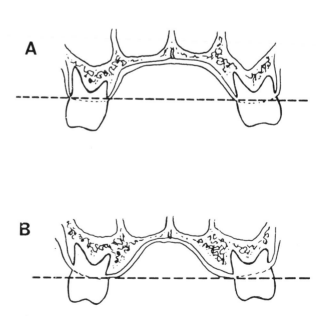

Figure 4-16. Down syndrome palate and normal palate are of same height. Cross sections through palate. A: Normal. B: Narrow palate of trisomy 21 syndrome, giving illusion of being high. From Shapiro et al.[55]

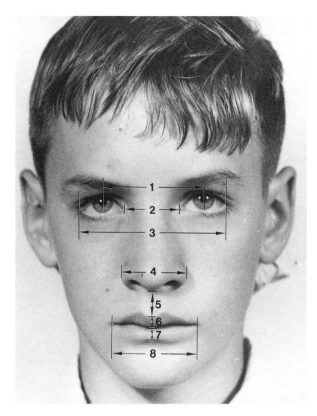

Figure 4-17. Examples of a few facial measurements. Many others are possible. (1) Interpupillary distance, (2) inner canthal distance, (3) outer canthal distance, (4) interalar distance, (5) philtral length, (6) upper lip thickness, (7) lower lip thickness, and (8) intercommissural distance. From Gorlin et al.[25]

The description of dysmorphic shape may be relatively simple in some instances, such as calvarial shape in craniosynostosis (Fig. 4-18),[10] or relatively complex, such as the helical rim of the ear in Down syndrome. DiLiberti[20] used the method of Fourier descriptors to identify geometric patterning by approximating the inner margin of the helix as a digitized two-dimensional contour from photographs of children with trisomy 21 syndrome and comparing them with a control group of normal children. Contours typical of trisomy 21 syndrome were divergent from those of the control group. DiLiberti[20] concluded that mathematical analysis of two-dimensional biological shapes was a promising analytical tool for dysmorphic studies and that three-dimensional patterns were also possible, but involved much greater computational complexity.

The use of composite imaging for facial dysmorphic diagnosis was discussed by Hogan and Pauli,[26] who noted that dysmorphic diagnosis was like signal detection, syndrome-specific traits being considered as the signal contaminated by familial and idiosyncratic noise. Signal averaging improves the signal-to-noise ratio by taking advantage of the fact that dysmorphic diagnostic signaling remains relatively constant whereas background noise always differs. Hogan and Pauli[26] produced a composite image of 15 adult achondroplastic facial photographs on a computer graphics terminal. Major facial features of achondroplasia were identifiable on the composite despite the fact that it did not closely resemble any particular patient. Signal averaging may be of use for syndrome-specific

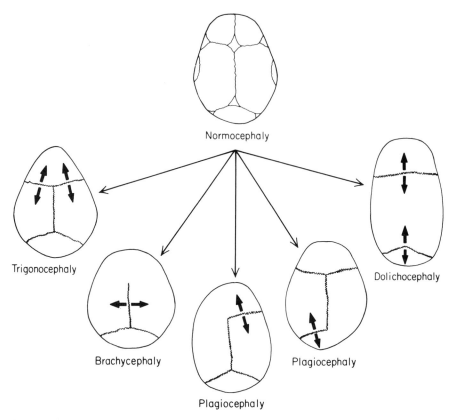

Figure 4-18. With premature craniosynostosis, skull shape depends on order and rate of progression of involved sutures. With single suture synostosis, growth restriction occurs at right angles to fused suture with compensatory expansion in same direction as fused suture. From Cohen.[10]

portraits in syndromology textbooks and may also be useful for evaluating craniofacial reconstruction and for research purposes.

Cephalometrics

The application of roentgencephalometry to the study of craniofacial anomalies has been exhaustively reviewed by Kreiborg.[32] Infant cephalometry has been discussed particularly well by Pruzansky and Lis,[51] Kreiborg et al.,[34] and Kreiborg.[32] The most sophisticated cephalometric unit for research and hospital environments has been designed by Solow and Kreiborg.[57] Cohen[11] critically reviewed cephalometric studies of dysmorphic syndromes.

Hohl et al.[27] developed a photocephalometric technique that allows transparent lateral and frontal photographs to be superimposed accurately over their corresponding cephalograms (Fig. 4-19); the technique permits pre- and postoperative comparison of soft tissue (Fig. 4-20) and skeletal changes.

Profile pattern analysis, a technique based on radiographs used extensively in the dysmorphic analysis of hand–wrist films,[48] has been applied to the craniofacial region by Garn and his coworkers.[24] Dimensions used are defined in Table 4-2 and illustrated in Figure 4-21. A craniofacial profile pattern of monozygotic twins with Robin sequence appears in Figure 4-22, showing close resemblance, extreme reduction in facial and cranial depths, and above-average facial heights. A craniofacial pattern of monozygotic twins with oto-palato-digital syndrome I is shown in Figure 4-23, indicating pronounced syndromic patterning with large discrepancies in a few of the cranial and facial depths.

Laser Scanning

Moss et al.[44] described a laser scanning system that is repeatable without danger to the patient since radiation is not involved; the system does not involve contact with the patient's face, yet permits three-dimensional visualization (Fig. 4-24). The image can be rotated and viewed from any perspective and can be shaded in as a solid image. Laser scanning is useful for longitudinal studies of soft tissue during growth and for comparison of pre- and postoperative surgical states.

Three-Dimensional Craniofacial Surface Imaging from CT Scans

Vannier et al.,[61] Marsh et al.,[39] and Marsh and Vannier[37,38] developed a computer method that reconstructs three-dimensional bone and soft tissue sur-

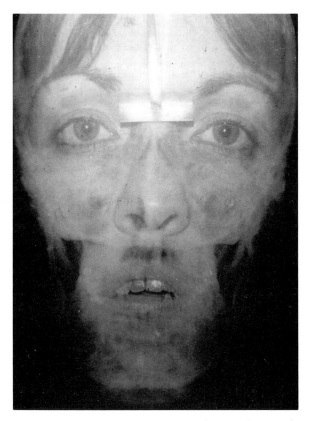

Figure 4-19. Photocephalometric technique showing frontal cephalogram with transparent photograph accurately superimposed. From Hohl et al.[28]

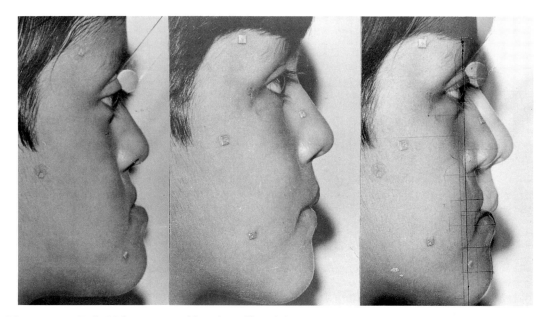

Figure 4-20. Left: Male, 14 years old, with midface deficiency and mild ocular proptosis. Center: Profile change following Le Fort III advancement procedure. Right: Pre- and postsurgical views compared by superimposing transparent facial photographs. From Hohl et al.[28]

Table 4-2. Dimensions Used in Craniofacial Profile Pattern Analysis

Dimension	Abbreviation	Landmarks	Landmark Numbers
Posterior skull base length	PS	Opisthion–sella	8–7
Total skull base length	TS	Opisthion–glabella	8–6
Anterior skull base length	AS	Sella–glabella	7–6
Sella–nasion	SN	Sella–nasion	7–5
Facial depth	FD	Condylion–nasion	9–5
Palatal length	PL	Anterior–Posterior nasal spines	4–11
Superior ramus length	SR	Condylion–coronoid process	9–17
Mandibular corpus length	MC	Gnathion–gonial intersection	1–16
Ramus height	RH	Condylion–gonial intersection	9–16
Mandibular height	MH	Distal M_1 CEJ Point 15[a]	14–15
Symphyseal height	SH	Gnathion–infradentale	1–2
Alveolar height	AH	Supradentale–anterior nasal spine	3–4
Anterior dental height	AD	Infradentale–supradentale	2–3
Posterior dental height	PD	Distal M^1 CEJ–distal M_1 CEJ	12–14
Palate–mandible height	PM	MH line extended to alveolar plane	13–15
Gonion–sella	GS	Gonial intersection–sella	16–7
Posterior facial height	PF	Distal M^1 CEJ–point 10[a]	12–10
Superior facial height	SF	Anterior nasal spine–nasion	4–5

From Garn et al.[24]

[a]Denotes points defined by intersections. Landmark 10 is a point on the condylion-nasion line from which a perpendicular intersects the distal cemento-enamel junction of the maxillary first molar (Distal M^1 CEJ). Landmark 15 is a point on the inferior mandibular plane from which a perpendicular intersects the distal cemento-enamel junction of the mandibular first molar (Distal M_1 CEJ).

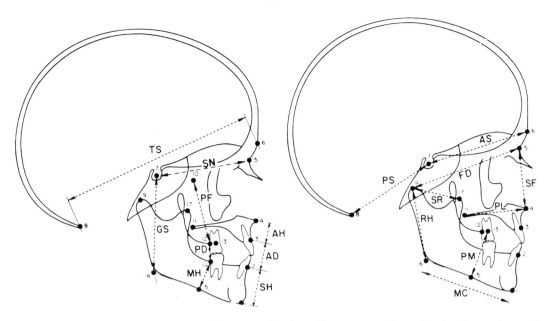

Figure 4-21. Selected dimensions used in craniofacial profile pattern analysis. Landmark numbers and dimensions correspond to description in Table 4-2. From Garn et al.[24]

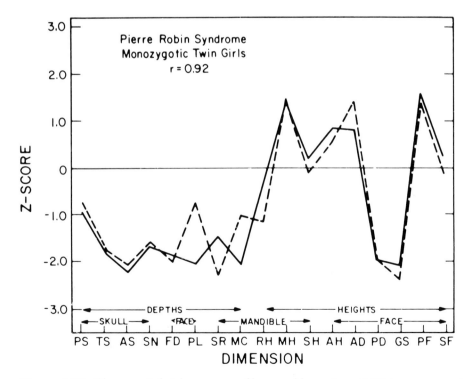

Figure 4-22. Close craniofacial pattern profile resemblance ($r_z = 0.92$) in monozygotic twin girls with clinical manifestations of Robin sequence (called Pierre Robin syndrome in this illustration). Extreme reduction of facial and cranial depths and above-average facial heights are clearly visible in this representation. From Garn et al.[24]

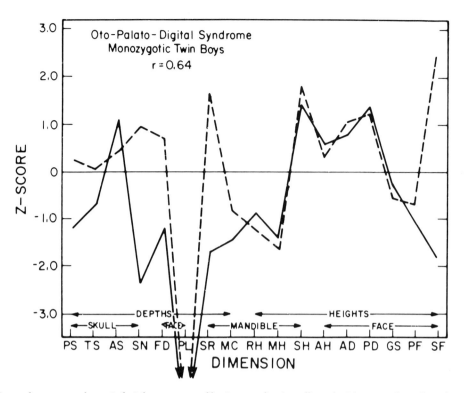

Figure 4-23. Strongly patterned craniofacial pattern profiles in set of twins affected with oto-palato-digital syndrome I. As shown, both twins are highly divergent from norms for age and sex. Twins show moderate resemblance to each other ($r_z = 0.64$), but large discrepancies in some cranial and facial depths (SN, SR, SF) indicate independent developmental dysmorphism. Both twins had surgical repair for soft palate clefts, but values for PL (palatal length) <5σ indicate that hard palate is also extremely underdeveloped. From Garn et al.[24]

faces from high-resolution computed tomography (CT) scans (Figs. 4-25, 4-26).[16,35] In contrast to other CT reconstruction methods, the Vannier-Marsh technique requires no additional hardware beyond the CT scanner that generated the original data. Thus, this type of surface imaging is practical because it is potentially available to any hospital with a third- or fourth-generation CT scanner. Three-dimensional views are constructed directly from the original CT scan slices. Although surface images are displayed in two dimensions, they represent three-dimensional data. The head or skull can be viewed from any perspective, and selected portions of the anatomy can be removed to facilitate study. For example, it is possible to remove the calvaria to study the cranial base (Fig. 4-27).[35] The Vannier-Marsh surface imaging technique is useful for studying dysmorphic conditions such as Apert syndrome, for surgical planning, and for comparing postoperative results with preoperative states. The best method for determining the presence or absence of individually synostosed calvarial sutures (short of histological interpretation, which is impractical) is to evaluate three-dimensional CT reconstructions that are known to have more diagnostic potential then either the CTs from which they were derived or from plain radiographs.[13,60]

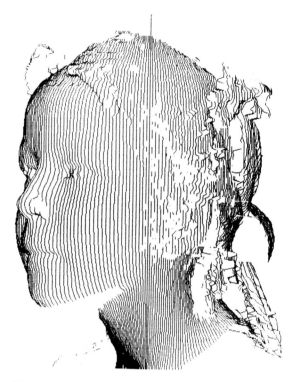

Figure 4-24. Three-dimensional visualization of face by laser scanning technique. Image can be rotated to be viewed from any perspective and can be shaded solid. Courtesy of S. Kreiborg, Copenhagen, Denmark.

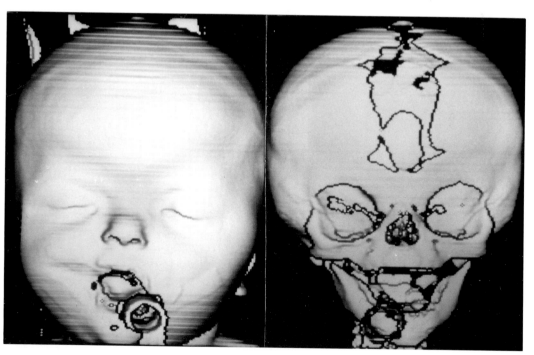

Figure 4-25. Three-dimensional surface imaging from CT scan. Frontal view of intubated 10-month-old infant with Apert syndrome. Left: Soft tissue. Right: Craniofacial skeleton. Note widely patent midline calvarial defect with island of bone present anteriorly. Courtesy of S. Kreiborg, Copenhagen, Denmark.

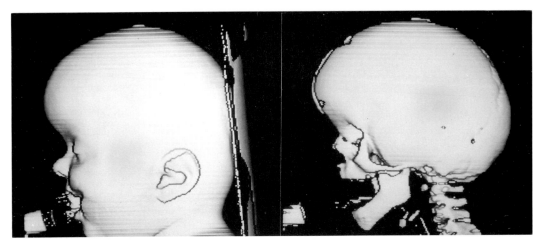

Figure 4-26. Three-dimensional surface imaging from CT scan. Lateral view of intubated 10-month-old infant with Apert syndrome. Left: Soft tissue. Right: Craniofacial skeleton. Courtesy of S. Kreiborg, Copenhagen, Denmark.

Magnetic Resonance Imaging

Images can be obtained and presented in the same planar format with magnetic resonance imaging (MRI) as with CT scan images. However, MR images of the head are often obtained and displayed in coronal and sagittal, rather than in axial, sections. With MRI, limited skeletal information is available, although

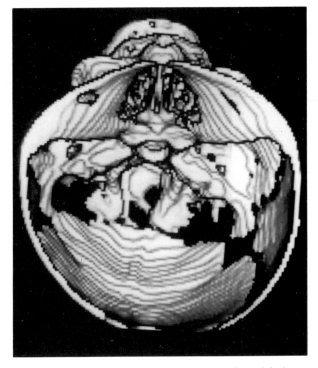

Figure 4-27. One-month-old girl with Apert syndrome. This cut of a three-dimensional model shows patent synchondroses in cranial base. Note asymmetry and extremely wide cribriform plate of ethmoid bone. From Kreiborg et al.[35]

soft tissue discrimination among various tissue types, such as fat and muscle, and within single types, such as gray matter versus white matter in the brain, far exceeds the discrimination available from CT scans.[39,45] Three-dimensional MRI of the brain with integration of the arterial and venous vascular trees has been discussed by Zonneveld.[64]

REFERENCES

1. Allanson JE: Rubinstein-Taybi syndrome: The changing face. *Am J Med Genet Suppl* 6:38–41, 1990.
2. Allanson JE, Cole TRP: Sotos syndrome: Evolution of facial phenotype. David W. Smith Workshop on Malformations and Morphogenesis, Wake Forest University, Winston-Salem, North Carolina, August 5–9, 1992.
3. Allanson JE, Hall JG, Hughes HE, Preus M, Witt RD: Noonan syndrome: The changing phenotype. *Am J Med Genet* 21:507–514, 1985.
4. Allanson JE, Hennekam RCM: Objective facial assessment of Rubinstein-Taybi syndrome. David W. Smith Workshop on Malformations and Morphogenesis, Big Sky, Montana, July 30 to August 3, 1995.
5. Allanson JE, Ireland M: Craniofacial measurement in Cornelia de Lange syndrome: Can the mild phenotype be defined? David W. Smith Workshop on Malformations and Morphogenesis, Tampa, Florida, August 4–9, 1994.
6. Allanson JE, O'Hara P, Farkas LG, Nair RC: Anthropometric craniofacial pattern profiles in Down syndrome. *Am J Med Genet* 47:748–752, 1993.
6a. Astley SJ, Clarren SK, Little RE, Sampson PD, Daling JR: Analysis of facial shape in children gestationally exposed to marijuana, alcohol, and/or cocaine. *Pediatrics* 89:67–77, 1992.
7. Breg WR, Steele MW, Miller OJ, Warburton D, de Capos A, Allderdice PW: The cri-du-chat syndrome in adolescents and adults: Clinical findings in 13 older patients with partial deletion of the short arm of chromosome no. 5 (5 "p minus"). *J Pediatr* 77:782–791, 1970.
8. Char F: The halo iris of the Noonan syndrome. *Proc Greenwood Genet Center* 6:159, 1987.
9. Clarren SK, Sampson PD, Larsen J, Donnell DJ, Barr HM, Bookstein FL, Martin DC, Streissguth AP: Facial effects of fetal alcohol exposure: Assessment by photographs and morphometric analysis. *Am J Med Genet* 26:651–666, 1987.
10. Cohen MM Jr: *Craniosynostosis: Diagnosis, Evaluation, and Management.* New York: Raven Press, 1986.
11. Cohen MM Jr: A critical review of cephalometric studies of dysmorphic syndromes. *Proc Finn Dent Soc* 77:17–25, 1981.
12. Cohen MM Jr: Dysmorphic growth and development and the study of craniofacial anomalies. *J Craniofac Genet Dev Biol Suppl* 1:43–55, 1985.
13. Cohen MM Jr: Letter to the editor: Lambdoid synostosis is an overdiagnosed condition. *Am J Med Genet* 61:98–99, 1996.
14. Cohen MM Jr: Perspectives on craniofacial asymmetry. II. Asymmetric embryopathies. *Int J Oral Maxillofac Surg* 24:8–12, 1995.
15. Cohen MM Jr: Syndromology: An updated conceptual overview. II. Syndrome classifications. *Int J Oral Maxillofac Surg* 18:223–228, 1989.
16. Cohen MM Jr: Syndromology: An updated conceptual overview. IX. Facial dysmorphology. *Int J Oral Maxillofac Surg* 19:81–88, 1990.
17. Cohen MM Jr: *The Child With Multiple Birth Defects.* New York: Raven Press, 1982.
18. Cohen MM Jr: Understanding Proteus syndrome, unmasking the Elephant Man, and stemming elephant fever. *Neurofibromatosis* 1:260–280, 1988.
19. Cohen MM Jr, Richieri-Costa A, Guion-Almeida M-L, Saavedra D: Hypertelorism: Interorbital growth, measurements, and pathogenetic considerations. *Int J Oral Maxillofac Surg* 24:387–395, 1995.

20. DiLiberti JH: Computerized analysis of two dimensional biological shapes: Applications to dysmorphology. *Proc Greenwood Genet Center* 6:132, 1987.
21. Farkas LG: *Anthropometry of the Head and Face in Medicine*. New York: Elsevier, 1981.
22. Farkas LG, Munro IR (eds): *Anthropometric Facial Proportions in Medicine*. Springfield, IL: CC Thomas, 1987.
23. Feingold M, Bossert WH: Normal values for selected physical parameters: An aid to syndrome delineation. *Birth Defects* 10(13):1–15, 1974.
24. Garn SM, Smith BH, LaVelle M: Applications of pattern profile analysis to malformations of the head and face. *Radiology* 150:683–690, 1984.
25. Gorlin RJ, Cohen MM Jr, Levin LS: *Syndromes of the Head and Neck*. Third edition. New York: Oxford University Press, 1990.
26. Hogan KJ, Pauli RM: Composite imaging in genetic diagnosis. *Proc Greenwood Genet Center* 6:133, 1987.
27. Hohl TH, Wolford LM, Epker BN, Fonseca RJ: Craniofacial osteotomies: A photocephalometric technique for the prediction and evaluation of tissue changes. *Angle Orthod* 48:114–125, 1978.
28. Höhler H: Changes in facial expression as a result of plastic surgery in mongoloid children. *Aesthetic Plast Surg* 1:245–250, 1977.
29. Huang C-C, Emanuel I, Huang S-W, Chen T-Y: Two cases of the de Lange syndrome in Chinese infants. *J Pediatr* 71:251–254, 1967.
30. Hunter AGW, Allanson JE: Follow-up study of patients with Wiedemann-Beckwith syndrome with emphasis on the change in facial appearance over time. *Am J Med Genet* 51:10–107, 1994.
31. Kopf HK: Ohrmuschel und Hand Wachstum (Verwendung bei den Operationen der angeborenen Missbildungen und Unfalls Folgen). *Acta Univ Carol [Med] (Praha)* 2–4:77–294, 1974.
32. Kreiborg S: The application of roentgencephalometry to the study of craniofacial anomalies. *J Craniofac Genet Dev Biol Suppl* 1:31–41, 1985.
33. Kreiborg S: Postnatal growth and development of the craniofacial complex in premature craniosynostosis. In Cohen MM Jr (ed): *Craniosynostosis: Diagnosis, Evaluation, and Management*. New York: Raven Press, 1986, pp 157–189.
34. Kreiborg S, Dahl E, Prydsoe U: A unit for infant roentgencephalometry. *Dentomaxillofac Radiol* 6:107–111, 1977.
35. Kreiborg S, Marsh JL, Cohen MM Jr, Liversage M, Pedersen H, Skovby F, Børgesen SE, Vannier MW: Comparative three-dimensional analysis of CT-scans of the calvaria and cranial base in Apert and Crouzon syndromes. *J Cranio-Max-Fac Surg* 21:181–188, 1993.
36. Ludman MD, Vincer MJ, Cron C, Aguiar M, Cohen MM Jr: Hypomandibular faciocranial dysostosis: Another case and review. *Am J Med Genet* 47:352–356, 1993.
37. Marsh JL, Vannier MW: Surface imaging from computerized tomographic scans. *Surgery* 94:159–165, 1983.
38. Marsh JL, Vannier MW: Three-dimensional surface imaging from CT scans for the study of craniofacial dysmorphology. *J Craniofac Genet Dev Biol* 9:61–75, 1989.
39. Marsh JL, Vannier MW, Stevens WG: *Comprehensive Care for Craniofacial Deformities*. Toronto: CV Mosby, 1985.
40. Martin R, Saller K: *Lehrbuch der Anthropologie*. Stuttgart: Fischer, 1962.
41. Meaney FJ, Farrer LA: Clinical anthropometry and medical genetics: A complication of body measurements in genetic and congenital disorders. *Am J Med Genet* 25:343–359, 1986.
42. Moore MH, David DJ, Cooter RD: Hairline indicators of craniofacial clefts. *Plast Reconstr Surg* 82:589–593, 1988.
43. Morris CA, Demsey SA, Leonard CO, Dilts C, Blackburn BL: Natural history of Williams syndrome: Physical characteristics. *J Pediatr* 113:318–326, 1988.
44. Moss JP, Linney AD, Grindrod SR, Arridge SR, Clifton JS: Three-dimensional visualization of the face and skull using computerized tomography and laser scanning techniques. *Eur J Orthod* 9:247–253, 1987.

45. Naidich TP, Zimmerman RA: Common congenital malformation of the brain. In Brant-Zawadzki M, Norman D (eds): *Magnetic Resonance Imaging of the Nervous System.* New York: Raven Press, 1987, pp 131–150.
46. Niebuhr E: Anthropometry in the cri-du-chat syndrome. *Clin Genet* 16:82–85, 1979.
47. Passarge E, Mercke S, Altrogge HC: Cornelia de Lange syndrome, evolution of the phenotype. *Pediatrics* 48:833–836, 1971.
48. Poznanski AK, Garn SM, Nagy JM, Gail JC Jr: Metacarpophalangeal pattern profiles in the evaluation of skeletal malformations. *Radiology* 104:1–11, 1972.
49. Pruzansky S: Roentgencephalometry of infants: 1949–1973. *Transactions of the Third International Orthodontics Congress.* London: Crosby Lockwood Staples, 1975, pp 101–117.
50. Pruzansky S: Radiocephalometric studies of the basicranium in craniofacial malformations. In JG Bosma (ed): *Development of the Basicranium.* Bethesda, MD: U.S. DHEW, Pub. No. (NIH) 76-989, 1976, pp 278–300.
51. Pruzansky S, Lis EF: Cephalometric roentgenography of infants: Sedation, instrumentation, and research. *Am J Orthod* 44:159–186, 1958.
52. Roche AF, Malina RM: *Manual of Physical Status and Performance in Childhood. Vol. 1A, Physical Status.* New York: Plenum Press, 1983.
53. Schwarzfischer F: Ohrmuschel. Becker PE (ed): In *Humangenetik.* Vol. 1/2. Stuttgart: Georg-Thieme, 1969.
54. Sedano HO, Cohen MM Jr, Jirasek J, Gorlin RJ: Frontonasal dysplasia. *J Pediatr* 76:906–913, 1970.
55. Shapiro BL, Gorlin RJ, Redman RS, Bruhl H: The palate and Down's syndrome. *N Engl J Med* 276:1460–1463, 1967.
56. Snyder RG, Schneider LW, Owings CL, Reynolds HM, Gollomb DH, Schork MA: *Anthropometry of Infants, Children, and Youths to Age 18 for Product Safety Design SP-450.* Worendale, PA: Society of Automobile Engineers, 1977.
57. Solow B, Kreiborg S: A cephalometric unit for research and hospital environments. *Eur J Orthod* 10:346–352, 1988.
58. Stengel-Rutkowski S, Schimanek P, Wernheimer A: Anthropometric definitions of dysmorphic facial signs. *Hum Genet* 67:272–295, 1984.
59. Tessier P: Anatomical classifications of facial, cranio-facial and laterofacial clefts. *J Max-Fac Surg* 4:69–92, 1976.
60. Vannier MW, Hildebolt CF, Marsh JL, Pilgram TK, McAlister WH, Shackelford GD, Offutt CJ, Knapp RH: Craniosynostosis: Diagnostic value of three-dimensional CT reconstruction. *Radiology* 173:669–673, 1989.
61. Vannier MW, Marsh JL, Warren JO: Three dimensional CT reconstruction images for craniofacial surgical planning and evaluation. *Radiology* 150:179–184, 1984.
62. Ward RE: Facial morphology as determined by anthropometry: Keeping it simple. *J Craniofac Genet Dev Biol* 9:45–60, 1989.
63. Zigelmayer G: Mund-Kinn-Region. In Becker PE (ed): *Humangenetik.* Vol. 1/2. Stuttgart: Georg-Thieme, 1969.
64. Zonneveld FW: A decade of clinical three-dimensional imaging: A review. Part III. Image analysis and interaction, display options, and physical models. *Invest Radiol* 29:716–725, 1994.

5

Guide to Physical Measurements

Grandmother, what low-set ears you have!
In relation to what, my dear?

From *The Revised Little Red Riding Hood*[34]

The wolf's question above expresses the difficulty in quantifying some traits. Low-set ears tend to be overdiagnosed on clinical examination, yet its quantitation is refractory to accurate measurement. Certainly there are known ways to measure low-set ears, although they are not entirely satisfactory. The ears may be evaluated by the point of attachment at the helix in relation to eye position. The ears can also be evaluated as low-set in relation to the cranial vault or mandibular ramus. The ears may appear to be low-set when the cranial vault is high, as in the Apert syndrome; when the mandibular ramus is short, as in Robin sequence; or when the neck is short, as with Klippel-Feil anomaly. Illusory low-set ears may occur with posteriorly angulated ears, small ears, dysplastic ears, protruding ears, or hyperextension of the head. In some cases, such ears may be low-set, but in other cases they may not.[3,34]

USEFUL PHYSICAL MEASUREMENTS

Physical measurements of the body and its parts and comparison to normal values are very useful in the study of dysmorphic syndromes. Besides standard height, weight, and head circumference values obtained during examination, many other measurements are available (Table 5-1). A number of syndromes with dysmorphic features have disturbed growth of the body or disproportionate growth of body parts. In some instances, measurements are available for specific syndromes such as Down syndrome,[4] Turner syndrome,[18,26,27] Noonan

Table 5-1. Guide to References for Useful Measurements

Encyclopedias of measurements	Craniofacial measurements
Hall et al.[10]	Anthropometric
Saul et al.[36]	Farkas[5]
Physical growth measurements	Farkas and Munro[6]
Hamill et al.[11]	Cephalometric
Tanner[39]	Broadbent 1975[2]
Tanner and Whitehouse[41]	Riolo et al.[33]
Tanner and Whitehouse[42]	Saksena et al.[35]
Newborn measurements	Prenatal measurements
Merlob et al.[23]	Ultrasound
Lubchenco et al.[20]	Hansmann[12]
Lubchenco et al.[21]	Organ weights
Radiographic measurements	Potter and Craig[27]
General	Shepard et al.[37]
Lusted and Keats[22]	Specific syndrome measurements
Hand	Hall et al.,[10] pp 443–468
Poznanski[29]	Saul et al.,[36] pp 169–210

syndrome,[32,43] Williams syndrome,[25] Prader-Willi syndrome,[14] Marfan syndrome,[31] achondroplasia,[15,17] and diastrophic dysplasia.[16]

Physical measurements and their analyses and interpretation make up a very complex and highly specialized field. On the other hand, many measurements may be taken in clinical situations, using simple techniques, and compared with normal values.

ASSESSMENT OF METRIC STUDIES

Many different methodologically sophisticated approaches to metric studies are known.[7-9] However, both the quality and significance of the data vary in published studies. Furthermore, the choice of measuring devices and the reproducibility of landmarks can affect the accuracy of presumably objective measurements.[13] The comments discussed below should be taken into consideration when measuring any patient. It is only necessary to be aware of the limitations of any particular measuring method and published metric study and interpret the results accordingly by not overreading differences if the method or the study lacks precision.

1. In a longitudinal study, the same children are measured at every age. Such studies are time consuming and expensive. If some children drop out of the study and others are added, the study is mixed-longitudinal in type. In a cross-sectional study, different children are used at different ages. Such studies are less expensive and can be carried out more rapidly. Longitudinal studies can be used to develop growth curves and growth rates. Cross-sectional studies cannot be used to generate growth rates.

2. Some studies use standard deviations; others use percentiles. Although percentiles are easy to read, differences between them are not easy to interpret. Small differences in the middle of the distribution tend to be exaggerated, and large differences at the extremes tend to be minimized. A second drawback is that percentiles *per se* are not useful for future statistical analysis; they cannot be used for correlational analysis or for testing standard statisti-

cal hypotheses, although a number of nonparametric tests may be used. On the other hand, because the standard deviation is a measure of variation, studies using it can be subjected to standard statistical analyses.

3. In comparing disproportionate growth of various body parts in a dysmorphic syndrome, it is important to recognize that different methodologies and different populations may have been used to define different body part measurements. Thus, comparing one body measurement in relation to another in the same patient may not have a high degree of validity. Nevertheless, such measurement studies may be the only ones available.

4. Sample size may be too small in some studies.

5. Population ascertainment is important: Were the subjects randomly chosen, or were they selected in some way that might bias the results? Is the study cross-sectional or longitudinal? How similar is the control population to the patient's own background? Measurement data are known to vary in different populations, in different geographic regions, and by socioeconomic status. For example, the height of Asians tends to be distinctly less than that of Europeans. Australian aboriginals tend to have longer legs than Africans, who, in turn, tend to have longer legs than Europeans.[38] A middle class, white population from Yellow Springs, Ohio, cannot be equated with a lower class white population from Boston, Massachusetts. Interocular measurements have been shown to differ among Japanese, Mexicans, American blacks, and American whites.[19,30]

6. Some studies fail to separate data on the basis of sex.

7. Age group categories may span too wide a range.

8. The time at which a particular study is carried out is important because of the secular trends that may occur. Mean height tends to increase from one generation to the next. Mean age at menarche tends to be earlier in the present generation than in the past generation.[40] Migration from small communities to large urban centers produces a change in head shape in the next generation.[1,24]

9. Measurements differ in accuracy depending on the type of measurement, the measuring device used, and the care taken in performing the measurements. Obviously, measurements from radiographs are more accurate than measurements taken on soft tissue because of greater precision in point location.

10. Finally, few clinical studies provide any indication of how reliable their measurements are. A reliability factor can be especially helpful in the interpretation of soft tissue measurements on various patients. In most anthropometric studies, replicate measures are averaged together in an attempt to improve the accuracy of the measurements. It is a relatively simple matter to provide an error factor by using the replicate measurements to calculate a correlation coefficient for each distinct measure given. If the correlation coefficient is high, the measurement is more reliable than if the coefficient is low. By listing such a correlation coefficient for each measure in the published study, the clinician knows how reliable each particular measurement is. If the measuring error is high, deviation of a specific patient measurement is probably not as important as if the measuring error is low. If the measuring error is greater than the difference being measured, the results are meaningless unless they differ drastically from the norm. Unfortunately, most clinical studies of various measurements are not published with correlation coefficients. Furthermore, the coefficients cannot be calculated

from the published data because the difference between the two replicate measures is lost in the averaging process.

REFERENCES

1. Boas F: *Changes in Bodily Form of Descendants of Immigrants.* Washington, DC: Government Printing Office, 1911.
2. Broadbent BH Sr, Broadbent BH Jr, Golden WH: *Bolton Standards of Dentofacial Developmental Growth.* St. Louis: CV Mosby, 1975.
3. Cohen MM Jr: The problem of low-set ears in clinical dysmorphology. *Birth Defects* 11(2):74–75, 1975.
4. Cronk C, Crocker AC, Pueschel SM, Shea AM, Zackai E, Pickens G, Reed RB: Growth charts for children with Down syndrome: 1 month to 18 years of age. *Pediatrics* 81:102–110, 1988.
5. Farkas LG: *Anthropometry of the Hand and Face in Medicine.* Amsterdam: Elsevier, 1981.
6. Farkas LG, Munro IR (eds): *Anthropometric Facial Proportions in Medicine.* Springfield, IL: CC Thomas, 1987.
7. Garn SM: Applications of pattern analysis to anthropometric data. *Ann NY Acad Sci* 63:537–552, 1955.
8. Garn SM: Patterning in ontogeny, taxonomy, phylogeny, and dysmorphogenesis. In Wetherington, RK (ed): *Colloquia in Anthropology.* Dallas: Fort Burgwin Research Center, Inc., Southern and Methodist University, 1977, pp 83–106.
9. Garn SM, Rohmann CG: Interaction of nutrition and genetics in the timing of growth and development. *Pediatr Clin North Am* 13:353–379, 1966.
10. Hall JG, Froster-Iskenius VG, Allanson JE: *Handbook of Normal Physical Measurements.* New York: Oxford University Press, 1989.
11. Hamill PV, Drizd TA, Johnson CL, Reed RB, Roche AF, Moore WM: Physical growth: National Center for Health Statistics percentile. *Am J Clin Nutr* 32:607–629, 1979.
12. Hansmann M: *Ultrasonic Diagnosis in Obstetrics and Gynecology.* Berlin: Springer, 1985.
13. Harvey EA, Hayes AM, Holmes LB: Lessons on objectivity in clinical studies. *Am J Med Genet* 53:19–20, 1994.
14. Holm VA, Nugent JK: Growth in the Prader-Willi syndrome. *Birth Defects* 18(3B):93–100, 1982.
15. Horton WA, Rotter JI, Rimoin DL, Scott CI, Hall JG: Standard growth curves for achondroplasia. *Pediatrics* 93:435–438, 1978.
16. Horton WA, Hall JG, Scott CI, Pyeritz RE, Rimoin DL: Growth curves for height for diastrophic dysplasia, spondyloepiphyseal dysplasia congenita, and pseudoachondroplasia. *Am J Dis Child* 136:316–319, 1982.
17. Hunter AGW, Hecht JT, Reid CS, Pauli RM, Scott CI: Standard curves of weight and chest circumference in achondroplasia. David W. Smith Workshop on Malformations and Morphogenesis, Big Sky, Montana, July 30–August 3, 1995.
18. Ikeda Y, Higurashi M, Egi S, Ohzeki N, Hoshina H: An anthropometric study of girls with the Ullrich-Turner syndrome. *Am J Med Genet* 12:271–280, 1982.
19. Juberg RC, Sholte FG, Touchstone WJ: Normal values for intercanthal distances of 5- to 11-year-old American blacks. *Pediatrics* 55:431–436, 1975.
20. Lubchenco LO, Hansmann C, Dressler M, Boyd E: Intrauterine growth as estimated from liveborn birthweight data at 24 to 42 weeks of gestation. *Pediatrics* 32:793–800, 1963.
21. Lubchenco LO, Hansmann C, Boyd E: Intrauterine growth in length and head circumference as estimated from livebirth at gestational ages from 26 to 42 weeks. *Pediatrics* 37:403–408, 1966.

22. Lusted LB, Keats TE: *Atlas of Roentgenographic Measurement.* Second Edition. Chicago: Year Book Medical, 1967.
23. Merlob P, Siva Y, Reisner SH: Anthropometric measurements of the newborn infant (27–41 gestational weeks). *Birth Defects* 20(7):1–32, 1984.
24. Montagu MFA: *An Introduction to Physical Anthropology.* Third Edition, Springfield, IL: CC Thomas, 1960.
25. Morris CA, Derusey SA, Leonard CO, Dilts C, Blackburn BL: Natural history of Williams syndrome: Physical characteristics. *J Pediatr* 113:318–326, 1988.
26. Park E, Bailey JD, Cowell CA: Growth and maturation of patients with Turner's syndrome. *Pediatr Res* 7:1–7, 1983.
27. Pelz VL, Sussmann S, Timm D, Rostock I: Ullrich-Turner-Syndrom. *Kinderärzt Prax* 49:206–212, 1981.
28. Potter EL, Craig JM: *Pathology of the Fetus and the Infant,* Third Edition. Chicago: Year Book Medical, 1975.
29. Poznanski A: *The Hand in Radiologic Diagnosis: With Gamuts and Pattern Profiles.* Second Edition. Philadelphia: WB Saunders, 1984.
30. Pryor HB: Objective measurement of interpupillary distance. *Pediatrics* 44:973–977, 1969.
31. Pyeritz RE: Growth and anthropometrics in the Marfan syndrome. *Prog Clin Biol Res* 200:355–366, 1985.
32. Ranke MB, Heidemann P, Knupfer C, Enders H, Schmaltz A, Bierich JR: Noonan syndrome: Growth and clinical manifestations in 144 cases. *Eur J Pediatr* 48:220–227, 1988.
33. Riolo ML, Moyers RE, McNamera JA Jr, Hunter WS: *An Atlas of Craniofacial Growth: Cephalometric Standards from the University School Growth Study, The University of Michigan.* Monograph No. 2, Craniofacial Growth Series. Center for Human Growth and Development, University of Michigan, 1974.
34. Robinow M, Roche AF: Low-set ears. *Am J Dis Child* 125:482–483, 1973.
35. Saksena SS, Walker GF, Bixler D, Yu PL: *A Clinical Atlas of Roentgencephalometry in Norma Lateralis.* New York: Alan R. Liss, 1987.
36. Saul RA, Stevenson RE, Rogers RC, Skinner SA, Prouty LA, Flannery DB: Growth references from conception to adulthood. *Proc Greenwood Genet Center,* Suppl. No. 1, 1988.
37. Shepard TH, Shi M, Fellingham GW, Fujinaga M, FitzSimmons JM, Fantel AG: Organ weight standards for human fetuses. *Pediatr Pathol* 8:513–524, 1988.
38. Smith DW: *Growth and Its Disorders.* Philadelphia: WB Saunders, 1977.
39. Tanner JM: Physical growth and development. In Forfar JO, Arneil GC (eds): *Textbook of Pediatrics.* Edinburgh: Churchill Livingstone, 1978, pp 253–303.
40. Tanner JM: *Fetus Into Man: Physical Growth From Conception to Maturity.* Cambridge, MA: Harvard University Press, 1978.
41. Tanner JM, Whitehouse RH: Height and weight charts from birth to 5 years allowing for length of gestation. *Arch Dis Child* 48:786–789, 1973.
42. Tanner JM, Whitehouse RH: Clinical longitudinal standards for height, weight, height velocity, weight velocity, and stages of puberty. *Arch Dis Child* 51:170–179, 1976.
43. Witt DR, Keena BA, Hall JG, Allanson JE: Growth curves for height in Noonan syndrome. *Clin Genet* 30:150–153, 1986.

6

Genetics

Medical genetics involves the application of genetics to medical practice and includes the inheritance of medical disorders in families, cytogenetics, mapping of gene disorders to specific locations on chromosomes, and analysis of molecular mechanisms by which genes causing genetic disorders act. This chapter briefly covers a variety of topics, including cytogenetics and chromosomal anomalies, contiguous gene syndromes, single gene inheritance, gene mapping, genetic heterogeneity, mosaicism, uniparental disomy, imprinting, mitochondrial inheritance, anticipation, "sporadicity," variant additive patterns, and multifactorial inheritance. Extensive coverage is available elsewhere.[7,8,19,31]

CYTOGENETICS

Chromosome analysis can be carried out in a variety of clinical situations. Chromosomes are visible only when cells divide in mitosis or meiosis. Cell culture methods have greatly extended the range of possible tissues and types of cells from which dividing cells can be obtained: small lymphocytes, fibroblasts, amnionic fluid cells, and even viable cells from spontaneous abortions, embryos, and fetuses for a number of hours after death. Cartilage cells are viable for karyotypes even several days after death.

Many techniques have revealed the underlying structural features of chromosomes. Human chromosomes are grouped by size and centromere location; the latter may be metacentric, submetacentric, or acrocentric (Fig. 6-1). Characteristic banding patterns of the chromosomes permit identification of each individual chromosome (Fig. 6-2, Table 6-1). The karyotype or chromosomal constitution of any cell is abbreviated by three symbolic parts, each separated by a comma; the number of chromosomes observed; the number of sex chromosomes and their type; and specific description of an unusual chromosome or

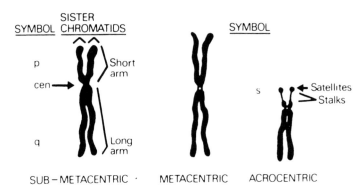

Figure 6-1. General morphology of human chromosomes. From Lubs and Ing.[21]

unusual chromosomes.[17,21] Table 6-2 lists the symbols commonly used. Numerical abnormalities reflect the total number of chromosomes (Fig. 6-3). Sex chromosome aneuploidy is described both numerically and in the sex chromosome constitution. Three examples are

46,XX	Normal female with 46 chromosomes and two X chromosomes
47,XXY	Klinefelter syndrome with 47 chromosomes, two X chromosomes, and one Y chromosomes
47,XY,+21	Trisomy 21 syndrome with 47 chromosomes, a normal male sex chromosome constitution, and one extra 21 chromosome

Structural abnormalities of chromosomes include deletions (Fig. 6-4), duplications, inversions, and translocations. The following is an example of a structural abnormality written in two ways—the short form and the detailed form:

Table 6-1. Chromosome Banding

Type	Stain	Area Stained	Effect
Q-banding	Quinacrine	Chromosome arms; mostly repetitive AT-rich DNA	Under UV light, distinct fluorescent banded pattern for each chromosome
G-banding	Giemsa	Chromosome arms; mostly repetitive AT-rich DNA	Distinct banded pattern for each chromosome; same as Q-banding pattern except single additional band near centromere of chromosomes 1 and 16
R-banding	Variety of techniques	Chromosome arms; mostly unique GC-rich DNA	Reverse banding pattern of that observed with Q- or G-banding
C-banding	Variety of techniques	Centromere region of each chromosome and distal portion of Y chromosome; highly repetitive, mostly AT-rich DNA	Largest bands usually on chromosomes 1, 9, 16, and Y; chromosomes 7, 10, and 15 have medium-sized bands; size of C-bands highly variable from person to person

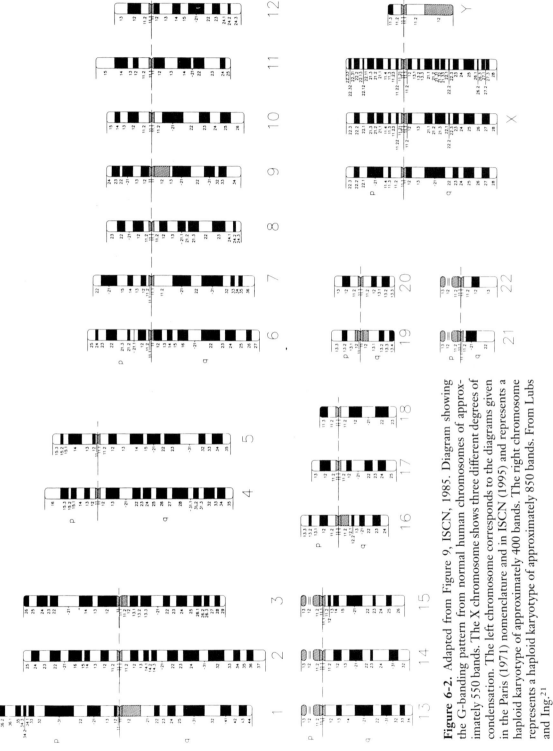

Figure 6-2. Adapted from Figure 9, ISCN, 1985. Diagram showing the G-banding pattern from normal human chromosomes of approximately 550 bands. The X chromosome shows three different degrees of condensation. The left chromosome corresponds to the diagrams given in the Paris (1971) nomenclature and in ISCN (1995) and represents a haploid karyotype of approximately 400 bands. The right chromosome represents a haploid karyotype of approximately 850 bands. From Lubs and Ing.[21]

Table 6-2. Symbols and Abbreviations Used in Cytogenetic Nomenclature

Symbol	Meaning
ace	Acentric fragment
→	(arrow) indicating 'from—to—'
*	(asterisk) used as a multiplication sign in describing variant or heteromorphic chromosomes
b	Break
cen	Centromere
chi	Chimera
:	(colon) used to describe a break
::	(double colon) describes breakage and reunion
,	(comma) separates chromosome number from sex chromosome constitution; separates sex chromosome constitution from description of unusual chromosome(s)
cs	Chromosome
csb	Chromosome break
csg	Chromosome gap
ct	Chromatid
ctb	Chromatid break
ctg	Chromatid gap
del	Deletion
der	Derivative chromosome
dic	Dicentric chromosome
dir	Direct
dup	Duplication
end	Endoreduplication
fra	Fragile site
g	Gap
h	Heteromorphic regions of 1q, 9q, and 16q
i	Isochromosome

(1) 46,XY,del(5)(p13)	Normal number of chromosomes with normal male
(2) 46,XY,del(5)(qter → p13:)	sex chromosome constitution and deletion of the short arm of chromosome 5

The first set of symbols (1) represents the short designation for the cri-du-chat syndrome. This form identifies the chromosome involved in the deletion and the breakpoint. The second set of symbols (2) represents the detailed designation and identifies the abnormal chromosome from end to end. The colon indicates that the segment closest to the 5p13 band is deleted. Both forms represent the same chromosomal anomaly. In publications, it has been recommended that the detailed form be given first, from then on using only the short form. In laboratory reports, the short form is used.[17,21]

Consider the symbols used for a Down syndrome translocation:

(1) 45,XX,t(14;21)(p11;q11)	One chromosome appears to be missing; the sex
(2) 45,XX,t(14;21)(14qter → 14p11:21q11 → qter)	constitution is female; and translocation between chromosomes 14 and 21 results in two chromosomes becoming one by centric fusion.

Table 6-2. (*Continued*)

Symbol	Meaning
ins	Insertion
inv	Inversion
mar	Marker chromosome
mat	Maternal origin
−	(minus) missing a whole (if before) or part of a (if after) chromosome
mos	Mosaic
p	Short arm
pat	Paternal origin
Ph[1]	Philadelphia chromosome
+	(plus) an additional whole (if before) or part of a (if after) chromosome
pcc	Premature chromosome condensation
pvz	Pulverization
q	Long arm
qr	Quadriradial
?	(question mark) unknown
r	Ring
rec	Recombinant
rob	Robertsonian translocation
s	Satellite
SCE	Sister chromatid exchange
;	(semicolon) separates different chromosomes (or parts) involved in rearrangements
/	(slash) separates different karyotypes in mosaics and chimeras
t	Translocation
tr	Triradial
ter	Terminal end of a chromosome (telomere)
var	Variant or heteromorphic chromosome

From Lubs and Ing.[21]

The first set of symbols (1) represents the short designation for the balanced translocation; the second set (2) represents the detailed designation.

CHROMOSOMAL ANOMALIES

Chromosome studies should be performed on all patients with a suspected chromosomal syndrome to confirm the diagnosis. Family studies may be indicated when structural rearrangements are present. For example, with translocation-type Down syndrome, it is important to know if the translocation arose *de novo* or if one parent is a translocation carrier. In the latter situation, the parent is at increased risk for having another child with translocation-type Down syndrome. Types of chromosome abnormalities are listed in Table 6-3, and mechanisms are summarized in Table 6-4.

Chromosome studies should also be carried out on any patient with multiple malformations when the overall diagnosis is unknown. The criteria listed in

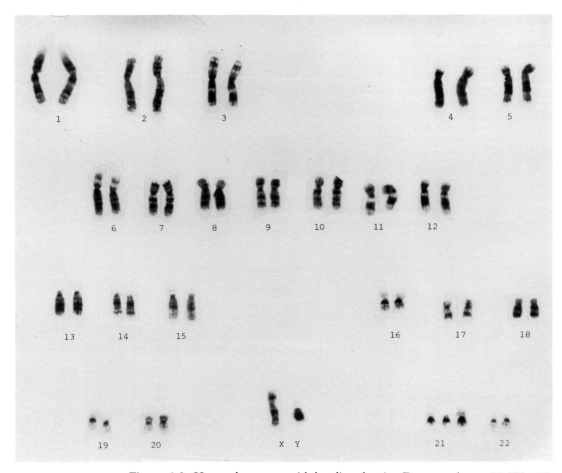

Figure 6-3. Human karyotype with banding showing Down syndrome (47,XY,+21).

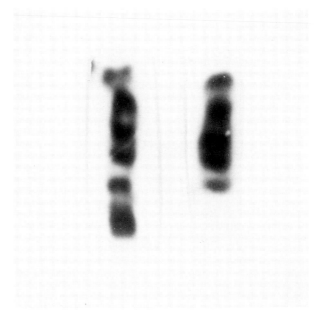

Figure 6-4. Deletion of long arm of chromosome 18 [right] del(18)(q22.1).

Table 6-3. Types of Chromosome Abnormalities

Numerical changes
   Involving whole sets: triploidy, tetraploidy
   Involving individual chromosomes: trisomy, double trisomy,
      monosomy, sex chromosome aneuploidy
   Mosaicism and chimerism
Structural changes
   Breaks and sister chromatid exchanges
   Deletions: terminal, interstitial, ring
   Duplications: tandem, inverted, isochromosome
   Translocations: centric fusion (Robertsonian), reciprocal,
      insertional, complex
   Inversions: paracentric, pericentric
   Duplication/deficiencies: partial trisomy/partial monosomy

From Miller.[23]

Table 6-5 may be used to help decide whether a chromosome study should be performed. The following generalizations should be kept in mind when using the criteria. First, chromosomal aberrations usually have adverse effects on *many* parts of the body. An individual with only two anomalies, such as an atrial septal defect and clinodactyly, is unlikely to have a chromosome problem. Second, most patients with unbalanced autosomes have growth deficiency of prenatal or postnatal onset and mental retardation. An individual with normal growth parameters and normal psychomotor development is not, as a rule, a candidate for chromosome study. Exceptions to both generalizations include some sex chromosome disorders that may have few recognizable anomalies. Other exceptions include very small deletions or duplications.[18] Specific autosomal and sex chromosomal aneuploidies, fragile X syndrome, deletions, duplications, and unusual chromosomal variants have been reviewed exhaustively elsewhere.[12]

Table 6-4. Mechanisms Leading to Chromosome Abnormalities

Mechanism	*Effect*
Nondisjunction, meiotic	Trisomy, monosomy (aneuploidy)
Nondisjunction, mitotic	Mosaicism, aneuploidy
Anaphase lag, meiotic	Monosomy
Anaphase lag, mitotic	Mosaicism
Double fertilization	Triploidy, tetraploidy
Retention of second polar body	Triploidy, tetraploidy
Fusion of twin zygotes	Conjoint twins, chimeras
Unequal crossing over	Deletion, duplication
Chromosome breakage and rejoining	Structural abnormalities
Aberrant segregation in translocation heterozygotes	Duplication/deficiencies (partial trisomy/partial monosomy)
Meiotic crossing over in inversion heterozygotes	Duplication/deficiencies, dicentric or acentric chromosomes

From Miller, 1990.[23]

Table 6-5. Indications for Chromosomal Studies[a]

Scalp
  Scalp defect (usually occipital) [tri-13, del(4p)]
  Posterior hair whorl over posterior fontanel [tri-21]

Ears (small) [tri-21, del(18q)]

Eyes
  Upslanting palpebral fissures [tri-21, del(18q)]
  Microphthalmia, anophthalmia [tri-13, del(13q)]
  Cyclopia or severe hypotelorism [tri-13, del(18q)]
  Coloboma (iris) [del(4p), cat eye syndrome]
  Retinoblastoma [del(13q)]

Nose (neonatal high nasal bridge)
  [tri-13,del(21q),del(13q)]

Philtrum (very short) [del(4p)]

Tongue
  Small hard-to-open mouth [tri-18]
  Downturned mouth [del(4p),del(5p),del(13q)]

Mandible (prominent) [multiple X syndromes, del(18q)]

Neck (webbed) [45,X Turner syndrome and multiple
  X syndromes, tri-8]

Sternum (short) [tri-18]

Abdomen
  Duodenal atresia [tri-21]
  Pyloric stenosis [del(21q)]
  Multicystic kidneys [45,X Turner]
  Polycystic kidneys [tri-13]
  Omphalocele [tri-18, triploidy]

Anus (atresia) [cat eye syndrome, del(13q), tri-18, tri-8]

External genitalia (scrotalization of phallus) [tri-13]

Extremities
  Edema [45,X Turner]
  Radial hypoplasia including thumb abnormalities
  [tri-18,del(13q),del(4p)]
  Radioulnar synostosis [multiple-X syndromes, XXY]
  Overlapping fingers with nail dysplasia [tri-18]
  Dermatoglyphics
    All low arches [tri-18]
    All ulnar loops [tri-21]
    Tibial arch [tri-21]
  Vertical sole creases [tri-8]
  Rocker-bottom feet with prominent heels [tri-13,
  tri-18]

Skin
  Keloids in whites [45,X, del(21q)]
  Hemagiomas in unusual places that persist [45,X
  Turner]

Vocalization
  Cat cry [del(5p)]

Miscellaneous (less specific but useful when combined
  with other features):
  Gynecomastia [XXY]
  Preauricular or helical pits [cat eye syndrome]
  Single umbilical artery [tri-18]
  Polydactyly [tri-13]
  Ambiguous genitalia [45,X/46,XY]

Courtesy of B. D. Hall (Lexington, Kentucky).

[a] Brackets enclose examples of chromosomal disorders that frequently have that particular feature.

CYTOGENETIC STUDIES

The field of human cytogenetics has passed through three phases. Chromosome analysis from 1956 to the late 1960s detected mostly abnormalities of chromosome number and a few structural aberrations. Discoveries during this period included conditions such as trisomies 13 (Fig. 6-5), 18, and 21; X-aneuploidy states such as Turner and Klinefelter syndromes; and deletions such as the cri-du-chat syndrome and deletion of the long arm of chromosome 18. In the 1970s, the introduction of banding techniques led to the discovery of a large number of interstitial and terminal deletions and duplications, double deletion, deletion-duplication, and double duplication. Examples include dup(5p) syndrome, del(11q) syndrome, mosaic tetrasomy 12p syndrome, del(16p) syndrome, and del(22q) syndrome, among many others (Fig. 6-6). While this phase continues to the present time, a third stage was introduced during the 1980s—prometaphase staining and combining cytogenetic and molecular methods for identifying microdeletions and for gene mapping. Fluorescent *in situ* hybridization (FISH) techniques were introduced in the late 1980s and early 1990s. FISH can be used to determine the origin of marker chromosomes and to detect

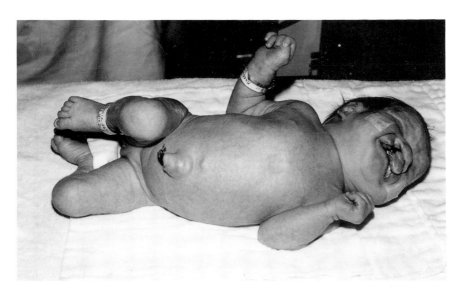

Figure 6-5. Trisomy 13 syndrome.

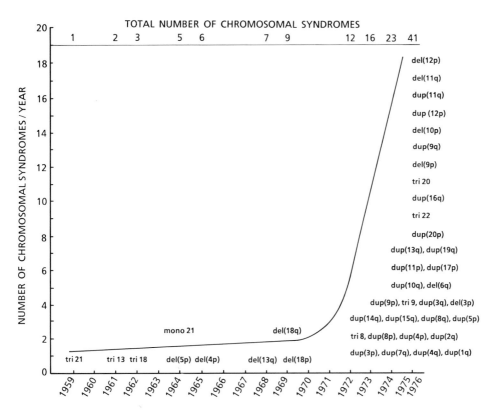

Figure 6-6. Dramatic increase in the number of identified chromosomal conditions with the introduction of banding techniques.

numerical aberrations, inversions, small translocations, deletions, and duplications. Clinical suspicion must be directed at a particular chromosome segment. The list of FISH applications is still growing and has penetrated the domain of single gene disorders.

CONTIGUOUS GENE SYNDROMES

Contiguous gene syndromes[33] (also known as *microdeletion syndromes*[32] and *small deletion syndromes*[9]) have extremely variable clinical manifestations because deletions and duplications are variable in degree. Some deletions are so small that they cannot be identified cytogenetically. Molecular techniques must be employed. Most cases appear sporadically, but some families simulate mendelian inheritance. The chromosomal banding patterns and microdeletions of four syndromes and one sequence are shown schematically in Figure 6-7, and the clinical characteristics of each are summarized in Table 6-6. Illustrations of two—the Langer-Giedion syndrome and the Prader-Willi syndrome—are shown in Figures 6-8 through 6-11. Another example of a contiguous gene syndrome is Alport syndrome with esophageal and genital leiomyomatosis [del(X)(q21.3–q22)].

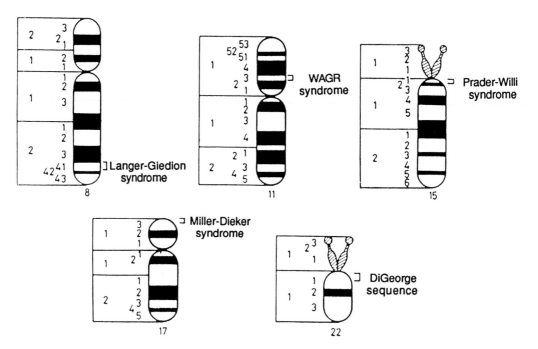

Figure 6-7. Schematic representation of banding patterns showing microdeletions for four syndromes and one sequence (see also Table 6-6). Chromosome number shown under each chromosome. First and second numbers on left side of chromosome are banding numbers that allow all chromosome bands to be described by region. Breakpoints for each of the four microdeletion syndromes and one microdeletion sequence shown on right side of chromosomes. From Schinzel.[32]

Table 6-6. Clinical Features of Selected Conditions with Microdeletions

Condition	Chromosome Micro-deletion Region	Clinical Characteristics
Langer-Giedion syndrome	del(8)(q24)	Multiple cone-shaped epiphyses, multiple exostoses, sparse scalp hair, mild mental deficiency, characteristic facial appearance (see Fig. 6-8)
WAGR syndrome	del(11)(p13)	Wilms tumor, aniridia, gonadoblastoma, mental retardation; other features include male genital hypoplasia of varying degree and characteristic facial dysmorphism consisting of long face, upslanting palpebral fissures, ptosis of the eyelids, blepharophimosis, beaked nose, and low-set malformed ears
Prader-Willi syndrome	del(15)(q11)	Hypotonia, mental deficiency, short stature, obesity, hypogonadism, and distinctive facial appearance (see Figs. 6-9 through 6-11)
Miller-Dieker syndrome	del(17)(p13)	Lissencephaly, profound mental retardation with seizures and EEG abnormalities, growth deficiency, an early demise, microcephaly, prominent occiput, wrinkled skin over glabella and metopic suture, narrow forehead, downslanting palpebral fissures, small nose and chin, cardiac malformations, hypoplastic male external genitalia
DiGeorge sequence	del(22)(q11)	Abnormalities of the third and fourth pharyngeal pouches. Absence or hypoplasia of parathyroids and/or thymus and cardiac defects, especially type B interrupted aortic arch and ventricular septal defect. Facial anomalies in some cases involving the branchial arches and ocular hypertelorism. Can be associated with velocardiofacial syndrome

DEVELOPMENTAL EFFECTS OF ANEUPLOIDY

In aneuploidy, the number of chromosomes is not a multiple of 23; trisomy and monosomy are examples. Growth deficiency of prenatal onset is frequently an associated feature of autosomal aneuploidy. Mittwoch[24] suggested that general effects resulted from a decreased rate of cell proliferation. More specific phenotypic effects were thought to be produced by gene dosage effects, which resulted in differential mitotic rates at certain developmental stages. Although decreased cellular proliferation has been suggested by cell cycle studies of trisomy 18 syndrome[29] and trisomy 21 syndrome,[14] other studies have failed to demonstrate cell cycle changes in aneuploidy.[16] Naeye[25] indicated that in some instances of trisomy 13, trisomy 18, and trisomy 21, abnormal growth patterns in individual organs appear to be as characteristic for each trisomic disorder as are body and organ malformations.

Opitz and Gilbert[28] discussed the developmental effects of aneuploidy. They considered a number of features to be typical: an increased frequency of minor

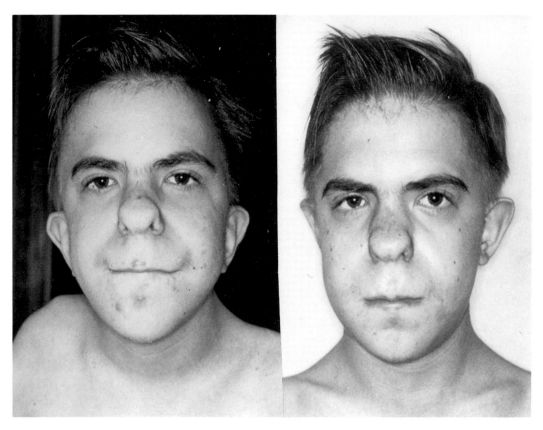

Figure 6-8. Langer-Giedion syndrome in twins with del(8)(q24). Note bulbous nasal tip, hypoplastic alar wings, long wide philtrum, thin upper lip, and protuberant ears.

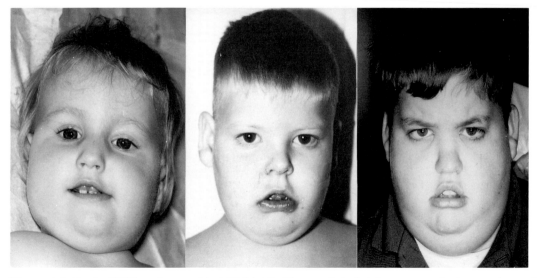

Figure 6-9. Prader-Willi syndrome with del(15)(q11). Characteristic facial appearance in three patients of different ages.

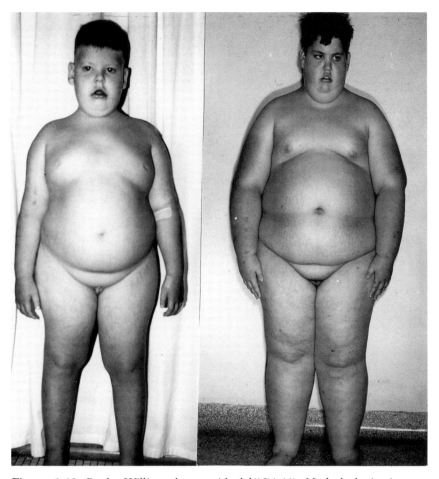

Figure 6-10. Prader-Willi syndrome with del(15)(q11). Marked obesity in two patients. Right, from Cohen and Gorlin.[6]

anomalies and less frequently occurring major malformations, growth and maturational disturbances, an increased frequency of neoplasia, structural and functional defects of the central nervous system, abnormal gonadal development with reduced numbers of germ cells, an increase in right–left asymmetry, an increased frequency of atavisms, and hyperreactivity to teratogens.

Epstein[9] developed seven principles governing the development of aneuploid phenotypes, including the following two: (1) Although aneuploid phenotypes have many overlapping nonspecific features, the phenotypes can be distinguished from one another; and (2) although any given aneuploidy syndrome may possess a great deal of variability in its phenotype, its overall pattern of defects is still specific.

Preus and Aymé,[30] using the methods of numerical taxonomy and cluster analysis to study del(4p) vs. dup(4p) and del(9p) vs dup(9p), rejected the syndrome/antisyndrome hypothesis because the proportion of significant differences between corresponding duplications and deletions was no greater than that observed between unrelated pairs of chromosomal syndromes. However, Epstein[9] suggested that a limited number of individual phenotypic features of

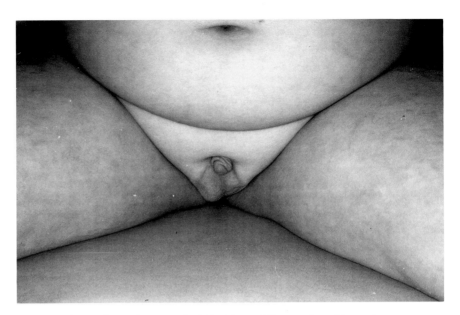

Figure 6-11. Prader-Willi syndrome with del(15)(q11). Micropenis and hypoplastic scrotum.

different pairs of duplications and deletions might still possibly represent real countercharacters. He proposed a mechanism by which such countercharacters could be generated, involving dose-dependent responses of tissues to growth-promoting or growth-inhibiting morphogens.

Lurie and Opitz[22] indicated that the deleterious effects of autosomal deletions may be explained by (1) aneuploidy effects; (2) hemizygosity of several genes within the homologous segment; (3) imprinting; or (4) a combination of these or possibly some as yet unknown mechanism(s). The phenotypic features of any autosomal deletion syndrome consist basically of two groups of abnormalities: specific and nonspecific. Nonspecific findings such as growth deficiency, microcephaly, and epicanthic folds are common to many different segmental autosomal aneuploidies. Only malformations specific for a given syndrome can be used for phenotypic mapping. Estabrooks et al.[10] used a complex of molecular probes to generate a preliminary phenotypic map of chromosome 4p16 based on 4p deletions.

SINGLE GENE INHERITANCE

An individual with an autosomal dominant disorder produces two kinds of gametes, one with a normal gene, one with an abnormal gene (Fig. 6-12). Thus, offspring of an affected individual have a 50% chance of being affected. An autosomal dominant pedigree is illustrated in Figure 6-13. Dominant disorders are transmitted from generation to generation without skips, and each sex has an equal chance of being affected. Notice that there are two instances of male-to-male transmission, which rule out X-linked inheritance. The ability of an autosomal dominant gene to be transmitted from generation to generation depends on the genetic fitness of the affected individual. A mother and child with autosomal dominant Crouzon syndrome are shown in Figure 6-14. In achondroplasia, the genetic fitness is reduced so that although some dominant

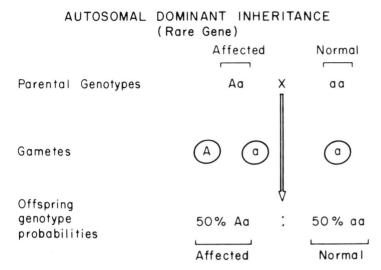

AUTOSOMAL DOMINANT INHERITANCE
(Rare Gene)

Figure 6-12. In autosomal dominant inheritance, an affected individual has a 50% chance of having an affected offspring.

pedigrees may be observed, many instances occur sporadically, resulting from new mutations. Most cases of Apert syndrome occur sporadically because the malformations and mental deficiency (present in some cases) diminish the patients' desirability as mates (Figs. 6-15, 6-16).[1]

Other features frequently found with autosomal dominantly inherited genes are incomplete penetrance and variable expressivity. *Penetrance* refers to the gene's ability to be expressed at all. In Figure 6-17, an autosomal dominant pedigree is shown with two instances of incomplete penetrance. Although incompletely penetrant individuals do not show the trait, they are carriers for the disorder, with a 50% risk of transmitting the gene to their offspring. A genetic trait may be variably expressed, ranging from mild to severe. For example, a parent with mandibulofacial dysostosis might exhibit only mildly downslanting palpebral fissures and mild zygomatic hypoplasia. On the other hand, her affected child might have severe downslanting of the palpebral fissures, absent zygomatic arches, and severe micrognathia.

With autosomal recessive inheritance, both parents are phenotypically nor-

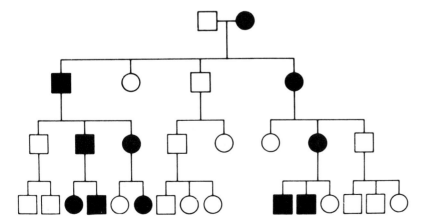

Figure 6-13. Autosomal dominant pedigree showing vertical transmission and male-to-male transmission.

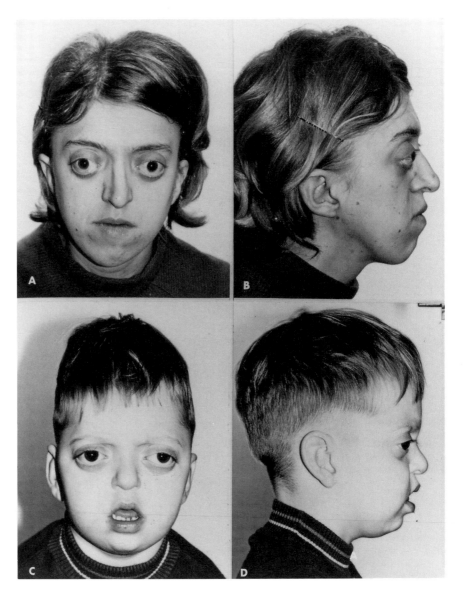

Figure 6-14. Autosomal dominant Crouzon syndrome in mother and son. From Cohen.[1]

mal but are heterozygous carriers for the abnormal gene. Parents produce two different kinds of gametes, one normal, one abnormal (Fig. 6-18). There is a 25% chance of having an affected child. Of the phenotypically normal children, some will be heterozygous carriers for the disorder, like their parents.

Because offspring have a 25% chance of being affected, sibships of two or more children may be found (Fig. 6-19). Both sexes have an equal chance of being affected. More remote ancestors as well as the parents are normal, as a rule. An increased percentage of pedigrees may have consanguinity. The rarer the gene is in the population, the more likely are consanguineous pedigrees to be found. Figure 6-20 shows how consanguinity increases the probability of homozygosity for the abnormal gene. Examples include Morquio syndrome and Ellis-van Creveld syndrome.

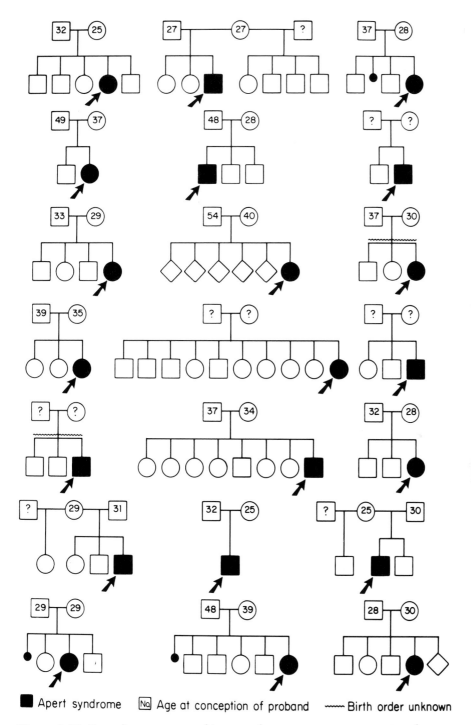

Figure 6-15. Sporadic occurrences of Apert syndrome represent new mutations for an autosomal dominant disorder in which the genetic fitness is dramatically reduced. From Cohen.[1]

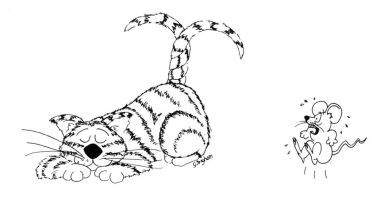

Mew-tation

Figure 6-16. "Sporadicity" *per se* does not necessarily mean that a condition is nongenetic. It could represent a new mutation for an autosomal dominant disorder.

In X-linked recessive inheritance, both parents are phenotypically normal. The mother is a carrier for the abnormal gene and is able to produce two kinds of gametes, one with a normal gene, one with the abnormal gene. Offspring genotype probabilities are illustrated in Figure 6-21. Half of the males are affected, and half of the females are phenotypically normal carriers for the gene. An X-linked recessive pedigree is shown in Figure 6-22A. The gene is transmitted from generation to generation in a diagonal pattern. Affected males do not produce affected offspring and are themselves the offspring of normal female carriers. In the population as a whole, more males tend to be affected. When females are affected, they are the offspring of an affected father and a normal carrier mother. In such instances, the parents are often related. It is also possible for affected females to have 45,X Turner syndrome or an X/autosomal translocation.

An example of an X-linked recessive disorder is the common type of hypo-

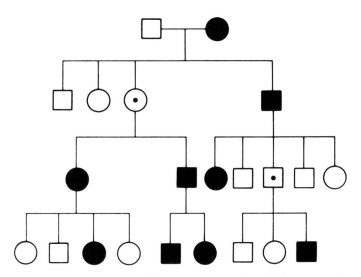

Figure 6-17. Autosomal dominant inheritance showing incomplete penetrance. Dots indicate genetic carriers for the abnormal gene who are phenotypically normal.

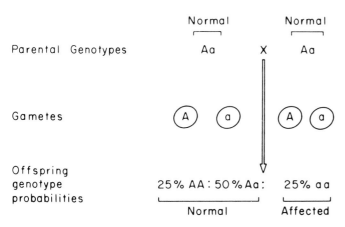

AUTOSOMAL RECESSIVE INHERITANCE
(Rare Gene)

	Normal		Normal
Parental Genotypes	Aa	X	Aa

Gametes (A) (a) | (A) (a)

Offspring genotype probabilities: 25% AA : 50% Aa : 25% aa

Normal — Affected

Figure 6-18. In autosomal recessive inheritance, both parents are phenotypically normal carriers who have a 25% risk of having an affected offspring.

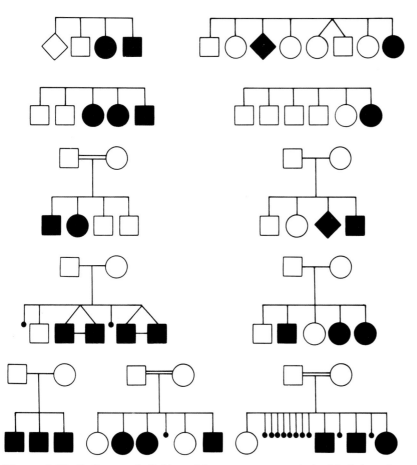

Figure 6-19. Pedigrees of sibships with recurrent cases of the Meckel syndrome. Affected siblings and consanguinity are consistent with autosomal recessive inheritance.

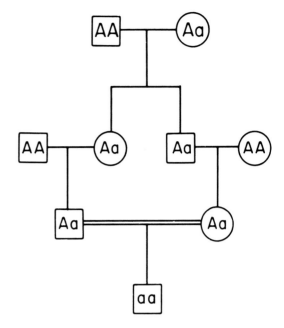

Figure 6-20. Affected homozygote (aa), parental consanguinity indicated by the double horizontal line between two heterozygous parents, two heterozygous grandparents who are brother and sister, and the heterozygous great grandmother.

hidrotic ectodermal dysplasia. A typical X-linked pedigree is found in Figure 6-22A, showing affected males and female carriers. The same pedigree is slightly altered in Figure 6-22B to look more like an X-linked dominant pedigree. This pattern fits if the disorder is defined as any degree of hypohidrosis. Since carrier mothers do have a patchy sweat gland distribution, they can be defined as being affected.

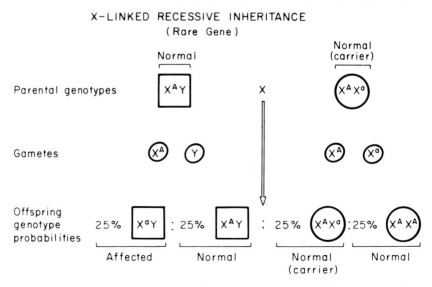

Figure 6-21. Parental genotypes, types of gametes, and offspring genotype probabilities in X-linked recessive inheritance.

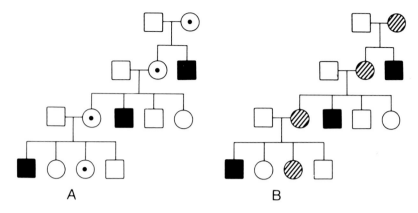

Figure 6-22. A: X-linked recessive pedigree (dots indicate female carriers). B: X-linked semidominant inheritance (disorder minimally defined so that female carriers are considered affected).

For X-linked dominant inheritance, parental genotypes, types of gametes, and offspring genotype probabilities are shown in Figures 6-23 and 6-24. A typical X-linked dominant pedigree is shown in Figure 6-25. Such a condition is transmitted from generation to generation without skips. All daughters of an affected male are affected. For affected females, offspring of either sex have a 50% chance of being affected. X-linked dominant conditions are usually more severely expressed in males than in females, and, in the population as a whole, more females tend to be affected. An example of an X-linked dominant condition is vitamin D–resistant rickets.

Finally, the parental genotypes, types of gametes, and offspring genotype probabilities for X-linked dominant inheritance, lethal in the male, are illustrated in Figure 6-26. Only females are affected. The deficiency of males is expressed as an excess number of abortions in the offspring of affected females. The condition is transmitted from mother to daughter. An example of an

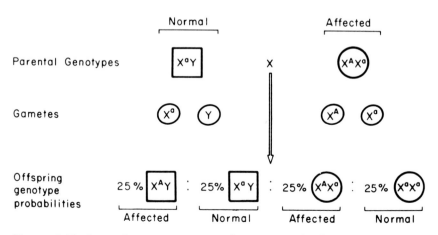

Figure 6-23. Parental genotypes, types of gametes, and offspring genotype probabilities in X-linked dominant inheritance (when the female is affected).

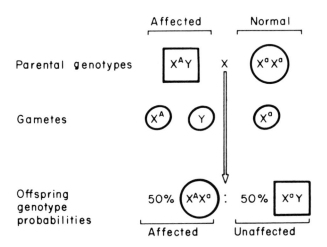

Figure 6-24. Parental genotypes, types of gametes, and offspring genotype probabilities in X-linked dominant inheritance (when the male is affected).

X-linked dominant condition, lethal in the male, is the oral-facial-digital syndrome, type I.

Bayesian methods of probability of recurrence have a number of uses in medical genetics, but the most important practical applications are for genetic counseling in autosomal dominant disorders with a variable age of onset or reduced penetrance and in X-linked disorders. Detailed consideration is beyond the scope of this chapter.[8,19]

GENE MAPPING

Genetic mapping makes use of linkage, in which different loci occupy the same region of a chromosome. Crossovers between loci on the same chromosome can

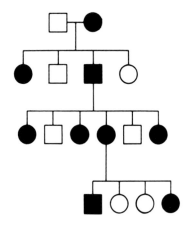

Figure 6-25. X-linked dominant pedigree. Note the vertical transmission and lack of male-to-male transmission. All daughters of an affected male are affected.

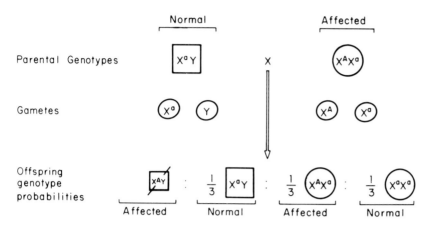

Figure 6-26. Parental genotypes, types of gametes, and offspring genotype probabilities in X-linked dominant inheritance (lethal in the male). Note that since the affected males are aborted, inheritance is from mother to daughter. An affected female has a one-third chance of having an affected daughter, a one-third chance of having a normal daughter, and a one-third chance of having a normal son.

result in recombination. The distance between two loci is estimated by how frequently recombinations occur in families. Crossovers are more likely to occur between loci when they are far apart on the chromosome than when loci are close together. If the recombination frequency is less than 50%, linkage is said to occur. In physical mapping, cytogenetic and molecular techniques are used to determine the actual physical location of genes on chromosomes.

Before the 1970s, gene linkage was attempted with polymorphisms such as blood group antigens, major histocompatibility locus antigens, polymorphic forms of enzymes, and known X-linked characteristics such as hemophilia and color blindness, among others.

Restriction fragment length polymorphisms (RFLPs) result from variations in DNA at specific restriction sites, producing variations in DNA-fragment lengths. These are sorted by electrophoresis and are visualized by using labeled probes. From the late 1970s to the present, the use of RFLPs has extended linkage studies to the entire genome. This allowed about 2,000 markers to be mapped. As powerful a technique as it was, it was limited by its use of a two-allele system, a marker being informative only when a parent was doubly heterozygous, i.e., being different at the disease gene locus and at the linked marker locus.

In the late 1980s, a class of markers with greater heterozygosity was discovered. These highly polymorphic single-locus probes were characterized by a varying number of tandem repeats (VNTR) of an oligonucleotide sequence. These markers were predominantly mapped to regions near the telomeres of chromosomes. Use of this technique greatly enhanced the ability to type the number of alleles at any one locus to many times the power of RFLPs. A special class of VNTRs, called CA-repeat markers, uniformly distributed over the entire genome, has come into use. This has been aided by the application of the

Table 6-7. Selected Genetic Disorders Localized to Specific Regions on Specific Chromosomes

Name	Chromosome and Region
van der Woude syndrome	1q32
Holoprosencephaly-2	2p21
Wardenburg syndrome, type 1	2q35
Morquio syndrome, type B (MPS IVB)	3p14.2–p21
Hurler, Hurler-Scheie, Scheie syndromes	4p16.3
Achondroplasia	4p16.3
Hypochondroplasia	4p16.3
Thanatophoric dysplasia, types 1 and 2	4p16.3
Rieger syndrome	4q25–q27
Diastrophic dysplasia	5q31–q34
Mandibulofacial dysostosis	5q32–q33.1
Saethre-Chotzen syndrome	7p21
Greig cephalopolysyndactyly	7p13
Split hand/split foot, type 1	7q11.2
Osteogenesis imperfecta, several forms	7q21.3–q22.1
Holoprosencephaly-3	7q36
Pfeiffer syndrome-1	8p11.2–p12
Branchio-oto-renal syndrome	8q13.3
Cleidocranial dysplasia	8q22
Cohen syndrome	8q22–q23
Nevoid basal cell carcinoma syndrome	9q31
Tuberous sclerosis-1	9q33–q34
Nail-patella syndrome	9q34
Apert syndrome	10q25.3–q26

polymerase chain reaction (PCR), which allows the use of a very small amount of DNA, e.g., buccal scrape, etc.

Gene mapping has been most successful with X-linked disorders because the X chromosome is a known site, while autosomal genes can be carried on any of the 22 pairs of chromosomes. Autosomal dominant disorders are more easily mapped than autosomal recessive conditions. With good fortune, a single large dominant family may provide sufficient data. With recessive inheritance, multiple families of affected siblings are necessary. Since families rarely have more than two or three affected siblings, 10 or more families may be required to establish linkage. If genetic heterogeneity is marked, the task is often impossible. Selected genetic disorders localized to specific regions on specific chromosomes are listed in Table 6-7. An extensive gene map of congenital malformations was published by Wilkie et al.[38]

GENETIC HETEROGENEITY

Genetic heterogeneity refers to clinical similarity produced by different genes. There may be many different mechanisms responsible. A single clinical disorder

Table 6-7. (*Continued*)

Name	Chromosome and Region
Crouzon syndrome	10q25.3–q26
Pfeiffer syndrome-2	10q25.3–q26
Stickler syndrome	12q13.1–q13.3
Spondyloepiphyseal dysplasia congenita	12q13.1–q13.3
Kniest syndrome	12q13.1–q13.3
Sanfilippo syndrome (MPS III)	12q14
Marfan syndrome	15q21.1
Rubinstein-Taybi syndrome	16p13.3
Tuberous sclerosis-2	16p13.3
Morquio syndrome, Type A (MPS IVA)	16q24.3
Neurofibromatosis, type I	17q11.2
Osteogenesis imperfecta, several forms	17q21.31–q22
Campomelic dysplasia-1	17q24.3–q25.1
Neurofibromatosis, type 2	22q11.21–q13.1
Focal dermal hypoplasia	Xp22.31
Chondrodysplasia punctata, X-linked recessive	Xp22.3
Kallmann syndrome	Xp22.3
Coffin-Lowry syndrome	Xp22.2–p22.1
Aicardi syndrome	Xp22
Cleft palate/ankyloglossia	Xq21.1–q21.31
Simpson-Golabi-Behmel syndrome	Xq26
Borjeson-Forssman-Lehmann syndrome	Xq26–q27
Fragile X syndrome	Xq27.3
Hunter syndrome (MPS III)	Xq27.3
Oto-palato-digital syndrome, type I	Xq28
Chondrodysplasia punctata, X-linked dominant type	Xq28

may be caused by two or more separately located genes, illustrated by tuberous sclerosis. The gene causing it may be located at 9q33–q34 or at 16p13.3. Intra-locus heterogeneity indicates that different mutations within a single gene may cause quite different phenotypes. Intra-family heterogeneity describes variable features and the variable course of a disorder even within a family with the same inherited gene defect.[11]

MOSAICISM

Mosaicism is a well-known concept in genetics. In reality, all humans are mosaics. Females are clearly mosaic with regard to their X chromosome (lyonization). However, recent evidence suggests that as many as 5% of all new mutations occur while the germ cell line is developing.[13] Thus, recurrence of new mutations may be much higher than previously thought. In some cases, affected siblings with normal parents may represent a dominant mutation in the germ cell line of one normal parent rather than representing autosomal recessive inheritance. Examples have been found in osteogenesis imperfecta, achondroplasia, Apert syndrome, Crouzon syndrome. Another example includes a parent with segmental neurofibromatosis with a fully affected offspring. About 7% of patients with Duchenne muscular dystrophy arise from germ line mosaicism.

UNIPARENTAL DISOMY

In uniparental disomy, two copies of a given chromosome or chromosome segment come from one parent, and none comes from the other parent. With DNA markers, it is possible to determine whether a chromosome pair is inherited biparentally or uniparentally. In the latter case, it is likely that the chromosome in question was trisomic to begin with, followed by loss of a chromosome, leaving uniparental disomy. For example, cystic fibrosis, an autosomal recessive disorder resulting from the homozygous state of the gene on chromosome 7, has been shown in 0.02% of cases to have both copies of the gene maternally derived. However, 20%–30% of cases of Prader-Willi syndrome have their origin in this way.[13] Other disorders that occur sporadically, such as the Hallermann-Streiff syndrome, should be tested with DNA markers for possible uniparental disomy. Using one informative DNA marker per chromosome, the uniparental disomy hypothesis could be tested; about ten Hallermann-Streiff patients, together with their parents, would be informative in this connection.

In classic genetics, the influence of a gene is said to be independent of the source, but that is not strictly true. For example, in triploidy, if there are two male chromosome complements (diandry), a hydatiform mole is produced; if two female sets are present, the placenta is underdeveloped and the embryo is growth retarded.

GENOMIC IMPRINTING

In genomic imprinting, modifications in the genetic material occur depending on whether genetic information is maternally or paternally derived. Alterations involving imprinted regions result in different phenotypes. For example, Prader-Willi syndrome and Angelman syndrome are caused by microdeletions in the same area of the long arm of chromosome 15. The deletions of the two syndromes are close to one another within the same band, but the phenotypes are very different. In Prader-Willi syndrome, chromosome-15 deletions are always paternally derived and in Angelman syndrome, maternally derived.[13] In the former, disomy is from the mother; in the latter, disomy is from the father.

IMPRINTING, UNIPARENTAL DISOMY, AND THE BECKWITH-WIEDEMANN SYNDROME

The Beckwith-Wiedemann syndrome is a complex disorder that can result from aberrations in imprinting, including uniparental disomy. Patients generally fit into one of three categories: (1) those that occur sporadically and who have normal chromosomes; (2) those with chromosome anomalies including paternally derived 11p15.5 duplications and maternally derived 11p15.5 translocations and inversions; and (3) those with autosomal dominant pedigrees and expression almost exclusively in individuals born to female carriers, involving paternal imprinting.[2,34,35]

Overexpression of insulin-like growth factor 2 (IGF2) has been implicated in several subsets of sporadic Beckwith-Wiedemann patients: (1) those with paternal uniparental disomy; (2) those with somatic mosaicism for partial paternal isodisomy, which can explain some instances of hemihyperplasia; and (3) those with disruption of maternal imprinting with both paternal and maternal alleles active, which can explain patients with and without hemihyperplasia and even patients with crossed hemihyperplasia. Embryonal tumors reported in Beckwith-Wiedemann syndrome (Wilms tumor, adrenal cortical carcinoma, hepatoblastoma, and rhabdomyosarcoma) retain paternal alleles but lose heterozygosity, specifically maternal alleles.[2,34,35]

Distinct clusters of 11p15.5 translocations have been identified in some Beckwith-Wiedemann syndrome patients.[36] Weksberg and coworkers[37] suggested that such translocations may cause the syndrome not by directly interrupting a gene but by modifying the expression of distantly located genes through cis-acting alterations to chromatin domains ("chromatin context").

MITOCHONDRIAL INHERITANCE

Mitochondrial inheritance is characterized by transmission of the disorder from a mother to all of her sons and daughters. However, only females transmit the condition, since mitochondria are contributed to the zygote only by the female. Male mitochondria, being located in the neck of the sperm, do not enter the zygote; only the head of the sperm does. Mitochondria replicate independently of their host cell and possess their own DNA, which differs from nuclear DNA.

However, we know that the expression of mitochondrially inherited disorders varies considerably and that not all of the children are affected. This has been explained by not all of the mitochondria having the mutation (heteroplasmia). If all of the mitochondria have the mutation, this is spoken of as homoplasmia. Another factor may be modifying nuclear genes.

Disorders that have mitochondrial inheritance include certain encephalomyopathies, Leber's optic atrophy, rare forms of isolated sensorineural hearing loss, and aminoglycoside sensitivity.

ANTICIPATION

Until recently, anticipation has been thought to be a genetic pseudophenomenon. Anticipation, the progressively earlier appearance and increasing severity of a disorder, has been shown to exist. It is caused by expansion of genes by the addition of repeated base sequences, resulting in gene instability. A mild increase (premutation) does not result in clinical findings, but above a critical level (mutation) the condition becomes clinically evident. The gene enlargement occurs during female meiosis in fragile X syndrome, myotonic dystrophy, and X-linked spinal/bulbar muscular atrophy.

"SPORADICITY"

Earlier, it was emphasized that sporadic occurrence *per se* does not necessarily indicate that the condition in question is nongenetic. Figures 6-27 and 6-28 show some examples of sporadic occurrence with autosomal dominant and autosomal recessive disorders. Sporadic occurrence is found most frequently with

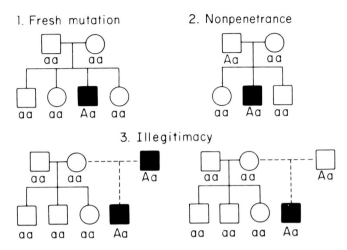

Figure 6-27. Examples of "sporadicity" in autosomal dominant inheritance.

multifactorial disorders. "Sporadicity" also occurs with variant additive patterns (Fig. 6-29).

VARIANT ADDITIVE PATTERNS

At times, it may be difficult to distinguish between a true multiple anomaly syndrome, which is a form of discontinuous variability with respect to normal first-degree relatives, and a variant additive pattern, which is a form of continuous variability with respect to such relatives. A *variant additive pattern* usually

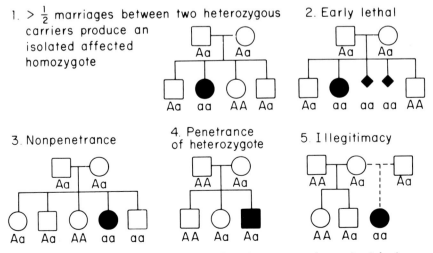

Figure 6-28. Examples of "sporadicity" in autosomal recessive inheritance.

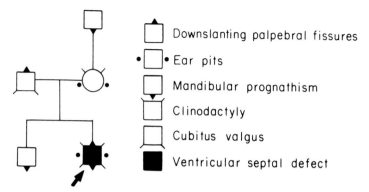

Figure 6-29. Variant additive pattern. Note that all features of the pattern observed in the proband except the ventricular septal defect are dispersed in various members of the family. From Cohen.[3]

consists of several minor anomalies and often a major anomaly in the same individual so that the pattern of morphologic findings in that individual is statistically unusual for the general population but biologically normal for the individual's family, with the possible exception of the major anomaly. A variant additive pattern is an unusual chance pattern that can be identified in the population because the minor anomalies that make up the pattern in the proband may be observed separately in various relatives. Thus, the pattern is not caused by a monogenic or chromosomal abnormality, but by a variety of different genes acting independently. In this context, the minor anomalies in the proband and his or her family should be regarded as normal, morphologic variants.[3,4,15,26]

The parents often explain that their child is not at all abnormal but simply resembles other members of the family. Facial comparison may be particularly telling. Many variant additive patterns do not have a major anomaly. When a major anomaly occurs in addition by chance, the likelihood of referral to a syndromologist increases. Care must be taken not to overdiagnose a variant additive pattern as a true multiple anomaly syndrome of presumed unitary etiology.[3,4,15,26]

A typical example of a variant additive pattern is a proband with downslanting palpebral fissures, ear pits, mandibular prognathism, clinodactyly, cubitus valgus, and ventricular septal defect. In the examination of the proband's relatives (Fig. 6-27), the father is noted to have downslanting palpebral fissures and cubitus valgus, the mother is found to have ear pits and clinodactyly, and both the brother and the maternal grandfather are observed to have mandibular prognathism. Thus, all the features except the ventricular septal defect are dispersed in various members of the family as minor anomalies. They happen to come together in the proband by chance in addition to one major anomaly—a ventricular septal defect. The probability of all these anomalies coming together in future offspring in this family is slight, although various individual anomalies or combinations of anomalies may recur. For example, of three future offspring, a first might have ear pits; a second, ventricular septal defect, clinodactyly, and downslanting palpebral fissures; a third, mandibular prognathism and cubitus valgus. Thus, a variant additive pattern may be considered unique to an affected individual or to an affected family. In this particular family, genetic counseling should take into account a multifactorial recurrence risk of a ventricular septal defect.[4]

MULTIFACTORIAL INHERITANCE

Multifactorial inheritance results from a combination of genetic and environmental factors. Such traits are primarily quantitative and continuous in nature. In the threshold model of multifactorial inheritance, the total liability of expression of the trait in question is reflected in the population as a normally distributed curve. Expression of the trait is restricted to those individuals who exceed a threshold of liability. Examples of multifactorial inheritance include cleft lip/palate and anencephaly.

Multifactorial traits have a number of characteristics. First, the risk in relatives is greater than the frequency of the disorder in the general population. The magnitude of the difference in the risk is less as the frequency of the malformation increases in the population. Thus, first-degree relatives such as siblings and offspring are most likely to be affected since, on the average, they share 50% of their genes. Second-degree relatives such as aunts, uncles, nieces, and nephews are less likely to be affected since they share only 25% of their genes. Third-degree relatives such as first cousins are even less likely to be at risk since they share only 12.5% of their genes.

Second, the risk of the trait in question increases with each additional family member affected. The recurrence risk for a second affected child with a cleft lip/palate is approximately 4% if both parents are normal; the risk increases to approximately 16% if one parent is also affected. Third, the more severe the malformation, the greater the risk to the relatives. The risk for a second affected child is higher if the proband has bilateral cleft lip-palate than if the proband has unilateral cleft lip. Fourth, if sex differences exist in the frequency of the trait in question, the risk to relatives is greater when the trait occurs in the less frequently affected sex. For example, cleft palate occurs less frequently in males than in females. The risk for cleft palate is greater in siblings of males with cleft palate than in siblings of females with cleft palate. Finally, an increase in parental consanguinity is to be expected with multifactorial causation.

CHANCE AND SINGLE GENE STOCHASTIC MODEL

Recently, Kurnit et al.[20] revolutionized our thinking about the role that chance may play in the occurrence of malformations. Their model may be applicable to malformations that are presently thought to have "low risk multifactorial recurrence." Multifactorial explanations depend on the interaction between genetic and environmental factors. Thus, high discordance in monozygotic twins for major malformations such as ventricular septal defect (only 2/26 concordant)[27] has been ascribed to subtle environmental influences for want of a better explanation. Kurnit et al.[20] suggested that this variability may be inherent in the role that chance itself plays in the process of development. Using computer simulations to describe endocardial cushion outgrowth and fusion, randomly walking cells were allowed to migrate, divide, and adhere with preset probabilities. Based on these simulations, a stochastic single gene model generated a continuous liability curve resembling that obtained from a multifactorial threshold model. Outcomes were quite variable despite using identical genotypes and environments. Thus, segregation of a given malformation may be explained by a single defective gene that predisposes to, but does not necessarily result in, the malformation. Furthermore, the low penetrance and remarkably variable expressivity that characterize a number of presumed autosomal dominant malformation syndromes are possibly reflections of specific stochastic influences that are intrinsic to the embryonic process itself. Future studies may demonstrate that such syndromes arise predictably as a single gene disorder modified by the stochastic laws that govern growth.[5]

REFERENCES

1. Cohen MM Jr: *Craniosynostosis: Diagnosis, Evaluation and Management*. New York: Raven Press, 1986.
2. Cohen MM Jr: Letter to the Editor: Wiedemann-Beckwith syndrome, imprinting, IGF2 and H19: Implications for hemihyperplasia, associated neoplasms, and overgrowth. *Am J Med Genet* 52:233–234, 1994.
3. Cohen MM Jr: On the nature of syndrome delineation. *Acta Genet Med Gemellol* 26:103–119, 1977.
4. Cohen MM Jr: *The Child With Multiple Birth Defects*. New York: Raven Press, 1982.
5. Cohen MM Jr, Cole DEC: Origins of recognizable syndromes: Etiologic and pathogenetic mechanisms and the process of syndrome delineation. *J Pediatr* 115:161–164, 1989.
6. Cohen MM Jr, Gorlin RJ: The Prader-Willi syndrome. *Am J Dis Child* 117:213–218, 1969.
7. Emery AEH, Mueller RF: *Elements of Medical Genetics*. Eighth Edition. Edinburgh: Churchill Livingstone, 1992.
8. Emery AEH, Rimoin DL, Pyeritz RE (eds): *Principles and Practice of Medical Genetics*. 3rd Ed. Edinburgh: Churchill Livingstone, 1996.
9. Epstein CJ: *The Consequences of Chromosome Imbalance: Principles, Mechanisms, and Models*. Cambridge: Cambridge University Press, 1986.
10. Estabrooks LL, Rao KW, Driscoll DA, Crandall BF, Dean JCS, Ikonen E, Korf B, Alysworth AS: Preliminary phenotypic map of chromosome 4p16 based on 4p deletions. *Am J Med Genet* 57:581–586, 1995.
11. Evans DGR, Harris R: Heterogeneity in genetic conditions. *Q J Med* 84:563–565, 1992.
12. Gorlin RJ, Cohen MM Jr, Levin LS: *Syndromes of the Head and Neck*. 3rd Ed. New York: Oxford University Press, 1990.
13. Hall JG: Nontraditional inheritance. *Growth Genet Hormones* 6:1–4, 1990.
14. Heidemann A, Schmalenberger B, Zankl H: Sister chromatid exchange and lymphocyte proliferation in a Down syndrome mosaic. *Clin Genet* 23:139–142, 1983.
15. Herrmann J, Opitz JM: Naming and nomenclature. *Birth Defects* 10(7):69–86, 1974.
16. Hoehn H, Simpson M, Bryant EM, Rabinovitch PS, Salk D, Martin GM: Effects of chromosome constitution on growth and longevity of human skin fibroblast cultures. *Am J Med Genet* 7:141–154, 1980.
17. ISCN 1995: *An International System for Human Cytogenetics Nomenclature*. Basel: Karger, 1995.
18. Jones KL, Jones MC: A clinical approach to the dysmorphic child. In Emery AEH, Rimoin DL (eds): *Principles and Practice of Medical Genetics*. 2nd Ed. Edinburgh: Churchill Livingstone, Vol 1. 1983, pp 215–224.
19. Jorde LB, Carey JC, White RL: *Medical Genetics*. St. Louis: Mosby, 1995.
20. Kurnit DM, Layton WM, Matthysse S: Genetics, chance, and morphogenesis. *Am J Hum Genet* 41:979–995, 1987.
21. Lubs HA, Ing PS: Human cytogenetic nomenclature. In Emery AEH, Rimoin DL (eds): *Principles and Practice of Medical Genetics*. 2nd Ed. Edinburgh: Churchill Livingstone, Vol I. 1990, pp 237–245.

22. Lurie IW, Opitz JM: Phenotypic mapping and clinical ideology. *Am J Med Genet* 57:587, 1995.

23. Miller OJ: Chromosomal basis of inheritance. In Emery AEH, Rimoin DL (eds): *Principles and Practice of Medical Genetics.* 2nd Ed. Edinburgh: Churchill Livingstone, Vol I. 1990, pp 77–93.

24. Mittwoch U: Mongolism and sex: Common problem of cell proliferation? *J Med Genet* 9:82–85, 1971.

25. Naeye RL: Prenatal organ and cellular growth with various chromosomal disorders. *Biol Neonat* 11:248–260, 1967.

26. Neuhauser G, Opitz JM: Studies of malformation syndrome in man XXXX: Multiple congenital anomalies/mental retardation syndrome or variant familial developmental pattern; differential diagnosis and description of the McDonough syndrome (with XXY son from XY/XXY father). *Z Kinderheilkd* 120:231–242, 1975.

27. Newman TB: Etiology of ventricular septal defects: An epidemiologic approach. *Pediatrics* 76:741–749, 1985.

28. Opitz JM, Gilbert EF: Pathogenetic analysis of congenital anomalies in humans. In Ioachim HL (ed): *Pathobiology Annual.* Vol 12. New York: Raven Press, 1982, pp 301–349.

29. Pious D, Millis AJT, Sabo K: *In vitro* growth rates in primary cellular growth deficiency syndromes. *Pediatr Res* 9:279, 1975.

30. Preus M, Aymé S: Formal analysis of dysmorphism: Objective methods of syndrome definition. *Clin Genet* 23:1–16, 1983.

31. Raskó I, Downes CS: *Genes in Medicine.* London: Chapman and Hall, 1995.

32. Schinzel A: Microdeletion syndromes, balanced translocations, and gene mapping. *J Med Genet* 25:454–462, 1988.

33. Schmickel RD: Contiguous gene syndromes: A component of recognizable syndromes. *J Pediatr* 109:231–241, 1986.

34. Viljoen D, Ramesar R: Evidence for paternal imprinting in familial Beckwith-Wiedemann syndrome. *J Med Genet* 29:221–225, 1992.

35. Weksberg R, Shen DR, Fei YL, Song QL, Squire J: Disruption of insulin-like growth factor 2 imprinting in Beckwith-Wiedemann syndrome. *Nature Genet* 5:143–150, 1993.

36. Weksberg R, Teshima I, Williams BRG, Greenberg CR, Pueschel SM, Chernos JE, Fowlow SB, Hoyme E, Anderson IJ, Whiteman DAH, Fisher N, Squire J: Molecular characterization of cytogenetic alterations associated with the Beckwith-Wiedemann syndrome (BWS) phenotype refines the localization and suggests the gene for BWS is imprinted. *Hum Mol Genet* 2:549–556, 1993.

37. Weksberg R, Perlikowski S, Squire J: "Chromatin context" as a mechanism of abnormal morphogenesis in human disease: The human equivalent of variegated position effect. XVI David W. Smith Workshop on Malformations and Morphogenesis, Big Sky, Montana, July 30–August 3, 1995, p 25.

38. Wilkie AOM, Amberger JS, McKusick VA: A gene map of congenital malformations. *J Med Genet* 31:507–517, 1994.

7

Teratogens

In this chapter principles of teratogenesis are reviewed and human teratogenic conditions are then discussed. The word *teras* is derived from Greek and means *monster.* Teratology means literally "the study of monsters," which, of course, is not an appropriate concept for anomalies that occur in humans. The study of teratology deals with environmental causes of birth defects—experimental in animals, descriptive and epidemiologic in humans.

ADVERSE ENVIRONMENTAL FACTORS
AND THE GENOTYPE

Susceptibility to teratogenesis depends on the genotype of the conceptus. Some species respond to a given teratogen more readily then others do. For example, humans and other higher primates are exquisitely sensitive to thalidomide, whereas lower primates are highly resistant. There are also differences in the teratogenic response of various animal strains within the same species.[35,36] For example, Fraser and Fainstat[17] reported birth prevalence differences in cleft palate in several strains of mice treated with cortisone. Finally, individual genetic differences result in variable teratogenic effects in littermates.

Interaction between genetic and environmental factors has been demonstrated in some experimental animal studies. For example, Warkany and Schraffenberg[33] observed that rat embryos at the cephalic end of the uterine horns were more susceptible to the teratogenic effects of X-radiation than more caudally situated littermates.

TIMING OF EXPOSURE

Susceptibility to teratogenesis varies during intrauterine development. The period from fertilization to differentiation of the three germ layers is a refractory

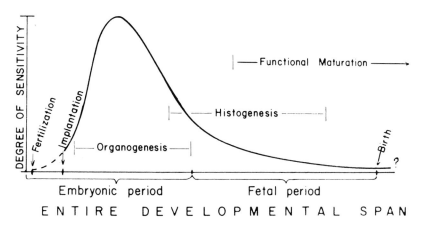

Figure 7-1. Curve approximating susceptibility of human embryo to teratogenesis from fertilization until after birth. From Wilson.[36]

period when little teratogenesis occurs, but appreciable lethality may occur. A high degree of sensitivity occurs during organogenesis from about days 18 to 60. Peak susceptibility to anatomic defect occurs at approximately 30 days (Fig. 7-1). During advanced organogenesis, resistance to teratogenesis increases with age, and larger doses of a teratogen are required to produce comparable manifestations, if they can be produced at all. Because the fetal period (second to ninth months) is characterized by histogenesis (refined cellular and tissue changes) and functional maturation, teratogenic interference at this time consists mainly of growth retardation and functional disturbances (such as mental retardation).[35,36]

Figure 7-2 shows a group of susceptibility curves of particular organs and organ systems to a hypothetical teratogen in the rat. If a teratogen is administered on the tenth day, the vertical line (arrow) that intersects the curves indi-

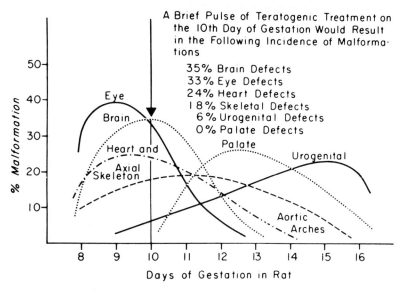

Figure 7-2. Group of curves representing susceptibility of organs and organ systems to hypothetical teratogenic agent in the rat. From Wilson.[36]

cates the birth prevalence of various malformations that occur in a series of newborn rat pups. The composition of the syndrome could be altered both qualitatively and quantitatively by shifting the administration of the hypothetical teratogen to another day.[35,36]

MECHANISMS AND PATHOGENESIS

The process of teratogenesis can be summarized in three sequential categories: causes, mechanisms, and manifestations (Fig. 7-3). Causes of teratogenesis are located in the environment and act directly or indirectly on germ cells, embryos, or fetuses. Note that the environment can include maternal metabolic states, such as diabetes mellitus. These causes produce various reactions or mechanisms such as mitotic interference, altered nucleic acid integrity, or enzyme inhibition. Such mechanisms lead to abnormal developmental events (pathogenesis) in which the demonstrable aspects of teratogenesis (manifestations) occur. These include cell death, failed cell interactions, or impeded morphogenetic movement and their final expression: intrauterine death, malformation, growth retardation, and/or functional deficit.[35]

NATURE OF TERATOGENIC AGENTS

Many different categories of teratogens are known (Fig. 7-3), and, even within various categories, teratogens may have different natures. It is generally agreed that developing tissues are more sensitive to environmental factors than mature somatic tissues. Maternal defense against chemical agents consists of reducing the dosage received by the embryo through the bloodstream by (1) homeostatic processes such as catabolism in the liver, excretion by the kidney, protein binding, and tissue storage; and (2) the rate of placental transfer (Fig. 7-4). The

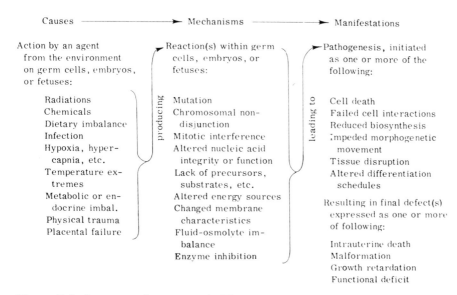

Figure 7-3. Summary of teratogenesis. Three categories: causes, mechanisms, and manifestations. From Wilson.[35]

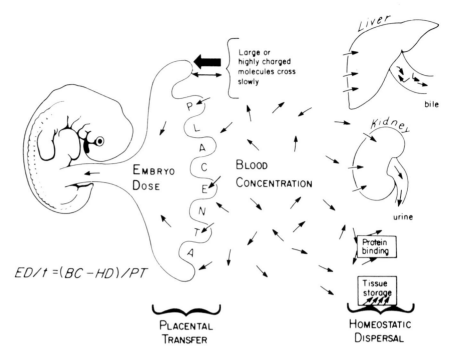

Figure 7-4. Maternal defense against chemical agents consists of reducing dosage received by embryo through bloodstream by (1) homeostatic processes such as catabolism in the liver, excretion by the kidney, protein binding, and tissue storage; and (2) rate of placental transfer. The formula ED/t = (BC − HD)/PT, although not a precise mathematical one, indicates that embryo dose (ED) over a given time (t) depends on maternal blood concentration (BC), which constantly tends to be reduced by homeostatic dispersal (HD) and placental transfer (PT). From Wilson.[35]

formula ED/t = (BC − HD)/PT, although not a precise mathematical one, indicates that the embryo dose (ED) over a given time (t) depends on the maternal blood concentration (BC), which constantly tends to be reduced by homeostatic dispersal (HD) and placental transfer (PT).[35]

TERATOGENIC MANIFESTATIONS OF DEVIANT DEVELOPMENT

Teratogens are capable of producing one or more of the four types of developmental deviation: (1) death of the developing organism, (2) structural abnormality or malformation, (3) growth deficiency, and/or (4) functional deficit. These deviations are not equally likely to occur at all teratogenic exposure times, and one or another is likely to predominate at different intervals during development. For example, radiation administered during the cleavage and blastocyst stages in the mouse embryo causes death, whereas, if administered just prior to differentiation, growth deficiency is found in some instances; malformations are rare. When most teratogenic agents are administered during early organogenesis, however, both embryonic death and malformations are induced. As development progresses, death and malformations become less likely to occur, and the probability of growth retardation and functional deficit increases.[35,36]

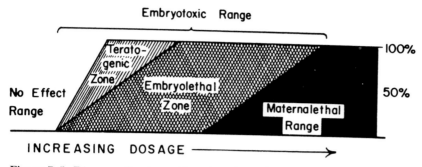

Figure 7-5. Diagram of toxic manifestations shown by embryo and maternal organism as dosage of drug or chemical increases. From Wilson.[36]

DOSAGE

Most experimental evidence indicates the existence of a threshold for embryotoxic manifestations (Fig. 7-5). There is a no-effect dosage range below the threshold at which embryotoxic effects begin to appear. Teratogenic effects and embryolethality frequently begin at about the same threshold and increase at approximately parallel rates as the dosage increases up to the point at which all conceptuses are affected. Larger dosages result in embryolethality, and still larger doses produce maternal lethality. The ratio of embryolethal to maternal lethal dosage is highly variable and depends on the type of drug or chemical.[35,36] *It should be carefully noted that the actual teratogenic range is very narrow.* It appears to be easier to produce no effect, an embryolethal effect, or a maternal lethal effect than it is to produce a teratogenic effect.

As already indicated, no standard ratio exists between maternal lethal and embryotoxic dosage ranges, except that the latter is almost always some fraction of the former. The curve in Figure 7-6 spans one-half to one-fourth of the

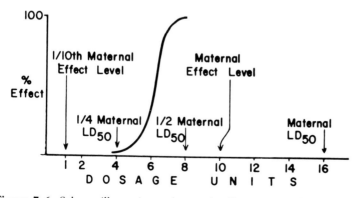

Figure 7-6. Scheme illustrating embryotoxic effects as some fraction of dosage that causes maternal toxic or pharmacologic effects. From Wilson.[36]

Table 7-1. Summary of Some Human Teratogens

Agents	*Most Common Major Defects*
Drugs	
Alcohol	Growth retardation
	Reduced palpebral fissures, facial dysmorphism
	Microcephaly, mental retardation
	Cardiovascular defects
Hydantoin	Growth retardation
	Facial dysmorphism
	Microcephaly, mental retardation
Valproate	Spina bifida
	Craniofacial dysmorphism
Trimethadione	Developmental delay
	Growth deficiency
	V-shaped eyebrows, ear anomalies
	Cardiovascular defects
Retinoids	Abortion
	Craniofacial dysmorphism
	Various CNS anomalies
Warfarin	Hypoplasia of nasal cartilages
	Various CNS defects
	Stippled epiphyses
Cocaine	Vascular disruptions
Angiotensin-converting enzyme inhibitors	Renal tubular dysgenesis
	Oligohydramnios sequence
	Hypocalvaria
Methimazole	Symmetric skull defect
	Urachal malformations
Misoprostol	Scalp-cranial defect
Aminopterin and methotrexate	Abortion
	Hydrocephalus
	Growth retardation, mental retardation
Lithium	Ebstein heart anomaly
	Other cardiac defects
Thalidomide	Limb reduction defects
	Girdle hypoplasia
	Ear anomalies
Diethystilbesterol	Vaginal adenosis
	Cervical erosion and ridges
	Adenocarcinoma of the vagina
Tetracycline	Stained teth
	Hypoplasia of enamel
Streptomycin	Hearing loss
Androgens and high dosages of masculinizing progestigens	Masculinization
Environmental chemicals	
Lead	CNS effects
Toluene	Microcephaly
	CNS dysfunction
	growth deficiency
	Minor anomalies

Table 7-1. (*Continued*)

Agents	Most Common Major Defects
Smoking	Abortion Perinatal mortality Growth retardation
Methylmercury	Cerebral atrophy Spasticity, seizures Mental retardation
Polychlorinated biphenyls (PCBs)	Growth retardation Skin discoloration
Infectious agents	
Rubella	Deafness Cataracts Heart defects
Cytomegalovirus	Growth retardation Mental retardation Hearing loss
Toxoplasmosis	Hydrocephalus Blindness Mental retardation
Varicella	Skin scarring Muscle atrophy Mental retardation
Venezuelan equine encephalitis	Brain destruction Cataracts Death
Syphilis	Abnormal teeth and bones Mental retardation
Maternal metabolic factors	
Diabetes	Congenital heart defects Caudal dysgenesis Other anomalies
Phenylketonuria	Abortion Microcephaly Mental retardation
Physical agents	

Ionizing radiation (exposures above the diagnostic range)	Dependent on stage of pregnancy:
	  Abortion
	  Major organ malformations, 18–36 days
	  Microcephaly and mental retardation, 8–15 weeks

Hyperthermia	Neural tube defects Other CNS anomalies Mental retardation
Nutritional Factors	
Iodine deficiency	Goiter Mental retardation Growth retardation

maternal lethal dose (LD$_{50}$). The dose–response curve for teratogenicity is usually very steep and may rise from the no-effect level to the 100%-effect level by doubling the dose,[35,36] as represented in Figure 7-6.

HUMAN TERATOGENS

Teratogenic agents based on experimental work in laboratory animals number in the hundreds.[35] In contrast, relatively few human teratogens are known because they are based on clinical reports and epidemiologic surveys. A brief summary of some human teratogens known to date[7,12,15,19,23,29,30] appears in Table 7-1. Agents include drugs, environmental chemicals, infectious agents, maternal metabolic factors, physical agents, and nutritional factors.

Fetal Alcohol Syndrome

The fetal alcohol syndrome (FAS) is the most important human teratogenic condition known today. It occurs with a birth prevalence of 1 in 500 in the United States. One in 30 pregnant women abuse alcohol and about 6% of children born to women within this group have clinically recognizable FAS.

Major features include growth deficiency of prenatal onset persisting into postnatal life, developmental delay, microcephaly, short palpebral fissures, epicanthal folds, midface hypoplasia, short nose, long flat philtral area, convex upper lip with thin vermilion border (Figs. 7-7, 7-8), micrognathia in some cases, joint abnormalities, alterations of the palmar creases, and cardiac defects, especially atrial and ventricular septal defects. Hypoplastic labia may occur, and

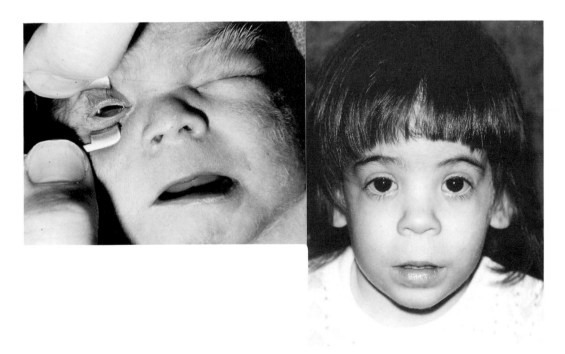

Figure 7-7. Fetal alcohol syndrome. Left: Note short palpebral fissures. Right: Characteristic facial appearance with short palpebral fissures, short nose, long philtral area, smooth philtrum, thin upper lip, and midface hypoplasia. Left, courtesy of D.W. Smith, Seattle, Washington. Right, from Clarren and Smith.[8]

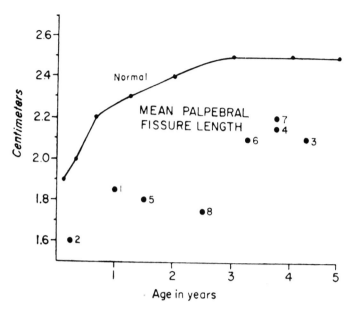

Figure 7-8. Palpebral fissure length in eight patients with fetal alcohol syndrome compared with mean normal value. From Jones et al.[26]

hypospadias and renal malformations are less common. In early life, poor coordination, hypotonia, neonatal irritability, and hyperactivity are characteristic. Ptosis and strabismus may also be observed, and approximately 15% have cleft palate. Embryonal tumors have been noted on occasion.[8,11,22,24–26]

The term *fetal alcohol effects* (FAE) has been used to refer to children who appear to have a form fruste of FAS. Unfortunately, FAE has been applied somewhat indiscriminately to children with a variety of problems, including simple growth deficiency or isolated behavioral aberrations based on knowledge—or suspicion—that their mother drank alcohol during pregnancy. Thus, it has been suggested by some that clinical use of the term FAE be abandoned and that simple *verifiable facts* be recorded.[1]

Pearson et al.[29] observed overlap in the facial features of FAS and toluene embryopathy. They suggested that the mechanisms of craniofacial teratogenesis may be nonspecific, a *variety of teratogens giving rise to facial abnormalities similar to those found in FAS.*

Fetal Hydantoin Syndrome

The fetal hydantoin syndrome consists of growth deficiency of prenatal onset persisting into postnatal life, microcephaly, developmental delay with dull mentality or frank mental retardation, and dysmorphic features including short nose, low nasal bridge, mild ocular hypertelorism, ptosis of the eyelids, strabismus, wide mouth, sutural ridging, and a short neck with mild webbing. Less commonly observed are limb anomalies such as hypoplastic nails and short distal phalanges, finger-like thumbs, and low-arch dermal ridge patterns on the fingers. Congenital heart defects (especially ventricular septal defect), renal malformations, and hypospadias have been observed in some patients. Cleft lip with or without cleft palate occurs in some instances (Figs. 7-9, 7-10). A number of embryonal neoplasms have been reported.[11,20,21]

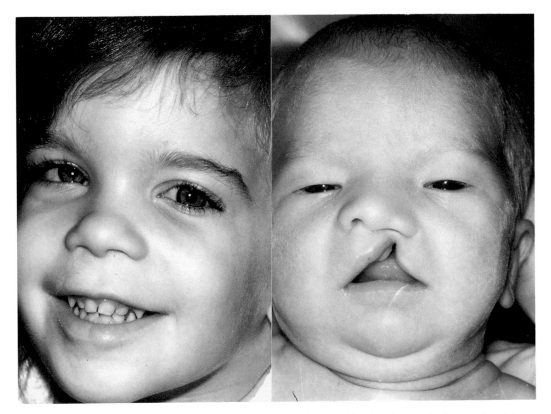

Figure 7-9. Fetal hydantoin syndrome. Left: Short nose, low nasal bridge, hypertelorism, and strabismus. Right: Cleft lip. Courtesy of J.W. Hanson, Iowa City, Iowa.

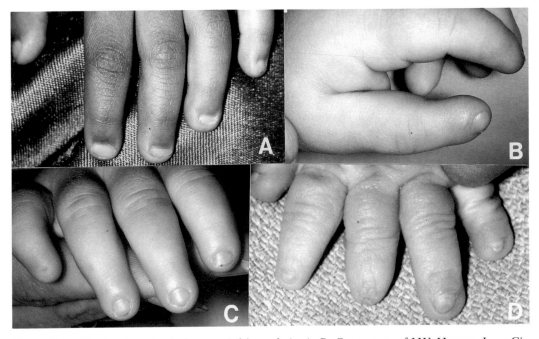

Figure 7-10. Fetal hydantoin syndrome. Nail hypoplasia. A, B, C, courtesy of J.W. Hanson, Iowa City, Iowa.

Of mothers taking Dilantin for the control of seizures, only 5%–10% of newborn infants exhibit fetal hydantoin syndrome. However, at least 30% of cases have some fetal hydantoin effect or effects.[20] Epoxide hydrolase activity has been shown to be an enzymatic biomarker for prenatal risk prediction of the fetal hydantoin syndrome (Fig. 7-11).[6]

Fetal Trimethadione Syndrome

Major features of the fetal trimethadione syndrome include mental deficiency, speech disorders, prominent forehead, V-shaped eyebrows, epicanthic folds, low-set ears with anteriorly folded helices, highly arched palate, and micrognathia. In some instances, features may include intrauterine growth retardation, short stature, microcephaly, cardiac defects, ambiguous genitalia, hypospadias, strabismus, ptosis of the eyelids, and single palmar creases. The diagnosis should be considered in any infant prenatally exposed to trimethadione or any other oxazolidine type of anticonvulsant.[13,37]

Fetal Valproate Syndrome

The fetal valproate syndrome phenotype consists of developmental delay or neurologic abnormality, midface hypoplasia, short nose with broad or flat nasal bridge, epicanthic folds, minor anomalies of the ear, long or flat philtrum, thin vermilion border, and micrognathia. Prominent metopic ridge (Fig. 7-12) and outer orbital ridge deficiency or bifrontal narrowing and various major anomalies such as tracheomalacia, talipes equinovarus, and lumbrosacral meningomyelocele (Fig. 7-13) seem peculiar to infants with valproic acid exposure *in utero.*[2]

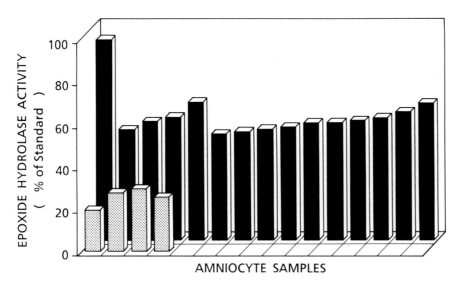

Figure 7-11. Epoxide hydrolase activity in amniocyte samples from 19 prospectively monitored fetuses. Samples from 4 fetuses subsequently given diagnosis of fetal hydantoin syndrome are indicated by stippled bars, and 15 samples from fetuses subsequently confirmed not to have characteristic features of syndrome are indicated by black bars. From Buehler et al.[6]

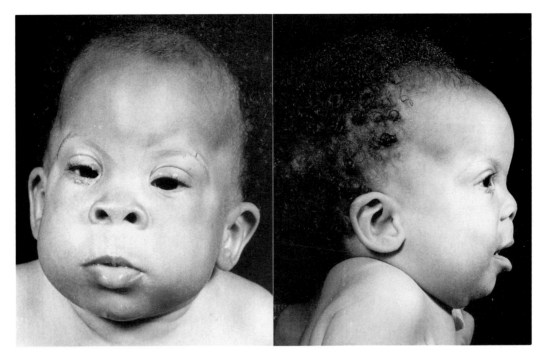

Figure 7-12. Fetal valproate syndrome. Note prominent metopic ridge, outer orbital ridge deficiency, and midface hypoplasia with short nose, broad nasal bridge, anteverted nostrils, long flat philtrum, and posterior angulation of ears. From Ardinger et al.[2]

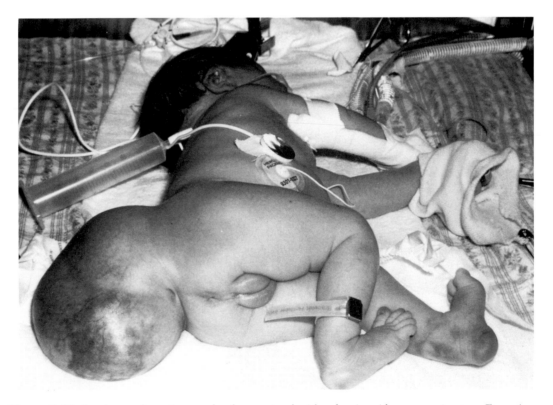

Figure 7-13. Lumbosacral meningomyelocele associated with valproic acid exposure *in utero*. From Ardinger et al.[2]

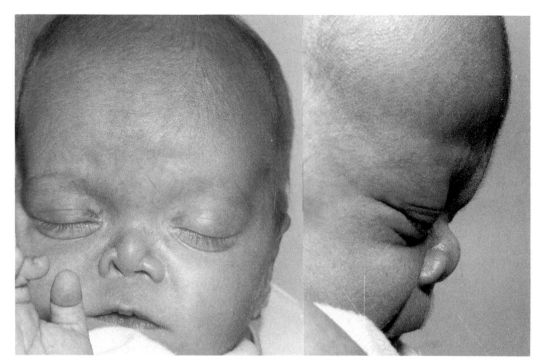

Figure 7-14. Warfarin embryopathy. Hypoplastic nose. Courtesy of J.G. Hall, Vancouver, British Columbia, Canada.

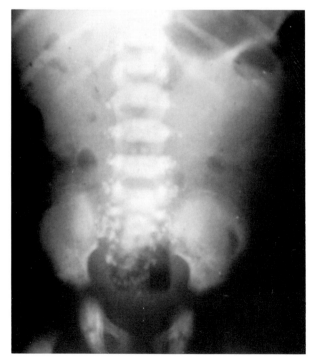

Figure 7-15. Warfarin embryopathy. Note stippling around vertebral column. Courtesy of J.G. Hall, Vancouver, British Columbia.

Warfarin Embryopathy

Characteristic features of warfarin embryopathy include chondrodysplasia punctata with stippling of uncalcified epiphyses radiographically, nasal hypoplasia, low nasal bridge, and deep groove between the alae nasi and the nasal tip (Fig. 7-14). Stippled epiphyses are also observed (Fig. 7-15). Growth deficiency of prenatal onset, developmental delay, mental retardation, and other neurological abnormalities may be present. Most characteristic are central nervous system anomalies that result in microcephaly. Pathogenesis is based on inhibition of vitamin K reductase by warfarin, which results in undercarboxylation of osteocalcin and matrix Gla protein.[11a,18,28,34]

Retinoic Acid Embryopathy

Retinoic acid, an analog of vitamin A, has long been known to be teratogenic in laboratory animals. Human teratogenicity has occurred from treatment of severe recalcitrant cystic acne with isotretinoin in women who were pregnant or who became pregnant while on medication. By 1985, 154 human pregnancies with fetal exposure to isotretinoin were known.

Characteristic features of retinoic acid embryopathy include central nervous system abnormalities such as hydrocephalus, lissencephaly, cerebral dysgenesis, and heterotopias. Other findings include small malformed ears, micrognathia, ocular abnormalities and cleft palate in some instances, conotruncal heart defects and aortic arch abnormalities, and DiGeorge sequence.[14,27]

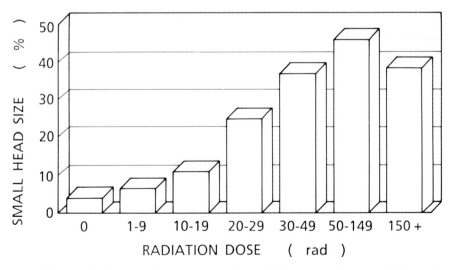

SMALL HEAD CIRCUMFERENCE AMONG HIROSHIMA CHILDREN EXPOSED IN UTERO BEFORE THE 18TH WEEK OF GESTATION

Figure 7-16. Relation of dose to head circumference in Hiroshima children exposed *in utero* before 18th week of gestation. Heads considered small were those with circumference 2 or >2 SD below age- and sex-specific mean on at least one medical examination and 1 or >1 SD below average at all other examinations during ages (10–19 years) studied. From Blot.[4]

Table 7-2. Significant Malformations in Infants of Diabetic Mothers

Central nervous system
  Microcephaly
  Anencephaly/spina bifida
  Holoprosencephaly
	Gastrointestinal
	  Neonatal small left colon
	  Malrotation of bowel
	  Anal/rectal atresia

Craniofacial
  Ear anomalies
  Cleft lip/palate
	Genitourinary
	  Renal agenesis
	  Multicystic dysplasia
	  Hypospadias
	  Cryptorchidism

Cardiovascular
  Ventricular septal defect
  Transposition of the great vessels
  Situs inversus
  Single umbilical artery
	Skeletal
	  Caudal dysgenesis
	  Rib and/or vertebral anomalies

*From Cohen.[9]

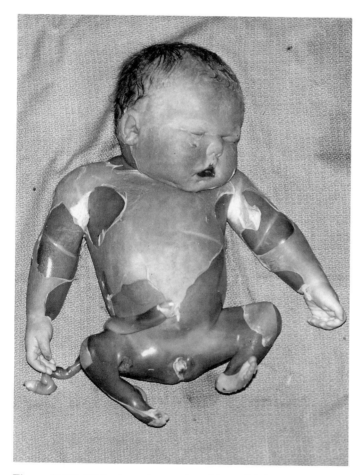

Figure 7-17. Diabetic embryopathy with caudal dysgenesis. From Cohen.[9]

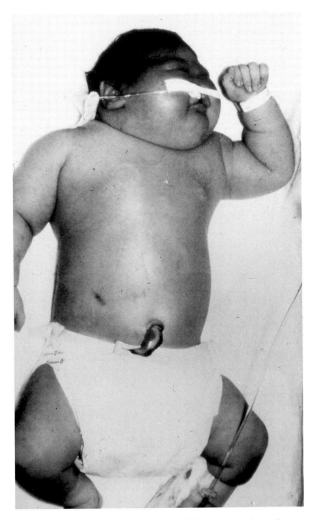

Figure 7-18. Macrosomia, holoprosencephaly, and facial dysmorphism in infant of diabetic mother. Courtesy of B.D. Hall, Lexington, Kentucky.

Congenital Rubella Syndrome

Clinical manifestations of congenital rubella syndrome are widespread and have been noted in the cardiovascular system, central nervous system, eyes, ears, blood, liver, and bones. Features include intrauterine growth retardation, microcephaly, mental deficiency, cataracts, microphthalmia, deafness, patent ductus arteriosus, septal defects, thrombocytopenia, and osteolytic metaphyseal lesions.[32]

Radiation

Severe radiation effects (see Table 7-1) include malformations, particularly microcephaly and eye defects, intrauterine growth retardation, and embryonic death.[5] In Nagasaki, fetuses exposed to irradiation showed increased mortality. Pregnant women with acute radiation symptoms who were within 2 km of the hypocenter had a higher percentage of abortions and stillbirths than a control

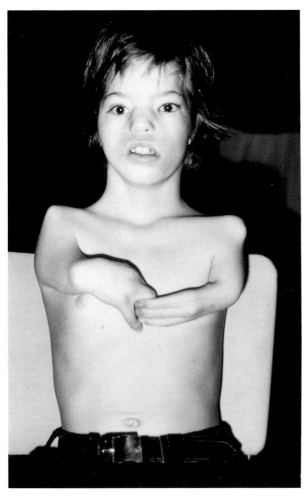

Figure 7-19. Thalidomide embryopathy. Phocomedia of both arms and absent ears. Courtesy of P.J.W. Stoelinga, Arnhem, The Netherlands.

group. Prospective studies in Hiroshima and Nagasaki established a definite relationship between irradiation and microcephaly (Fig. 7-16). The highest frequency of microcephaly was found in those individuals who had been exposed before the 18th week of intrauterine life, particularly between the 3rd and 15th weeks; associated mental deficiency was common. A dose–response relationship was dramatically shown by Blot.[4]

Diabetic Embryopathy

Many investigators have shown that congenital malformations occur with increased frequency in the offspring of diabetic mothers. The most important ones are listed in Table 7-2. Neave[27a,b] showed that anomalies with greater frequency in offspring of diabetic mothers include microcephaly, ear anomalies, ventricular septal defect, single umbilical artery, and malformations of the ribs and/or vertebral column. An increase in deformations can be expected with major malformations or with fetal macrosomia.[31a] Two startling anomalies that may occur, albeit with low frequency, in diabetic embryopathy are caudal dys-

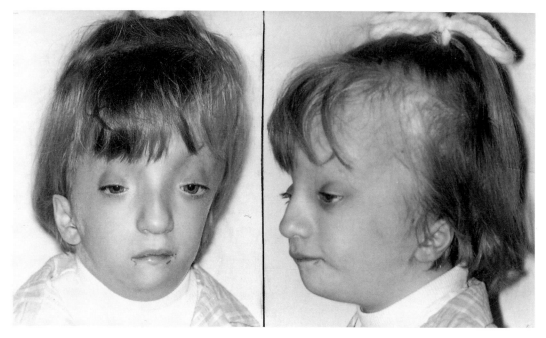

Figure 7-20. Folic acid antagonist–induced syndrome caused by methotrexate, a methyl derivative of aminopterin. From Cohen.[11]

genesis (Fig. 7-17) and holoprosencephaly (Fig. 7-18).[3,9] The efficacy of diabetic control on the incidence of birth defects is a complex subject beyond the scope of this chapter.

Thalidomide Embryopathy

Thalidomide resulted in the most dramatic epidemic of birth defects ever recorded. It has been estimated that more than 10,000 babies were affected between 1958 and 1963. Anomalies include phocomelia, other limb reduction defects, malformed ears, facial hemangiomas, esophageal or duodenal atresia, tetralogy of Fallot, and renal agenesis (Fig. 7-19).[19,31]

Aminopterin Syndrome

On occasion, aminopterin, a folic acid antagonist, has been used as an abortifacient during the first trimester of pregnancy and has resulted in miscarriages, fetal death, and fetal anomalies. Infants after unsuccessful abortifacient use have been reported, and survivors have had marked dysmorphic similarities both clinically and radiologically. Normal infants have also been reported. Methotrexate, a methyl derivative of aminopterin, is known to cause a similar pattern of defects.[10]

Central nervous system anomalies have been observed, including anencephaly, meningoencephalocele, and hydrocephaly. Common craniofacial features include brachycephaly, bitemporal flattening, hypoplastic supraorbital ridges, ocular hypertelorism, prominent eyes, micrognathia, and posteriorly angulated and low-set hypoplastic ears. The hairline frequently shows bitem-

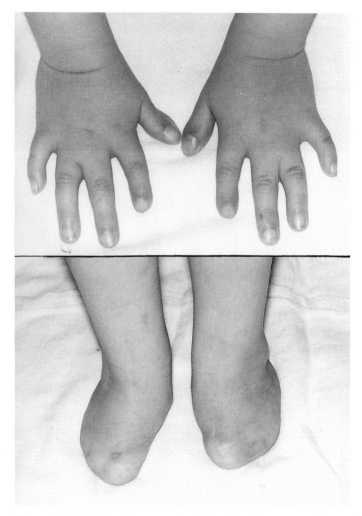

Figure 7-21. Folic acid antagonist–induced syndrome caused by methotrexate. Upper: Brachydactyly and partial soft tissue syndactyly involving digits three and four. Lower: Absence of toes. From Cohen.[11]

poral recession, and the eyebrows may be prominent medially and absent laterally (Fig. 7-20). Ossification defects of the parietal and frontal bones appear as radiolucencies on radiographs. Other anomalies include variably brachydactyly, syndactyly, and hypoplasia or absence of digits (Fig. 7-21).[10] Fraser et al.[16] described a patient with some similarities to the aminopterin syndrome and coined the term *aminopterin-like syndrome sine aminopterin* (ASSA).

REFERENCES

1. Aase JM, Jones KL, Clarren SK: Do we need the term "FAE"? *Pediatrics* 7:428–430, 1990.
2. Ardinger HH, Atkin JF, Blackston RD, Elsas LJ, Clarren SK, Livingstone S, Flannery DB, Pellock JM, Harrod MJ, Lammer EJ, Majewski F, Schinzel A, Toriello HV, Hanson JW: Verification of the fetal valproate syndrome phenotype. *Am J Med Genet* 29:171–185, 1988.

3. Barr M, Hanson JW, Currey K, Sharp S, Toriello H, Schmickel RD, Wilson GH: Holoprosencephaly in infants of diabetic mothers. *J Pediatr* 102:565–568, 1983.

4. Blot WJ: Growth and development following prenatal and childhood exposure to atomic radiation. *J Radiat Res* 16(Suppl):82–88, 1975.

5. Brent RL: Radiation teratogenesis. In Sever JL, Brent RL (eds): *Teratogen Update: Environmentally Induced Birth Defect Risks*. New York: Alan R. Liss, 1986, pp 145–163.

6. Buehler BA, Delimont D, Van Wales M, Finnell RH: Prenatal prediction of risk of the fetal hydantoin syndrome. *N Engl J Med* 322:1567–1572, 1990.

7. Castilla EE, Orioli IM: Letter to the Editor: Teratogenicity of Misoprostol: Data from the Latin-American collaborative study of congenital malformations (ECLAMC). *Am J Med Genet* 51:161–162, 1994.

8. Clarren SK, Smith DW: The fetal alcohol syndrome. *N Engl J Med* 298:1063–1067, 1978.

9. Cohen MM Jr: A comprehensive and critical assessment of overgrowth and overgrowth syndromes. *Adv Hum Genet* 18:181–303, 373–376, 1989.

10. Cohen MM Jr: *Craniosynostosis: Diagnosis, Evaluation, and Management*. New York: Raven Press, 1986.

11. Cohen MM Jr: Neoplasia and the fetal alcohol and hydantoin syndromes. *Neurobehav Toxicol Teratol* 3:161–162, 1981.

11a. Cole DEC, Hanley DA: Osteocalcin, in *Bone. Volume 3. Bone Matrix and Bone Specific Products*, Boca Raton: CRC Press, 1991, Ch. 7, pp. 239–294.

12. Delgado-Escueta AV, Janz D: Consensus guidelines: Preconception counseling, management, and care of the pregnant woman with epilepsy. *Neurology* 42(Suppl 5):149–160, 1992.

13. Feldman GL, Weaver DD, Lourien EW: The fetal trimethadione syndrome. *Am J Dis Child* 131:1389–1392, 1977.

14. Fernhoff PM, Lammer EJ: Craniofacial features of isotretinoin embryopathy. *J Pediatr* 105:595–597, 1984.

15. Fonseca W, Alencar AJC, Pereira RMM, Misago C: Congenital malformation of the scalp and cranium after failed first trimester abortion attempt with Misoprostol. *Clin Dysmorphol* 2:76–80, 1993.

16. Fraser FC, Anderson RA, Mulvihill JI, Preus M: An aminopterin-like syndrome without aminopterin (ASSAS). *Clin Genet* 32:28–34, 1987.

17. Fraser FC, Fainstat TD: Production of congenital defects in the offspring of pregnant mice treated with cortisone. *Pediatrics* 8:527–533, 1951.

18. Hall JG, Pauli RM, Wilson KM: Maternal and fetal sequelae of anticoagulation during pregnancy. *Am J Med* 68:122–140, 1980.

19. Hanson JW: Teratogenic agents. In Emery AEH, Rimoin DL (eds): *Principles and Practice of Medical Genetics*. Vol 1. 2nd Ed. New York: Churchill Livingstone, pp 183–213, 1990.

20. Hanson JW, Myrianthopoulos NC, Harvey MAS, Smith DW: Risks to the offspring of women treated with hydantoin anticonvulsants with emphasis on the fetal hydantoin syndrome. *J Pediatr* 89:662–668, 1976.

21. Hanson JW, Smith DW: The fetal hydantoin syndrome. *J Pediatr* 87:285–290, 1975.

22. Hanson JW, Streissguth AP, Smith DW: The effects of moderate alcohol consumption during pregnancy on fetal growth and morphogenesis. *J Pediatr* 92:457–460, 1978.

23. Hoyme HE, Jones KL, Dixon SD, Jewett T, Hanson JW, Robinson LK, Msall ME, Allanson JE: Prenatal cocaine exposure and fetal vascular disruption. *Pediatrics* 85:743–747, 1990.

24. Jones KL, Smith DW: Recognition of the fetal alcohol syndrome in early infancy. *Lancet* 2:999–1001, 1973.

25. Jones KL, Smith DW, Hanson JW: The fetal alcohol syndrome: Clinical delineation. *Ann NY Acad Sci* 273:130–139, 1976.

26. Jones KL, Smith DW, Ulleland CN, Streissguth AP: Pattern of malformation in offspring of chronic alcoholic mothers. *Lancet* 1:1267–1271, 1973.

27. Lammer EJ, Chen DT, Hoar RM, Agnish ND, Benke PJ, Braun JT, Curry CJ, Fernoff PM, Grix AW, Lott IT, Richard JM, Sun SC: Retinoic acid embryopathy. *N Engl J Med* 313:837–841, 1985.

27a. Neave C: *Congenital Malformations in Offspring of Diabetics.* Doctoral thesis, Harvard University School of Public Health, Cambridge, Massachusetts, 1967.

27b. Neave C: Congenital malformations in offspring of diabetics. *Perspect Pediatr Pathol* 8:213–222, 1984.

28. Pauli RM, Madder JD, Kranzler J, Culpepper W, Port R: Warfarin therapy initiated during pregnancy and phenotypic chondrodysplasia punctata. *J Pediatr* 88:506–508, 1976.

29. Pearson MA, Hoyme HE, Seaver LH, Rimsza ME: Toluene embryopathy: Delineation of the phenotype and comparison with fetal alcohol syndrome. *Pediatrics* 93:211–215, 1994.

30. Sever JL, Brent RL: *Teratogen Update: Environmentally Induced Birth Defect Risks.* New York: Alan R. Liss, 1986.

31. Smithells RW, Newman CGH: Recognition of thalidomide defects. *J Med Genet* 29:716–723, 1992.

31a. Van Allen MI, Brown ZA, Plovie B, Hanson ML, Knopp RH: Deformations in infants of diabetic and control pregnancies. *Am J Med Genet* 53:210–215, 1994.

32. Warkany J: *Congenital Malformations: Notes and Comments.* Chicago: Year Book Medical Publishers, 1971.

33. Warkany J, Schraffenberger E: Congenital malformations induced in rats by roentgen rays. *Am J Roentgenol* 57:455–463, 1947.

34. Whitfield MF: Chondrodysplasia punctata after warfarin in early pregnancy. *Arch Dis Child* 55:139–141, 1980.

35. Wilson JG: *Environment and Birth Defects.* New York: Academic Press, 1973.

36. Wilson JG: Principles of teratology. In Perrin EV, Finegold MJ (eds): *Pathobiology of Development or Ontogeny Revisited.* Baltimore: Williams & Wilkins, 1973.

37. Zackai EH, Mellman WJ, Niederer BA, Hanson JW: The fetal trimethadione syndrome. *J Pediatr* 87:280–284, 1975.

8

Syndrome Classifications

There are many possible ways to classify syndromes for different purposes.[1–3,5,15,16] Only a few categories are considered here: etiologic, embryonic, germ layer based, monothetic, polythetic, mixed, and prototypic.

ETIOLOGIC CLASSIFICATIONS

Syndromes can be classified according to broad etiologic categories such as monogenic, chromosomal, and environmentally induced. Such classifications usually require supplementary categories, e.g., multifactorial, disruptive, and unknown. Besides general etiologic categories, narrow and specific categories may be useful for some purposes, e.g., mucolipidoses or fibroblast growth factor receptor mutations.

EMBRYONIC CLASSIFICATIONS

The understanding of mechanisms of normal and abnormal development is based on detailed observations of normal embryos and malformations. Technical advances have permitted meaningful comparison between humans and experimental animals, particularly mice. Embryonic classifications of various malformations and more extensive developmental fields are commonplace.

Classifications of multiple anomalies are more challenging. A good example is the work of Van Allen[13] on renal anomalies. A classification is proposed in which kidney anomalies are divided into four main categories: (1) errors of organogenesis, (2) errors of position/fusion, (3) errors of histogenesis, and (4) obstruction. Associated anomalies are common in disorders with errors of organogenesis. More discrete anomalies result from disorders of histogenesis. Contiguous anomalies in the caudal part of the embryo provide evidence for developmental fields. Finally, noncontiguous anomalies most likely represent the expression of genes important for development at different times during embryogenesis.

CLASSIFICATION BY GERM LAYERS

Developmental disturbances of tissue structure are the basis of some classifications. Thus, hamartoneoplastic syndromes are sometimes classified on the basis of the germ layer involved; multiple osteochondromas involve only one layer—the mesoderm. On the other hand, Gardner syndrome—consisting of polyposis of the colon, osteomas, desmoid tumors, leiomyomas, lipomas, odontomas, and redundancy of retinal epithelium—involves all three germ layers. Nosologic subgroups for the many forms of ectodermal dysplasia have been proposed. For example, the well-known X-linked form of ectodermal dysplasia has been assigned to the tricho-odonto-onycho-dyshidrotic subgroup.[4]

There are dangers in overclassifying on the basis of germ layer involvement, however, because of interactions between tissue layers. For example, not all defects in type I neurofibromatosis are attributable to the neural crest. Many features such as café-au-lait spots, neurofibromas, sphenoid bone dysplasia, and pheochromocytoma are, in fact, of neural crest origin. Other findings such as cerebral cortical heterotopias and optic gliomas appear to be derived from the neural tube itself. Still other findings such as pseudoarthrosis, coarctation of the aorta, renal artery stenosis, rhabdomyosarcoma,* and leukemia* appear to be of mesodermal origin. Finally, findings such as generalized short stature at present defy explanation.[10,11,14]

MONOTHETIC CLASSIFICATIONS

In a monothetic classification, syndromes are grouped together because they share a single feature such as polydactyly or cleft palate. Such groupings are often used as an aid in differential diagnosis. Examples of monothetic classifications include syndromes with arthrogryposis, syndromes with craniosynostosis, or syndromes with a propensity for Wilms tumor.

POLYTHETIC CLASSIFICATIONS

In a polythetic classification, syndromes are grouped together because they share a large proportion of their principal anomalies. Such groupings are even better aids in differential diagnosis. If the anomalies share close dysmorphic similarities, making up a tightly overlapping phenotypic spectrum, then the developmental pathways of the syndrome group possibly may be similar or even the same. Such a group is known as a *community of syndromes*, a concept pioneered and developed by Pinsky.[7–9] An example of a syndrome community involving müllerian ducts, distal extremities, urinary tract, and ears is presented in Table 8-1.

---

*Both rhabdomyosarcoma and leukemia occur with low frequency in type I neurofibromatosis, but with higher frequency than as isolated neoplasms in the general population.

Table 8-1. A Community of Malformation Syndromes Involving Müllerian Ducts, Distal Extremities, Urinary Tract, and Ears

Syndrome	Hand-Foot-Uterus Syndrome	Vaginal Atresia-Polydactyly Syndrome	Camptobrachydactyly	Rudiger Syndrome	Winter Syndrome	Cryptophthalmos Syndrome
Distal extremities	Short first metacarpals and metatarsals, fusion of carpal and tarsals, short calcaneus	Polydactyly, metacarpal dysplasia	Short metacarpals, short metatarsals, brachymesophalangy, polymetatarsalism, polydactyly	Brachydactyly	Fifth finger clinodactyly	Syndactyly, osseous phalangeal anomalies
Internal genitalia	Duplication of uterus, subseptate vagina	Vaginal atresia, vaginal duplication, urogenital sinus	Septate vagina	Bicornuate uterus, cystic ovaries	Vaginal atresia	Vaginal atresia, bicornuate uterus
Urinary tract	—	Ureteral stenosis, double ureter, polycystic kidney	Urinary incontinence, bladder neck dysmorphism?	Ureterovesical junction stenosis	Renal dysgenesis	Renal dysgenesis
Ears	—	—	—	Lack of cartilage in pinna	External and middle ear anomalies	External and middle ear anomalies
Mode of inheritance	Autosomal dominant	Autosomal recessive	Autosomal dominant	Autosomal recessive?	Autosomal recessive?	Autosomal recessive

Modified from Pinsky.[7]

A syndrome community permits description of a phenotypic class as a whole. Such a class can act as a repository in which certain patients can be placed for later retrieval who cannot be diagnosed with certainty as having a specific syndrome within the class, but whose overall pattern of anomalies clearly belongs to the syndrome community. Syndrome communities can also facilitate bibliographic retrieval and computer manipulation of various conditions. This is particularly useful for poorly delineated or rare syndromes. A syndrome community can aid in the recall of various syndromes and their features, which is helpful in differential diagnosis.[9]

The idea that syndromes are lumped together because they are phenotypically similar is not incompatible with the idea that the same syndromes are split apart because they are etiologically heterogeneous. Disorders that are etiologically heterogeneous may have pathogenetically similar mechanisms. Because syndrome communities are heuristic, they stimulate hypotheses about relationships among various members of the group. The syndrome community concept is not that all members of the community are necessarily pathogenetically similar. Some members of the group may be spurious. The syndrome community concept simply raises the question in the same way that the original grouping of the mucopolysaccharidoses led to the perception of their differences as well as their similarities.[9]

MIXED CLASSIFICATIONS

Mixed classifications are used for several purposes, most commonly as methods for organizing syndromology textbooks. The arbitrary nature of some syndrome categories may be a perfectly reasonable way to organize a large number of syndromes. For example, Smith[12] uses categories such as osteochondrodysplasias, face–limb defects as a major component, unusual neuromuscular findings with associated defects, and the hamartoses. Similarly, Gorlin et al.[5] classify

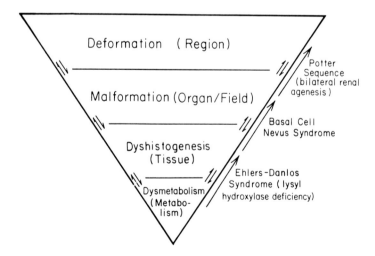

Figure 8-1. Stratification of syndrome prototypes as dysmetabolic, dyshistogenetic, malformational, and deformational, representing expression at the metabolic, tissue, organ, and regional levels, respectively. Examples of compound syndromes that express themselves at more than one level appear on the right. From Cohen.[1]

Table 8-2. Syndrome Prototypes

Type	Level of Disturbance	Features	Examples
Dysmetabolic syndrome	Metabolism	Often normal at birth with generalized progressive disturbances after birth Clinical features relatively uniform compared with other types of syndromes Not associated with congenital malformations Biochemically defined or potentially so Commonly recessive mode of inheritance	Hurler syndrome, Lesch-Nyhan syndrome, Tay-Sachs disease
Dyshistogenetic syndrome	Tissues	Simple dyshistogenetic syndrome Characterized by involvement of only one germ layer Inheritance may be dominant or recessive	Marfan syndrome, achondroplasia
		Hamartoneoplastic syndrome Characterized by hamartomas, hyperplasias and a propensity for neoplasia May involve one, two, or all three germ layers Inheritance is commonly dominant	Gardner syndrome, Peutz-Jeghers syndrome
Malformation syndrome	Organs or fields	Several noncontiguous malformations in the same patient Characterized by embryonic pleiotropy in which the several malformation sequences are developmentally unrelated at the embryonic level Lack of biochemical definition,[a] highest state of definition is a known-genesis syndrome of the chromosomal or pedigree type	Trisomy 13 syndrome, Meckel syndrome, Rubinstein-Taybi syndrome
Deformation syndrome	Regions	Characterized by changes in the shape or structure of previously normal parts Most important cause is lack of fetal movement, whether the cause be a mechanical, functional or malformational disturbance Commonly affects musculoskeletal system	Potter sequence based on a non-malformational cause such as amniotic rupture, Rosenmann-Arad syndrome[b]

From Cohen.[1]

[a] Lack of biochemical definition in the dysmetabolic sense. Molecular definition (specific mutations) is possible in an increasing number of malformation syndromes.

[b] Most multiple deformations are based on malformational or deformational sequences.

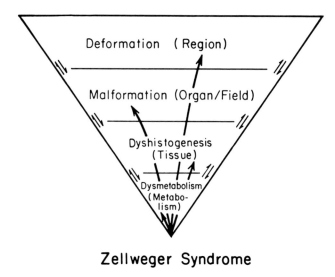

Zellweger Syndrome

Figure 8-2. Zellweger syndrome showing clinical expression at all four levels. From Cohen.[1]

syndromes under headings such as metabolic syndromes, branchial arch and oral–acral syndromes, syndromes of postnatal onset obesity, and syndromes of orofacial clefting.

SYNDROME PROTOTYPES

Syndromes can be analyzed at different levels of organization. In the broadest possible context, four general classes of syndromes can be defined: the dysmetabolic syndrome, the dyshistogenetic* syndrome, the malformation syndrome, and the deformation syndrome, and these have been discussed elsewhere.[1,3,6] They represent disturbances in metabolism, tissues, organs, and regions, respectively. The four types of syndromes and their relationships are illustrated by the inverted triangle shown in Figure 8-1. It will be observed that the syndromes are stratified. For example, a malformation syndrome has underlying dyshistogenetic and dysmetabolic levels, but the condition expresses itself ultimately at the level of organ formation.†

Four different syndrome prototypes and their characteristics together with examples are shown in Table 8-2. Syndrome prototypes provide a framework for analyzing various types of syndromes by giving us convenient points of reference in our thinking. Some syndromes closely fit the syndrome prototypes; others have features overlapping between one type and another.

For example, on the right in Figure 8-1 are shown some representative syn-

*Many authorities use the term *dysplasia*. However, the term has been used in so many different ways in medicine and pathology that I prefer the term *dyshistogenesis*, which I find less ambiguous although perhaps more cumbersome. See discussion on dysplasia in Chapter 2 under the heading Other Definitions.

†Many malformations are morphologic defects of organ structure, but some affected areas, both large, e.g., a defect of blastogenesis, and small, e.g., cleft lip, cannot properly be described as defects of organ structure.

dromes that each express themselves at two levels. Bilateral renal agenesis results in oligohydramnios, producing the Potter sequence. The nevoid basal cell carcinoma syndrome has dyshistogenetic features such as basal cell carcinomas, keratocysts, and medulloblastoma; true malformations such as ocular hypertelorism, bifid ribs, cervical spina bifida occulta, and, occasionally, cleft lip, may also occur. In one of the autosomal recessive forms of the Ehlers-Danlos syndrome, lysyl hydroxylase deficiency results in dyshistogenetic skin changes. Figure 8-2 shows that the Zellweger syndrome expresses itself at all four levels. Patients have a progressive downhill course with an early demise typical of a dysmetabolic syndrome. The brain exhibits neuronal malmigration, which is dyshistogenetic. Patent ductus arteriosus and patent foramen ovale are often present, representing malformations. Finally, clubfoot and flexion contractures of the fingers represent deformations.

REFERENCES

1. Cohen MM Jr: *The Child With Multiple Birth Defects.* New York: Raven Press, 1982.
2. Cohen MM Jr: Dysmorphic syndromes with craniofacial manifestations. In Stewart RE, Prescott, GH (eds): *Oral Facial Genetics.* St. Louis: CV Mosby, pp 500–662, 1976.
3. Cohen MM Jr: Syndromology: An updated conceptual overview. II. Syndrome classifications. *Int J Oral Maxillofac Surg* 18:223–228, 1989.
4. Freire-Maia, Pinheiro M: *Ectodermal Dysplasias: A Clinical and Genetic Study.* New York: Alan R. Liss, 1984.
5. Gorlin RJ, Cohen MM Jr, Levin LS: *Syndromes of the Head and Neck.* Third Edition, New York: Oxford University Press, 1990.
6. Herrmann J, Opitz JM: Naming and nomenclature of syndromes. *Birth Defects* 10(7):69–86, 1974.
7. Pinsky L: A community of human malformation syndromes involving the müllerian ducts, distal extremities, urinary tract, and ears. *Teratology* 9:64–80, 1974.
8. Pinsky L: The community of human malformation syndromes that shares ectodermal dysplasia and deformities of the hands and feet. *Teratology* 11:227–242, 1975.
9. Pinsky L: The polythetic (phenotypic community) system of classifying human malformation syndromes. *Birth Defects* 13(3A):13–30, 1977.
10. Riccardi VM, Eichner JE: *Neurofibromatosis, Phenotype, Natural History and Pathogenesis.* Baltimore: Johns Hopkins University Press, 1986.
11. Riccardi VM, Mulvihill JJ (eds): *Neurofibromatosis (von Recklinghausen Disease).* Advances in Neurology, Genetics, Cell Biology, and Biochemistry, Vol. 29. New York: Raven Press, 1981.
12. Smith DW: *Recognizable Patterns of Human Malformation.* Third edition. Philadelphia: WB Saunders, 1982.
13. Van Allen M: Cited in Cohen MM Jr: Intermediate mesoderm: Kidneys and gonads. Summary of the Fourth Robert J. Gorlin Conference on Dysmorphology. *Clin Dysmorphol* 4:178–180, 1995.
14. Wander JV, Das Gupta TK: Neurofibromatosis. In *Current Problems in Surgery.* Vol XIV. Chicago: Year Book Medical Publishers, February 1977.
15. Warkany J: Overview of malformation syndromes. *Birth Defects* 10(7):1–5, 1974.
16. Warkany J: Syndromes. *Am J Dis Child* 121:364–370, 1971.

9

Syndrome Delineation

The process of syndrome delineation was first articulated by Opitz and his colleagues.[21] I later used similar concepts with different terminology.[9,10,14]

KNOWN AND UNKNOWN GENESIS SYNDROMES

The process of syndrome delineation can be divided into the following stages: (1) unknown genesis syndromes, including provisionally unique pattern syndromes and recurrent pattern syndromes; and (2) known genesis syndromes, including pedigree syndromes, chromosomal syndromes, biochemical defect syndromes, and environmentally induced syndromes.[10,14]

In an unknown genesis syndrome, the cause is simply not known. In a *provisionally unique pattern syndrome*, several anomalies are observed in the same patient such that the clinician does not recognize the overall pattern of defects from his or her own experience, nor from searching the literature, nor from consultation with the most learned colleagues in the field.

Two different examples of provisionally unique pattern syndromes are briefly presented here. The first of these is illustrated in Figure 9-1 and consists of sagittal synostosis, mental deficiency, strabismus, micrognathia, anomalous pulmonary venous return, umbilical hernia, complete anterior dislocation of the tibiae and fibulae with absent patellae (allowing the knees to be flexed against the ventral surface of the body), obvious foot deformities, camptodactyly and ulnar deviation of fingers two through five bilaterally, and short first metacarpals with proximally placed thumbs.[6,7]

The second example of a provisionally unique pattern syndrome (Figs. 9-2 to 9-4) consists of a dysmorphic face with prominent square forehead and Robin sequence; broad proximally placed thumbs, hypoplasia of the third and fifth middle phalanges, and absent middle phalanges in the second fingers; broad

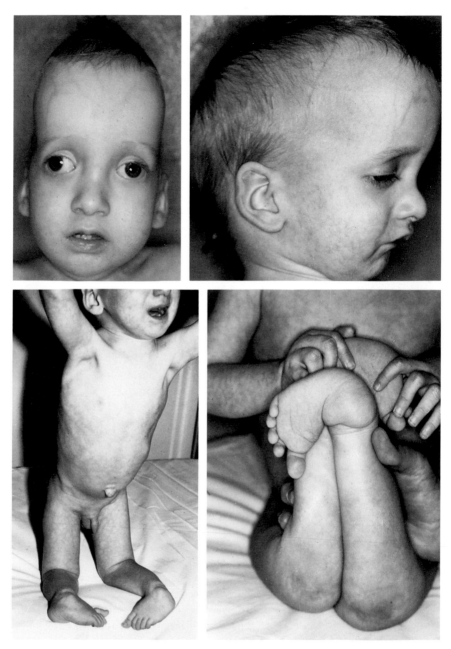

Figure 9-1. Provisionally unique pattern syndrome consisting of sagittal synostosis, scaphocephaly, mental deficiency, strabismus, micrognathia, anomalous pulmonary venous return, umbilical hernia, complete anterior dislocation of tibiae and fibulae with absent patellae (allowing the knees to be flexed against the ventral surface of the body), obvious foot deformities, camptodactyly and ulnar deviation of fingers two through five bilaterally, and short first metacarpals with proximally placed thumbs. From Cohen.[6,7]

halluces and postaxial polydactyly; rhizomelic short stature and radiographic abnormalities of the spine and pelvis.[19]

Most likely the anomalies in each of the two provisionally unique pattern syndromes have a common cause, though unknown, rather than having different causes acting independently. The probability that such anomalies occur in the

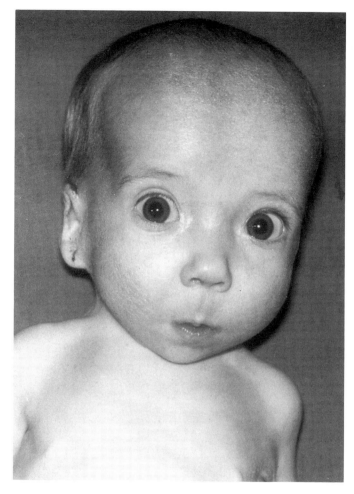

Figure 9-2. Dysmorphic face with Robin sequence. Martsolf et al.[19]

same patient by chance becomes less likely the more anomalies the patient has and the rarer these anomalies are individually in the general population.[14]

Obviously, if a second example of either syndrome comes to light, the condition is no longer unique. A provisionally unique pattern syndrome is a one-of-a-kind syndrome to a particular observer at a particular point in time (Figs. 9-5, 9-6). There may be a nineteenth century description of a similar instance that escapes his or her attention. There may also be some instances of the syndrome in different parts of the world that remain as yet unrecognized. Thus, many syndromes appear to be unique at the time the initial patient is discovered, but are no longer unique when two or more examples become known.[14]

A *recurrent pattern syndrome* can be defined as a similar or identical set of anomalies in two or more unrelated patients. The three patients whose findings are summarized in Table 9-1 have a recurrent pattern syndrome known as Gomez-López-Hernández syndrome.[14,18] Findings include mental deficiency, cerebellar ataxia, parietal alopecia, corneal opacities, and other abnormalities (Fig. 9-7). The same abnormalities in two or more patients suggest, but do not prove, that the pathogenesis in both cases may be the same. At the recurrent pattern stage of syndrome delineation, the etiology is still not known. In gener-

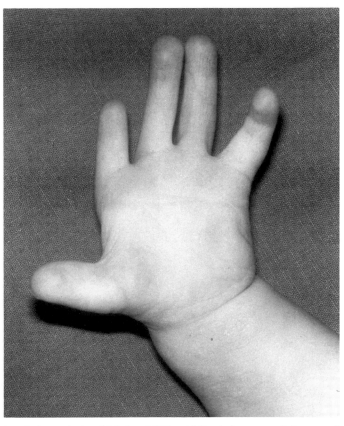

Figure 9-3. Broad proximally placed thumb, hypoplasia of third and fifth middle phalanges, and absence of middle phalanx of index finger. Martsolf et al.[19]

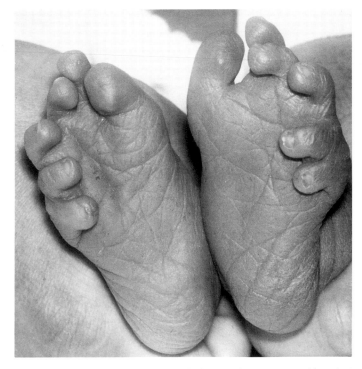

Figure 9-4. Postaxial hexadactyly and abnormal toes. Martsolf et al.[19]

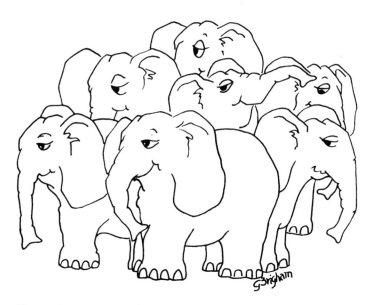

Figure 9-5. Many syndromologists belong to the *it-takes-two-or-more-to-make-a-syndrome* school. Such syndromologists would look at this cartoon and exclaim, *Hey! Look at all the elephants.* See Fig. 9-6. From Cohen.[14]

al, the validity of a recurrent pattern syndrome increases with the more abnormalities found in the condition and the more patients recognized as having the syndrome.[14] A more well-delineated recurrent pattern syndrome with at least 20 reported examples is the Weaver syndrome.[1] Features are listed in Table 9-2 and illustrated in Figure 9-8. To date, all instances have occurred sporadically except for one presumed instance in affected siblings.[1,2]

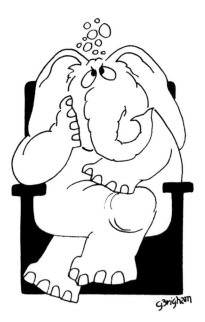

Figure 9-6. Syndromologists who belong to the *it-takes-two-or-more-to-make-a-syndrome* school would look at this cartoon and exclaim, *It can't be an elephant! There's only one.* The logic of the situation is inescapable. There can be a one-of-a-kind syndrome. From Cohen.[14]

Table 9-1. Gomez-Lopéz-Hernández Syndrome

Findings	López-Hernández (1982)		Gomez (1979)
	Case 1	Case 2	Case 3
Demographics			
Sex	Female	Female	Female
Population	Mexico	Mexico	USA
Growth			
Short stature	+	+	?
Performance			
Mental deficiency	+	+	+
Central nervous system			
Pons-vermis fusion	+	+	?
Atresia of fourth ventricle	+	+	?
Cerebellar ataxia	+	+	+
Trigeminal anesthesia	+	+	+
Craniofacial			
Cranisynostosis	+	+	−
Parietal alopecia	+	+	+
Ocular hypertelorism	+	−	+
Corneal opacities	+	+	+
Midface deficiency	+	+	+
Low-set, posteriorly angulated ears	+	+	?
Limbs			
Clinodactyly	+	+	?
Genitalia			
Hypoplastic labia majora	+	+	?

Modified from Cohen.[6]

At the recurrent pattern stage of syndrome delineation, the number of find-ings is usually expanded as the number of patients increases. However, because the etiology remains unknown at this time, other examples of the syndrome tend to be selected because they most closely resemble the first case. This results in an artificial homogeneity of cases that emphasizes the most severe aspects of the syndrome. Thus, we should be wary of estimated frequencies given in review articles and textbooks for various anomalies that occur in a recurrent pattern syndrome; they tend to be overestimates that can affect the prognostic risk counseling for possibly developing some features of the syndrome such as mental retardation.[14]

A *known genesis syndrome* can be defined as several anomalies causally related on the basis of (1) occurrence in the same family or, less conclusively, the same mode of inheritance in different families; (2) a chromosomal defect; (3) a specific defect in an enzyme or structural protein; or (4) an environmental factor.[14,17] The term *pedigree syndrome* refers to known genesis on the basis of pedigree evidence alone; the basic defect itself remains undefined, although the condition

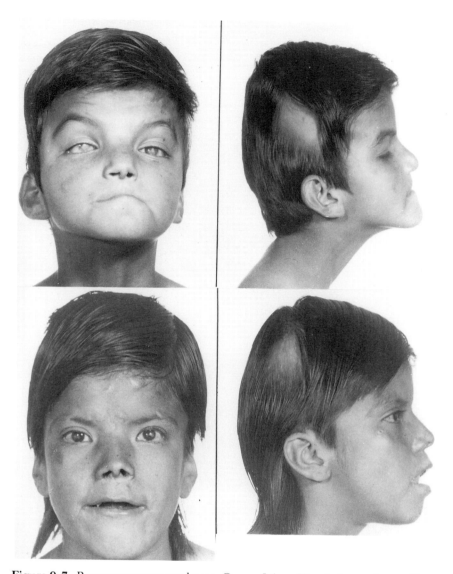

Figure 9-7. Recurrent pattern syndrome. Gomez-López-Hernández syndrome. Two patients with parietal alopecia, corneal opacities, pons-vermis fusion, trigeminal anesthesia, cerebellar ataxia, and mental deficiency. From López-Hernández.[18]

is known to represent a monogenic disorder. Examples include autosomal dominantly inherited branchio-oto-renal syndrome, autosomal recessively inherited Meckel syndrome, and oral-facial-digital syndrome I, which has X-linked dominant inheritance, lethal in the male. Chromosomal syndromes are cytogenetically determined such as trisomy 13 syndrome, del(18q) syndrome, and 49,XXXXY syndrome. In a *biochemical defect syndrome*, specific enzymatic defects are known in recessive syndromes. Examples include the autosomal recessively inherited Hurler syndrome and the X-linked recessive Lesch-Nyhan syndrome. The term is also meant to include specific defects in structural proteins in some of the dominant disorders, such as defective fibrillin-1 in Marfan syndrome, as well as other types of molecular defects, such as fibroblast growth factor receptor mutations in some of the craniosynostosis syndromes. An *environmentally*

Table 9-2. Features of Weaver Syndrome

Findings	Frequencies
Growth	
Prenatal growth excess	16/20
Postnatal growth excess	19/20
Accelerated osseous maturation	19/19
Performance	
Hypertonia	10/18
Hypotonia	5/18
Developmental delay	19/19
Hoarse, low-pitched cry	14/17
Craniofacial	
Broad forehead	18/19
Flat occiput	6/11
Large ears	15/17
Ocular hypertelorism	19/19
Prominent or long philtrum	10/14
Relative micrognathia	17/19
Limbs	
Camptodactyly	11/16
Prominent fingerpads	6/9
Thin, deeply set nails	9/10
Broad thumbs	4/6
Clinodactyly, toes	4/5
Limited elbow or knee extension	10/13
Widened distal long bones	16/18
Foot deformities[a]	7/10
Other	
Excess loose skin	11/12
Umbilical hernia or diastasis recti	12/17
Inguinal hernia	4/14
Inverted nipples	3/4

From Cohen.[2]

[a] Talipes equinovarus, talipes calcaneovalgus, metatarsus adductus.

induced syndrome is defined in terms of the environmental factor or causative teratogen such as retinoids, hydantoins, coumarin anticoagulants, trimethadione, and valproic acid.

COMMENTS ON THE PROCESS OF SYNDROME DELINEATION

The process of syndrome delineation is summarized in Figure 9-9. Generally, a syndrome can be placed into one of the categories previously discussed. Occa-

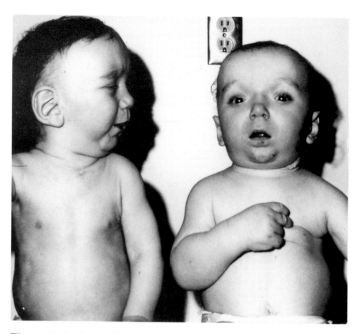

Figure 9-8. Example of a recurrent pattern syndrome in two patients with Weaver syndrome. Note similarity. From Weaver et al.[23]

sionally, a syndrome may be delineated in a one-step delineation, thus bypassing several of the stages mentioned earlier. For example, if a new chromosomal abnormality is discovered during the laboratory investigation of a patient clinically defined as having a provisionally unique pattern syndrome, the patient represents a known genesis syndrome of the chromosomal type in a one-step delineation. However, the variability of the clinical expression must await the discovery of more patients. In other instances, such as a large dominant pedigree with many affected individuals, a known genesis syndrome of the pedigree type and much of its phenotypic variability can be determined in one step.

Provisionally unique pattern syndromes occur with some frequency. Further delineation will often occur, given sufficient time. A truly unique pattern syndrome may occur with a chromosomal anomaly involving two or more breaks. The condition may be sporadic or segregate within a family. Since the chance of an identical duplication-deficiency syndrome occurring in another family is very slight, the syndrome may be considered unique to an affected individual or an affected family.[17]

The multiple anomalies that make up any syndrome are thought to be pathogenetically related. However, anomalies may concur either by chance or as a

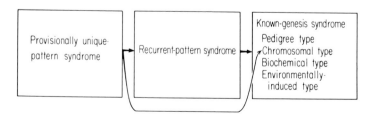

Figure 9-9. Summary of the process of syndrome delineation. See text. From Cohen.[14]

Table 9-3. Syndrome Delineation Involving Orofacial Clefting

Etiology	1971[a]	1978[b]	1990[c]
Monogenic	39	79	193
Autosomal dominant	(17)	(35)	(69)
Autosomal recessive	(18)	(39)	(104)
X-linked	(4)	(5)	(20)
Environmentally induced	0	6	10
Chromosomal	15	29	49
Unknown cause[d]	18	40	90
Total	72	154	342

From Cohen and Bankier.[15]

[a]Based on Gorlin et al.[16]

[b]Based on Cohen.[12]

[c]Based on POSSUM.[20]

[d]Includes distinctive syndromes of unknown genesis and associations.

statistically related association in the same patient. Some associations are well-stocked pools for future syndrome delineation.*

Syndrome delineation and the use of the delineation terms proposed should be thought of as a dynamic, flexible, and continually changing framework in which to view various syndromes. These categories should never be thought of as static or immutable, even at the higher stages of syndrome delineation. Etiologic and clinical heterogeneity is common and should be expected to occur even when not readily apparent. Moreover, we should not confuse syndrome delineation with understanding of the syndrome's pathogenesis, even at the higher stages of delineation. In a pedigree syndrome such as the autosomal recessively inherited Meckel syndrome, we know nothing about how the homozygous state of the Meckel gene produces such diverse features as encephalocele, polydactyly, and polycystic kidneys.

PACE OF SYNDROME DELINEATION

Syndrome delineation is proceeding at a very rapid pace. Tables 9-3, 9-4, and 9-5 illustrate syndrome delineation through the years with respect to orofacial clefting, craniosynostosis, and holoprosencephaly. Toriello[22] has estimated that newly recognized syndromes are being described at the rate of one or more per week, and, although some represent variable expression of previously recorded conditions, many actually represent newly recognized syndromes.

SIGNIFICANCE OF SYNDROME DELINEATION

The significance of syndrome delineation cannot be overestimated. As an unknown genesis syndrome becomes delineated, its phenotypic spectrum, its natu-

*Associations have been dealt with more fully in both Chapter 1 and Chapter 2.

Table 9-4. Syndrome Delineation Involving Craniosynostosis

Etiology	1975	1979	1986	1991
Chromosomal	0	11	14	16
Monogenic	12	26	31	40
Autosomal dominant	(5)	(12)	(13)	(15)
Autosomal recessive	(7)	(12)	(13)	(16)
X-linked	(0)	(2)	(2)	(3)
Inheritance pattern unclear	(0)	(0)	(3)	(6)
Environmentally induced	1	2	3	4
Unknown genesis	5	18	10	24
Miscellaneous	—	—	6	6
Total syndromes	18	57	64	90

From Cohen.[3,5,6,13]

ral history, and its inheritance pattern or risk of recurrence become known, allowing for better patient care and family counseling. If the phenotypic spectrum is known, the clinician can search for suspected defects that may not be immediately apparent but that may produce clinical problems at a later date, such as a hemivertebra in the Goldenhar syndrome. If a certain complication can occur in a given syndrome, such as a Wilms tumor in the Beckwith-Wiedemann syndrome, the clinician is forewarned to monitor the patient for possible development of neoplasia. Finally, if the recurrence risk is known, the parents can be counseled properly about future pregnancies. This is particularly important if the risk is high and the disorder is severely disabling or disfiguring,

Table 9-5. Syndrome Delineation Involving Holoprosencephaly (and Arhinencephaly) from 1971 to 1989

Etiology	1971	1982	1989
Chromosomal	8	21	35
Holoprosencephaly	8	17	29
Well-established types	(4)	(5)	(7)
Uncommon, less consistent types	(1)	(7)	(17)
Prebanding era karyotypes	(3)	(5)	(5)
Arhinencephaly	0	4	6
Monogenic	5	12	18
Holoprosencephaly	2	5	8
Autosomal dominant	(0)	(1)	(4)
Autosomal recessive	(2)	(4)	(3)
X-linked recessive	—	—	(1)
Arhinencephaly	3	7	10
Autosomal dominant	(1)	(2)	(3)
Autosomal recessive	(0)	(2)	(4)
X-linked recessive	(2)	(3)	(3)
Environmental	0	1	1
Unknown causes	0	2	8
Associations	0	3	4
Total	13	39	66

From Cohen.[4,8,11]

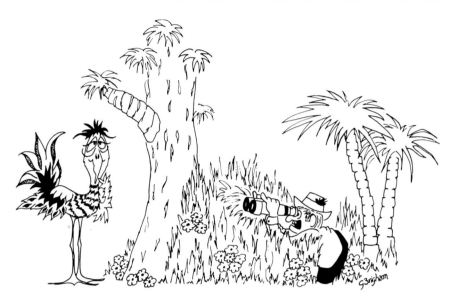

Figure 9-10. Some doctors think of syndromologists as bird watchers. This is a misconception because bird watching is a passive endeavor. Since syndrome delineation and syndrome diagnosis foster good patient care, the syndromologist is not passive, but is actively involved in patient care. From Cohen.[14]

has mental deficiency as one component, or has a dramatically shortened life span. For example, Stickler syndrome is an autosomal dominant disorder with a 50% recurrence risk when one parent is affected. Retinal detachment occurs in 20% of reported cases, and blindness affects 15%. Genetic counseling is important because the risk of developing serious ocular problems is high. This relatively common condition also illustrates the importance of syndrome delineation because the entity was unrecognized before 1965, although clearly it had existed before then. Thus, syndrome delineation fosters good patient care (Fig. 9-10). The overall treatment program gains rationality. In contrast, with a provisionally unique pattern syndrome, the treatment program and overall management frequently leave something to be desired.[14]

REFERENCES

1. Ardinger HH, Hanson JW, Harrod MJE, Cohen MM Jr, Tibbles JAR, Welch JP, Young-Wee T, Sommer A, Goldberg R, Shprintzen RJ, Sidoti EJ, Leichtman LG, Hoyme HE: Further delineation of Weaver syndrome. *J Pediatr* 108:228–235, 1986.

2. Cohen MM Jr: A comprehensive and critical assessment of overgrowth and overgrowth syndromes. *Adv Hum Genet* 18:181–303, 373–376, 1989.

3. Cohen MM Jr: An etiologic and nosologic overview of craniosynostosis syndromes. *Birth Defects* 11(2):137–189, 1975.

4. Cohen MM Jr: An update on the holoprosencephalic disorders. *Pediatrics* 101:865–869, 1982.

5. Cohen MM Jr: Craniosynostosis and syndromes with craniosynostosis: Incidence, genetics, penetrance, variability, and new syndrome updating. *Birth Defects* 15(5B):13–63, 1979.

6. Cohen MM Jr: *Craniosynostosis: Diagnosis, Evaluation, and Management.* New York: Raven Press, 1986.

7. Cohen MM Jr: Genetic perspectives on craniosynostosis and syndromes with crani-osynostosis. *J Neurosurg* 47:886–898, 1977.
8. Cohen MM Jr, Jirasek JE, Guzman RT, Gorlin RJ, Peterson MQ: Holoprosen-cephaly and facial dysmorphia: Clinical, pathogenetic and etiologic consider-ations. *Birth Defects* 7(7):125–135, 1971.
9. Cohen MM Jr: Human dysmorphic syndromes with craniofacial abnormalities. In *Oral-Facial Genetics.* Stewart RE, Prescott G (eds): St. Louis: CV Mosby, 1976, pp 500–662.
10. Cohen MM Jr: On the nature of syndrome delineation. *Acta Genet Med Gemellol* 26:103–119, 1977.
11. Cohen MM Jr: Perspectives on holoprosencephaly. Part I. Epidemiology, genetics, and syndromology. *Teratology* 40:211–235, 1989.
12. Cohen MM Jr: Syndromes with cleft lip and cleft palate. *Cleft Palate J* 15:306–328, 1978.
13. Cohen MM Jr: Sutural biology and the correlates of craniosynostosis. *Am J Med Genet* 47:581–616, 1993.
14. Cohen MM Jr: *The Child with Multiple Birth Defects.* New York: Raven Press, 1982.
15. Cohen MM Jr, Bankier A: Syndrome delineation involving orofacial clefting. *Cleft Palate Craniofacial J* 28:119–120, 1991.
16. Gorlin RJ, Cervenka J, Pruzansky S: Facial clefting and its syndromes. *Birth Defects* 7(7):3–49, 1971.
17. Herrmann J, Opitz JM: Naming and nomenclature. *Birth Defects* 10(7):69–86, 1974.
18. López-Hernández A: Craniosynostosis, ataxia, trigeminal anesthesia and parietal alopecia with pons-vermis fusion anomaly (atresia of the fourth ventricle). Report of two cases. *Neuropediatrics* 13:99–102, 1982.
19. Martsolf JT, Reed MH, Hunter AGW: Case report 56. Skeletal dysplasia, Robin anomalad, and polydactyly. *Syndrome Ident* 5(1):14–18, 1977.
20. Murdoch Institute: POSSUM Newsletter. September, 1987.
21. Opitz JM, Herrmann J, Dieker H: The study of malformation syndromes in man. *Birth Defects* 5(2):1–10, 1969.
22. Toriello HV: New syndromes from old: The role of heterogeneity and variability in syndrome delineation. *Am J Med Genet Suppl* 1:50–70, 1988.
23. Weaver DD, Graham CB, Thomas IT, Smith DW: A new overgrowth syndrome with accelerated skeletal maturation, unusual facies and camptodactyly. *J Pediatr* 84:547–552, 1974.

10

Etiologic and Pathogenetic Heterogeneity

In syndromology, a decision must be made whether similar patients have an identical disorder with slightly different manifestations or etiologically separate disorders with somewhat similar manifestations. Two basic principles used in clinical genetics are heterogeneity and pleiotropy. *Heterogeneity* refers to multiple causes resulting in the same effect. *Pleiotropy* means multiple effects from a single cause. *Splitting* occurs with genetic heterogeneity, and *lumping* occurs with pleiotropy (Fig. 10-1). Clinical, genetic, biochemical, and molecular methods are used to recognize genetic heterogeneity.[19]

Syndromologists are lumpers to the extent that they pull together pleiotropic effects of a single genetic disorder. On occasion, seemingly different entities have been lumped together as a single entity because the process of syndrome delineation has later judged them to be the same.

Many clinicians prefer the spectrum thinking of classic medicine to the discontinuous thinking of medical geneticists. The former emphasizes relationships and similarities between various disorders; the latter emphasizes differences and discontinuities of the same disorders. These seemingly different perspectives are actually compatible. Disorders that are etiologically heterogeneous (discontinuous) may have similar or identical pathogenetic pathways.[19]

MODELS OF ETIOLOGY, PATHOGENESIS, AND THE PHENOTYPE

Figure 10-2 shows the relationship between etiology, pathogenesis, and the phenotype (models I to V).[19] Etiologic and pathogenetic heterogeneity is common and should be expected even when not readily apparent. Unfortunately,

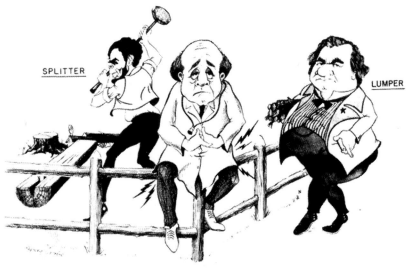

SPLITTER

LUMPER

FENCE-STRADDLER

Figure 10-1. In syndromology, a decision must be made whether similar patients have an identical disorder with slightly different manifestations or etiologically separate disorders with somewhat similar manifestations. Splitting occurs with genetic heterogeneity, and lumping occurs with pleiotropy. The cartoon indicates that splitting occurs with genetic heterogeneity and lumping occurs with pleiotropy. The cartoon indicates that splitting is harder work than lumping. With some conditions, it may be difficult to know whether to split or to lump. When this occurs, fence straddling is an appropriate position even though it may be uncomfortable. From Jackson et al.,[47] modified from McKusick.[60]

some discussions assume that there is one cause and one pathogenetic mechanism for a syndrome that need to be elucidated (Fig. 10-2, model I). However, this simplified view has little, if any, application to today's syndromes and their known complexity.

Model II shows a single disorder with a single pathogenetic mechanism re-

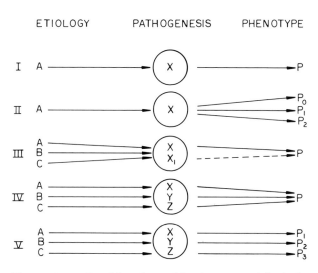

Figure 10-2. Possible relationships between etiologic factors, pathogenesis, and phenotype. See text. Modified from Cohen.[19]

sulting in variably expressed phenotypes. Although it is not difficult to imagine how this might apply to small phenotypic variations, such as the dermatoglyphic differences between identical twins,[42] it is much more difficult to explain discordance for major malformations, such as the high discordance for ventricular septal defect (only 2/25 concordant).[70] For want of a better explanation, this discordance has been ascribed to subtle environmental influences, but more recent analysis suggests that this variability may be inherent in the process of development itself. Using computer simulation techniques that assume a simple initial state and subsequent random motion of embryonal cells, Kurnit et al.[52] showed that postulating a single locus governing intercellular adherence is sufficient to generate a normal (i.e., parametric) liability curve for endocardial cushion defects that fits a threshold model and predicts a multifactorial pattern of inheritance. Thus, the reduced penetrance and remarkably variable expressivity that characterize a number of presumed autosomal dominant syndromes are possibly reflections of specific probabilistic or stochastic influences that are intrinsic to the embryonic process itself. Future studies may demonstrate that such syndromes arise predictably as a single gene disorder modified by the stochastic laws that govern growth.

Model III shows an etiologically heterogeneous phenotype with a single pathogenetic mechanism (X) or similar pathogenetic mechanisms (X, X₁). Let us deal with the former situation first. Oligohydramnios serves as an example of a single deformational pathogenesis with multiple etiologic factors, resulting in the Potter sequence. Intrauterine compression results in characteristic facial and limb deformities, pulmonary hypoplasia, wrinkled skin, and growth restriction. It may be caused by any condition that leads to oligohydramnios, such as bilateral renal agenesis, cystic dysplasia, severe polycystic disease of the kidneys, urinary tract obstruction, or amniotic leakage. Obstructive uropathy as a cause of oligohydramnios has several possible sites for obstruction, particularly in the male because of the more complex development of the male urethra. More extensive malformations may occur in some instances, sirenomelia with Potter facies and upper limb deformities being the most extreme example (see Chapter 2).[19]

Model III also illustrates an etiologically heterogeneous phenotype but with similar pathogenetic mechanisms (X, X₁). The DiGeorge sequence serves as an example; it may occur alone or as part of a broader pattern of abnormalities. Various syndromes and associations have been reported (Table 10-1). The idea has sometimes been expressed that the DiGeorge phenotype represents a contiguous gene syndrome in which del(22q11.2)* is found in some cases and that sporadic and familial cases (that simulate mendelian inheritance) represent undetectable submicroscopic deletions. However, if the syndrome delineation approach is focused on the problem, it is obvious that the DiGeorge sequence has too many known causes† to be reduced to a single chromosomal deletion.

*The acronym CATCH 22 has been used to refer to Cardiac defect, Abnormal facies, Thymic hypoplasia, Cleft palate, and Hypocalcemia, which may occur in variable combinations sometimes with del(22q). Sometimes DiGeorge sequence or velocardiofacial syndrome occur alone. Recent work has attempted to identify responsible genes, e.g., DGCR2/LAN, DGCR3, and IDD.[28]

†Chisaka and Capecchi[10] constructed a mouse model in which homeobox gene hox-1.5 was disrupted, producing hox-1.5/hox-1.5 mice. When the phenotypic findings were analyzed, by George, it looked like DiGeorge! Absent thymus, hypoplastic parathyroids, and cardiac anomalies were found. However, the cardiac anomalies were not of the conotruncal type seen in humans, and, furthermore, the mice had hypoplasia of the thyroid. Finally, the human equivalent of hox-1.5 maps to chromosome 7, not chromosome 22, where del(22q11.2) has been associated with some cases of velocardiofacial syndrome/DiGeorge sequence.

Table 10-1. Some Conditions with DiGeorge Sequence

Chromosomal	Velocardiofacial syndrome
dup(1q)	Zellweger syndrome
del(5p)	
dup(8q)	Teratogenic[b]
del(10p)	Diabetic embryopathy
del(17p)	Fetal alcohol syndrome
del(22q)[2]	Retinoid embryopathy
Mosaic triploidy	
	Associational
Monogenic	Arhinencephaly/DiGeorge sequence[c]
Isolated autosomal dominant[a]	CHARGE/DiGeorge sequence
Isolated autosomal recessive[a]	Hemifacial microsomia/DiGeorge sequence

Modified after Cohen and Cole[21]

[a] May possibly represent the same condition, i.e., an undetectable deletion may simulate mendelian inheritance

[b] Bisdiamine, a drug initially studied as a male contraceptive and not approved for human use in the United States, is known to produce a DiGeorge-like pattern of defects in experimental animals

[c] Inluding Kallmann syndrome

Although unknown at present, the pathogenetic mechanisms resulting from such diverse causes are probably similar (X, X_1) but not identical (X).

Model IV shows etiologically heterogeneous disorders with pathogenetically heterogeneous mechanisms resulting in the same phenotype. Consider holoprosencephaly, for example. The phenotype (P) (i.e., holoprosencephaly) is known to be etiologically heterogeneous (A,B,C) (e.g., may be caused in some cases by an autosomal recessive gene in the homozygous state, in other cases by trisomy 13, and in still other cases by maternal diabetes). Etiologic heterogeneity suggests that the pathogenesis may also be heterogeneous (X,Y,Z) (e.g., may be based on an insult to the prechordal mesoderm in some instances, a slightly later insult to the neural plate in other instances, or an insult producing decreased cellular proliferation of all three germ layers simultaneously in still other instances).[19]

In certain disorders, rapid progress in identification of the biochemical or molecular mechanism leads to identification of heterogeneous etiologic and pathogenetic mechanisms that share key phenotypic features (model V). The peroxisomal disorders serve as a striking example. Rhizomelic chondrodysplasia, neonatal adrenoleukodystrophy, Zellweger syndrome, and infantile Refsum disease are all characterized by generalized peroxisomal dysfunction and, as a result, share a distinctive biochemical phenotype that includes accumulation of very long chain fatty acids, phytanic acid, bile acid intermediates, pipecolic acid, and deficiency of plasmalogen synthesis. However, biochemical and genetic analysis indicates that some of these disorders are etiologically distinct. Moreover, variant forms with normal peroxisomal structure have come to light. Called pseudo-Zellweger syndrome and pseudoneonatal adrenoleukodystrophy, they clearly have an overlapping phenotype, but the peroxisomal defect is more circumscribed and the dysmorphic features are correspondingly milder.[21]

The elucidation of etiologic and pathogenetic mechanisms should be encouraged. Further syndrome delineation, biochemical phenotyping, and, eventually, molecular mapping will no doubt reveal even more etiologic and pathogenetic heterogeneity. A balanced approach includes both elucidation of basic mechanisms *and* the process of syndrome delineation.

SOME EXAMPLES OF ETIOLOGIC AND PATHOGENETIC HETEROGENEITY

We now turn to detailed analyses of the Robin sequence, hemifacial microsomia, and craniosynostosis to illustrate etiologic and pathogenetic heterogeneity.

ROBIN SEQUENCE

Robin sequence consists of micrognathia, cleft palate, and glossoptosis (Fig. 10-3A,B). Pathogenesis is usually thought to be based on a small mandible that prevents normal descent of the tongue. Thus, the tongue interferes with palatal fusion. The mandible is said to exhibit significant catch-up growth in time (Fig. 10-3C,D).

The syndromology perspective on the Robin sequence adds considerably to our understanding of the pathogenesis. Table 10-2 lists some representative syndromes in which Robin sequence may be a feature with variable frequency. The etiology of each condition is different.

In Stickler syndrome, Robin sequence occurs in some instances.[38] Since abnormalities of bones and joints are characteristic, the major pleiotropic effect is on connective tissue. Thus, in this condition, Robin sequence may result from intrinsic mandibular hypoplasia and failure of connective tissue penetration across the palate.[19]

Another condition that may have Robin sequence is dup(11q) syndrome.[6] With the hypoplastic growth that accompanies most chromosomal syndromes, there may not be significant mandibular catch-up growth in patients with dup(11q) syndrome who survive. Therefore, to include such patients in a mandibular growth study of Robin sequence would be to study *fruit*, since *oranges* are being confused with *apples*.[19]

Some instances of Robin sequence have been associated with oligohydramnios. It is thought that reduced amniotic fluid results in compression of the chin against the sternum, restricting mandibular growth and impacting the tongue between the palatal shelves. Because micrognathia is based on intrauterine molding, mandibular catch-up growth is expected after birth when intrauterine deforming forces are no longer acting. Poswillo[80] produced a phenocopy of Robin sequence in rats by puncturing the amnionic sac prior to palatal closure. Some experimental animals also had anomalies of the limbs, ranging from clubfoot to ring constrictions and intrauterine amputations. Such limb abnormalities have also been observed with Robin sequence in humans.

The association of amputations and/or limb reduction defects in some human cases suggests that Robin sequence may occur on a disruptive basis. For example, an amniotic tear may cause oligohydramnios, which can result in severe compressive disruption, causing limb reduction defects, and bands, producing amputations. Such primary disruption with oligohydramnios can also cause secondary deformation, e.g., mandibular constraint, leading to Robin sequence.

Finally, Robin sequence has been associated with congenital hypotonia. If neurogenic hypotonia occurred prior to complete closure of the palate, it is conceivable that Robin sequence might result from lack of mandibular exercise.[19] Thus, Robin sequence is not only etiologically heterogeneous but pathogenetically heterogeneous as well (Fig. 10-4).

Pathogenesis in Robin sequence can be understood at another level, thanks to

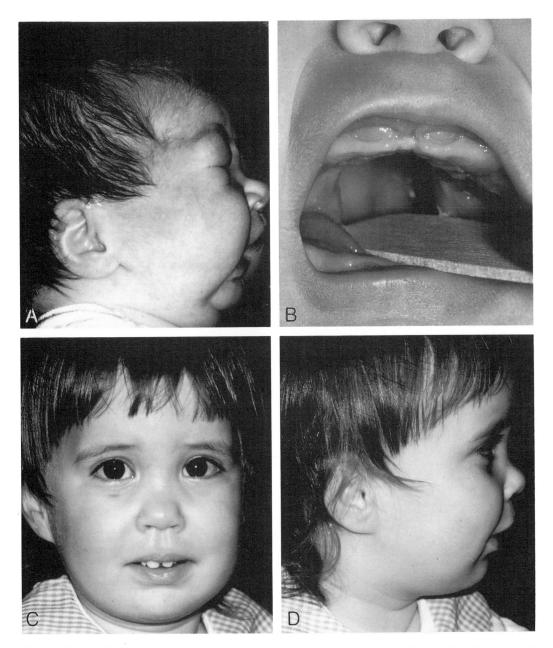

Figure 10-3. A,B: Patient with Robin sequence showing micrognathia and U-shaped cleft palate. C,D: Same patient showing mandibular catch-up growth. From Cohen.[19]

the brilliant work of Shprintzen.[104] Different mechanisms of obstruction found in Robin sequence are listed in Table 10-3. Analysis of the types of obstruction in Stickler syndrome, velocardiofacial syndrome, and mandibulofacial dysostosis are summarized in Table 10-4. Two conclusions are immediately apparent. First, *different mechanisms of obstruction can occur within the same syndrome.* Second, *glossoptosis is not the cause of upper airway obstruction in many cases* (6/11). A number of factors contribute to obstruction in Robin sequence (Table 10-5). In the velocardiofacial syndrome, hypotonia of the pharyngeal muscles is a key finding.[104]

Table 10-2. Some Syndromes with Robin Sequence[a]

Monogenic
  Abruzzo-Erickson syndrome
  Beckwith-Wiedemann syndrome
  Campomelic syndrome
  Carey neuromuscular syndrome
  Catel-Manzke syndrome
  Cerebrocostomandibular syndrome
  Chitayat syndrome
  Congenital myotonic dystrophy
  Diastrophic dysplasia
  Distal arthrogryposis-Robin syndrome
  Donlan syndrome
  Froster contracture-torticollis syndrome
  Mandibulofacial dysostosis
  Miller-Dieker syndrome
  Nager acrofacial dysostosis
  Otopalatodigital syndrome II
  PARC syndrome
  Persistent left superior vena cava syndrome
  Popliteal pterygium syndrome
  Postaxial acrofacial dysostosis
  Radiohumeral synostosis syndrome
  Richieri-Costa syndrome
  Robin-oligodactyly syndrome
  Sanderson-Fraser syndrome

Spondyloepiphyseal dysplasia congenita
Stickler syndrome
Stoll syndrome
Toriello-Carey syndrome
Velocardiofacial syndrome

Chromosomal
  del(4q) syndrome
  del(6q) syndrome
  dup(11q) syndrome

Teratogenically induced
  Fetal alcohol syndrome
  Fetal hydantoin syndrome
  Fetal trimethadione syndrome

Disruption
  Amniotic band disruption

Unknown genesis
  Bruce-Winship syndrome
  CHARGE association
  Femoral dysgenesis–unusual facies syndrome[b]
  Martsolf syndrome
  Möbius sequence
  Robin/amelia association
  Sickle-shaped scapulae and club feet

[a]Based on and modified from Cohen,[18-20] Updated from Shprintzen,[104] Carey et al.,[9] Chitayat et al.,[11] Richieri-Costa et al.,[90] Stoll et al.,[106] Verloes et al.,[118] Bruce and Winship,[7] Schimke et al.,[101] and Cohen.[14a]
[b]Some cases represent infants of diabetic mothers. However, in many cases the cause is unknown.

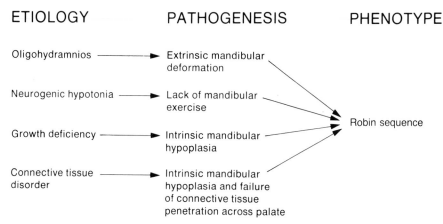

Figure 10-4. Etiologic heterogeneity suggests pathogenetic heterogeneity in the Robin sequence. The following pathogenetic possibilities should be considered. Oligohydramnios results in decreased amniotic fluid, compressing the chin against the sternum and thus restricting mandibular growth. If hypotonia restricts mouth opening during early fetal life prior to complete palatal closure, the Robin sequence might result from lack of mandibular exercise. Growth deficiency, as observed in chromosomal syndromes such as dup(11q) syndrome, may produce the Robin sequence by intrinsic mandibular hypoplasia. In a connective tissue disorder such as the Stickler syndrome, the Robin sequence may result from intrinsic hypoplasia and failure of connective tissue penetration across the palate. From Cohen.[19]

Table 10-3. Types of Obstruction in Robin Sequence

Type	Mechanism
1	True glossoptosis
2	Tongue retracts posteriorly with velum interposed between tongue and posterior pharyngeal wall
3	Medial movement of lateral pharyngeal wall
4	Pharynx constricts in sphincteric manner

Based on Shprintzen[104]

The shape of the mandible and the cranial base angle in three syndromes are summarized in Table 10-6. The velocardiofacial syndrome has a flattened cranial base angle (Fig. 10-5) that does not contribute to pharyngeal obstruction. On the other hand, an acute cranial base angle (flexion of the basicranium), found in both mandibulofacial dysostosis and Stickler syndrome to variable degrees, does contribute to pharyngeal obstruction. Finally, a specific mandibular shape is found in mandibulofacial dysostosis (Fig. 10-6).[5,27]

HEMIFACIAL MICROSOMIA

Hemifacial microsomia is a well-known condition affecting aural, oral, and mandibular growth (Fig. 10-7A,B). The disorder may be mild or severe, and involvement is limited to one side in most cases but bilateral involvement is also known to occur, with more severe expression on one side.[24] The condition overlaps with Goldenhar syndrome (oculoauriculovertebral dysplasia) in which cardiac, renal, and skeletal anomalies may be found. In the so-called expanded Goldenhar syndrome, a wide spectrum of central nervous system malformations has been added. The many terms used for this complex (Table 10-7) emphasize nosologic problems and indicate the wide spectrum of anomalies described by various authors. The confusion is best summed up by the Murphyism "Just because your doctor knows the name of your condition doesn't mean he knows what it is." Surgical treatment, however, is another matter. "Even though your doctor doesn't know what your condition is doesn't mean he can't do something about it."

Table 10-4. Pharyngeal Obstruction Type in Three Syndromes with Robin Sequence[a]

Syndrome	Number of Patients	Pharyngeal Obstruction Type			
		1	2	3	4
Stickler syndrome	6	2	3	0	1
Velocardiofacial syndrome	3	2	0	1	0
Mandibulofacial dysostosis	2	1	0	0	1

Based on Shprintzen[104]

[a]Although sample size is small, heterogeneous obstruction types are evident within the same syndrome. Also, glossoptosis is only responsible for 5 of 11 cases

**Table 10-5. Factors Contributing
to Obstruction in Robin Sequence
(Not Mutually Exclusive)**

Micrognathia (small mandible)

Retrognathia (retropositioned mandible)

Basicranial kyphosis (flexion of basicranium)

Pharyngeal hypotonia

Based on Shprintzen.[104]

The condition is obviously etiologically and pathogenetically heterogeneous. We have reviewed the condition extensively elsewhere,[24] commented on Goldenhar syndrome,[15] and proposed the term *oculoauriculovertebral spectrum.*[24]

A number of chromosomal anomalies have been associated, including del(5p), del(6q), trisomy 7 mosaicism, dup(7q), del(8q), trisomy 9 mosaicism, trisomy 18, trisomy 18 mosaicism, recombinant chromosome 18, ring 21 chromosome, del(22q), 49,XXXXY, 47,XXY, 47XXX, and 49,XXXXX. Some of these associations are meaningful, and some occur coincidentally. Meaningful chromosomal defects are likely to be those karyotypes observed repeatedly. Therefore, del(5q), trisomy 18, and perhaps dup(7q) may be significant associations. X chromosome aneuploidy states noted in several instances have been of different types and may not be significant.[23,34]

Several teratogenic agents have produced oculoauriculovertebral spectrum in humans. The phenotype has been observed in infants of diabetic mothers[35,48] and in infants born to pregnant women exposed to thalidomide,[58,62,96] primidone,[36] and retinoic acid.[54]

Most cases of oculoauriculovertebral spectrum are sporadic, but familial instances have been reported. Affected individuals in successive generations have been observed repeatedly.[33,39,87,93–95,103,109,111,114] The affected mother and daughter with radial limb defects noted by Moeschler and Clarren[64] may represent trisomy 18 mosaicism.[12] Within single families, expression has varied from complete hemifacial microsomia in severely affected individuals, to mild hemifacial microsomia in some relatives, and to simple preauricular tags or a mildly dysplastic ear in others.[24,93,94,112] Vertical transmission of the Goldenhar variant in some family members with lack of ocular involvement in others has been observed.[87,109]

We consider pathogenesis as it applies to hemifacial microsomia *per se.* Poswillo[81,82] reported a phenocopy of hemifacial microsomia in mice following

**Table 10-6. Mandibular Shape and Cranial Base
Angle in Robin Sequence**

Syndrome	Mandibular Shape	Cranial Base Angle Tendancy
Stickler syndrome	Nonspecific	Acute
Velocardiofacial syndrome	Nonspecific	Flat
Mandibulofacial dysostosis	Specific	Acute

Based on Shprintzen[104] and Glander and Cisnero[27]

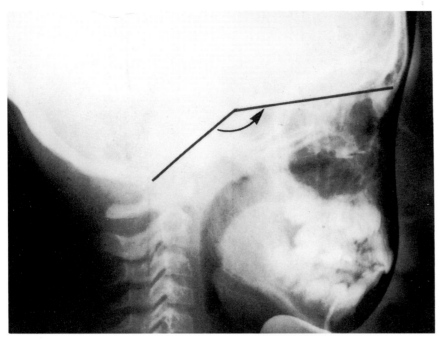

Figure 10-5. Velocardiofacial syndrome. Cephalogram showing flattened (increased) cranial base angle. From Arvystas and Shprintzen.[5]

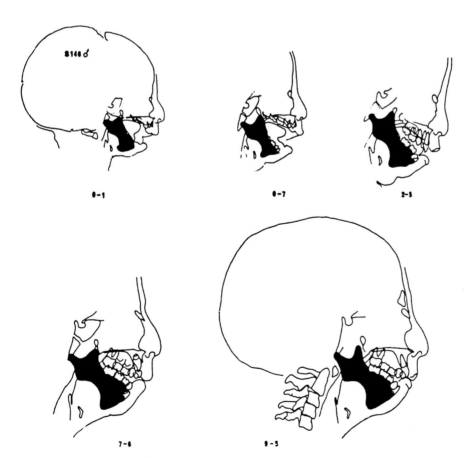

Figure 10-6. Mandibulofacial dysostosis. Serial cephalometric tracings. Note mandibular shape is retained from 1 month of age to 9 years 5 months. Shape persists into adulthood. From Pruzansky.[84]

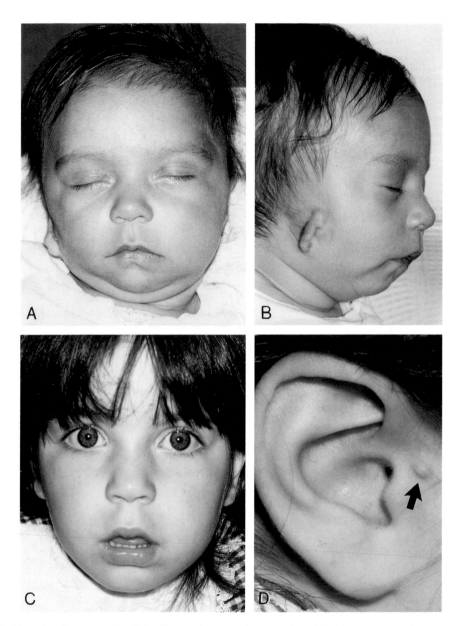

Figure 10-7. A,B: Hemifacial microsomia. C,D: Sister of patient shown in A and B. Note preauricular tag (arrow), representing an accessory auricular hillock. The ear is otherwise normal. From Cohen.[18,19]

maternal administration of triazene and in monkeys following maternal ingestion of thalidomide. He proposed that pathogenesis was based on embryonic
hematoma formation arising from the anastomosis that precedes formation of
the stapedial artery stem. Variation in the severity of hemifacial microsomia was
found to depend on the size and extent of hematoma formation, with large
hematomas interfering more severely with branchial arch growth by taking
longer to resolve than small hematomas.

Some cases of the amniotic band spectrum of disruptions have been noted to
simulate hemifacial microsomia.[37] In such instances, hemifacial microsomia may

Table 10-7. The Varied Nomenclature Applied to Oculoauriculovertebral Spectrum

Hemifacial microsomia	Unilateral craniofacial microsomia
Oculoauriculovertebral dysplasia	Otomandibular dysostosis
Goldenhar syndrome	Oral-mandibular-auricular syndrome
Goldenhar-Gorlin syndrome	Unilateral mandibulofacial dystosis
First arch syndrome	Unilateral intrauterine facial necrosis
First and second branchial arch syndrome	Auriculo-branchiogenic dysplasia
Lateral facial dysplasia	Facio-auriculo-vertebral malformation spectrum
Familial facial dysplasia	Oculoauriculovertebral spectrum

From Cohen et al.[24]

be caused by intrauterine compression secondary to oligohydramnios. Kennedy and Persaud[51] extracted amniotic fluid from pregnant rats at 16 days gestation and studied the embryos at various times thereafter. On histologic examination, hemorrhage and edema were found followed by tissue necrosis in the cartilage and mesenchymal preskeleton of the developing limbs. The observed reduction defects and amputations of the limbs resulted from venous stasis, hypervolemia, and embryonic oxygen deficiency caused by intrauterine compression. Kennedy and Persaud[51] did not give a detailed histologic evaluation of the branchial arch region, but they did note that micrognathia was observed in addition to subcutaneous hemorrhages in the head region. Thus, intrauterine compression might be construed as a possible mechanism for producing hematoma formation in the branchial arch region, thereby resulting in hemifacial microsomia. Because hemifacial microsomia in humans may occur with limb reduction defects in some cases, the association may be compatible with Poswillo's hypothesis. If hemifacial microsomia were to be observed with amniotic band–related limb abnormalities, this would also be compatible with Poswillo's hypothesis.

As previously indicated, hemifacial microsomia is both etiologically and pathogenetically heterogeneous. Hematoma formation itself has heterogeneous causes, including hypoxia, hypertension, pressor agents, salicylates, and anticoagulants.[82] It is also important to recognize that, although embryonic hematoma formation may explain some cases of hemifacial microsomia, it does not explain all cases. For example, in some familial instances, affected relatives may have only preauricular tags (Figs. 10-7C, D, 10-8). It is difficult to conceive of any basic mechanism causing hematoma formation that would explain these cases. In minimally affected individuals, the ear and mandible are well formed, and the preauricular tag seems to represent an accessory auricular hillock, an example of embryonic redundant morphogenesis. To postulate separate pathogenetic mechanisms to explain instances of hemifacial microsomia and accessory ear tags in the same family seems unnecessarily complicated. The most parsimonious hypothesis should take into account that the two pedigrees in Figure 10-8 represent a single entity that is variably expressed and genetically transmitted.

Another example that shows the limitations of the hematoma hypothesis is a true malformation syndrome in which hemifacial microsomia is only one component. The patient shown in Figure 10-9 has hemifacial microsomia, occipital encephalocele, hypoplastic lung, vertebral anomalies, and unilateral renal

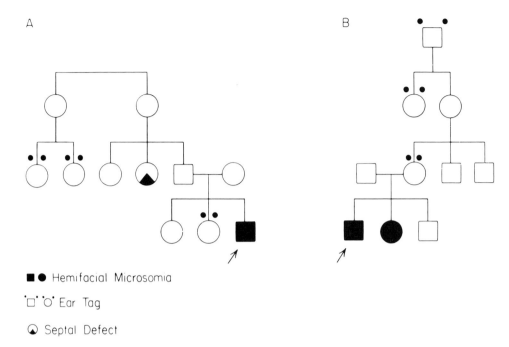

Figure 10-8. Pedigrees with hemifacial microsomia in which minimally affected relatives have only pre-auricular tags. From Cohen.[19]

agenesis. These anomalies most likely have a common cause (although unknown) rather than being caused by different factors acting independently. Whatever mechanism is responsible for one malformation should be responsible for the others. To date, there is no experimental evidence that hematoma formation can cause encephaloceles or renal agenesis. Therefore, it seems unlikely that hematoma formation has anything to do with the pathogenesis of this recurrent pattern syndrome.[19]

Other clinical reports have suggested the possibility of vascular pathogenesis. Gorlin et al.[31] noted that abnormal vascular supply to cephalic neural crest cells could impede embryonic development in the branchial arches. Robinson et al.[92] reported evidence of carotid artery occlusion in two cases. Moore et al.[65] demonstrated absence of the internal carotid artery in a severe case with hemifacial defects and unilateral hydranencephaly. In such cases it is not always clear whether vascular accidents or simply inadequate vascular supply is primary or whether craniofacial hypoplasia is primary, thereby resulting in diminished caliber of the vessels. Soltan and Holmes[105] proposed a hypothesis that links genetic causes and vascular disruption. For five relatives with different malformations usually attributed to vascular accidents (including one possible variant of oculoauriculovertebral spectrum), they suggested an underlying familial vascular anomaly predisposing to vascular accidents and resulting in various malformation complexes.

Various retinoic acid derivatives have been studied for their pathogenetic role in the production of branchial arch anomalies. Using vitamin A palmitate as a teratogen in pregnant rats, Poswillo[81] produced a Treacher Collins–like condition in the newborn rat pups resulting from early destruction of neural crest cells, which normally migrate into the branchial arches during early embryonic life. Sulik et al.,[107,108] using 13-*cis* retinoic acid as a teratogen in pregnant mice,

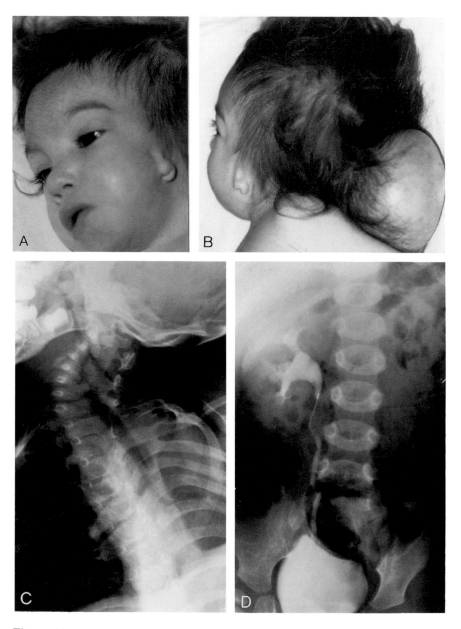

Figure 10-9. Patient with recurrent pattern syndrome consisting of hemifacial microsomia (A), occipital encephalocele (B), hypoplastic left lung, and vertebral anomalies (C), and unilateral renal agenesis (D). From Cohen.[18,19]

also produced a phenotype similar to Treacher Collins syndrome in mouse pups. The effects on first and second branchial arch ectodermal placodal cells following the release of neural crest cells from the neural folds into the developing cranial region were of major significance in the pathogenesis of the anomalies encountered. The fact that retinoic acid derivatives can affect not only the branchial arch region, but also the cardiovascular system, the axial skeleton, and the central nervous system[54,107,108] suggests that these teratogens should be studied further to determine whether an oculoauriculovertebral spectrum animal model can be produced.

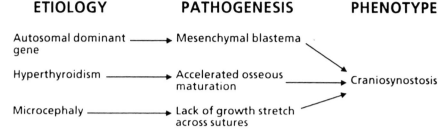

Figure 10-10. Etiologic and pathogenetic heterogeneity of craniosynostosis. From Cohen.[17]

CRANIOSYNOSTOSIS

Craniosynostosis is both etiologically and pathogenetically heterogeneous. It may be caused in some cases by an autosomal dominant gene, in other cases by hyperthyroidism, and in still other cases by microcephaly. The pathogenesis in these cases is heterogeneous (Fig. 10-10); there may be a defect in the mesenchymal blastema, accelerated osseous maturation, or lack of growth stretch across the sutures.* In some cases, there may be a common pathogenesis; microcephaly and low-pressure shunting for hydrocephalus both may occur with craniosynostosis secondary to lack of growth stretch across the sutures. In other cases, the pathogenesis may be similar; craniosynostosis may accompany α-L-iduronidase deficiency and also β-glucuronidase deficiency.[13,17]

Craniosynostosis may occur alone or together with other anomalies making up various syndromes. A great many such syndromes have been delineated to date (see Table 9-4).[17] Although most cases of simple craniosynostosis are sporadic, familial instances have been observed. Autosomal dominant inheritance has been identified most frequently. Some pedigrees have synostosis of a single suture such as the coronal, sagittal, or metopic. However, different sutures may be fused in affected relatives of the same family (Figs. 10-11, 10-12). Some known causes of craniosynostosis are listed in Table 10-8. Topics discussed below include (1) fetal head constraint, (2) lack of growth stretch across sutures, (3) metabolic and hematologic disorders, and (4) molecular mutations.

Fetal Head Constraint

Prenatal head constraint as a cause for some cases of craniosynostosis has received considerable attention. Clinical evidence is suggestive, but more definitive evidence was needed. Koskinen-Moffett and Moffett[51a] were able to demonstrate intrauterine constraint as an experimental cause of craniosynostosis. In a group of pregnant mice, the uterine cervix was closed off with a surgical clip to delay birth for 2 to 3 days, thereby crowding and constraining the growing fetuses. Of the 26 mouse pups from three experimental litters delivered by cesarean section, 91% had deformed bodies and plagiocephaly. The degree of plagiocephaly was greatest in those fetuses located proximally in the uterine horns, where crowding was most severe. Craniosynostosis, confirmed histologically, was found in 88% of the mouse pups, with fusion occurring in the coronal, squamosal, and/or squamosofrontal sutures.

---

*It is maintained by some that growth stretch across the sutures, which results from brain growth itself, keeps the sutures patent. Without significant brain growth, as in microcephaly, the sutures lack growth stretch and may close prematurely.

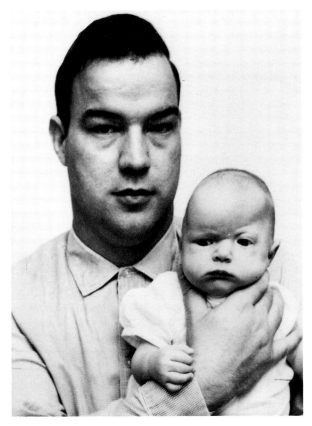

Figure 10-11. Dominantly inherited craniosynostosis. Father has sagittal synostosis. Infant has unilateral coronal synostosis. From Anderson and Geiger.[4]

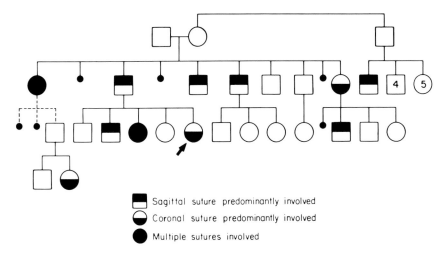

Sagittal suture predominantly involved
Coronal suture predominantly involved
Multiple sutures involved

Figure 10-12. Autosomal dominant inheritance of simple craniosynostosis illustrating variability of sutural fusion. Modified from Herrmann et al.[40]

Table 10-8. Some Conditions with Known Causes of Craniosynostosis

Monogenic	β-Glucuronidase deficiency
Autosomal dominant simple craniosynostosis[a]	Hematologic disorders
Apert syndrome	Thalassemias
Crouzon syndrome	Sickle cell anemia
Pfeiffer syndrome	Congenital hemolytic icterus
Jackson-Weiss syndrome	Polycythemia vera
Boston type craniosynostosis	Teratogens
Saethre-Chotzen syndrome[a]	Aminopterin
Greig cephalopolysyndactyly[a]	Diphenylhydantoin
Chromosomal syndromes	Retinoic acid
Numerous[17]	Valproic acid
Metabolic disorders	Malformations
Hyperthyroidism	Microcephaly
Rickets	Encephalocele
Mucopolysaccharidoses	Shunted hydrocephalus
Hurler syndrome	Holoprosencephaly
Morquio syndrome	

[a]Molecular defect not understood to date. Greig cephalopolysyndactyly was mapped to 7p13 by Vortkamp et al.[119] on the basis of three balanced translocations in different families. The translocation breakpoints disrupted the zinc finger gene GLI3. Saethre-Chotzen syndrome was mapped to 7p21.[8,55,86,88,116] Reid et al.[88] suggested that there may be more than one locus for Saethre-Chotzen syndrome on 7p.

Lack of Growth Stretch Across Sutures

Lack of growth stretch at the sutures may also be implicated in three malformations in which premature craniosynostosis may occur as a complicating feature. First, sutural fusion may accompany some cases of microcephaly. Lack of central nervous system growth may result in lack of growth stretch across the sutural areas, producing secondary craniosynostosis. Second, several reports have linked shunted hydrocephalus to craniosynostosis. Low pressure systems may be implicated, in which growth stretch across the sutural areas suddenly becomes deficient. Finally, some cases of encephalocele have been associated with craniosynostosis. Such *blow-out* lesions may sometimes result in lack of growth stretch across the sutures.[13]

Metabolic and Hematologic Disorders

Premature craniosynostosis may result from several dysmetabolic states. It has been observed to accompany hyperthyroidism during childhood. Sutural fusion may be caused by primary thyroid hyperplasia but more commonly results from excessive thyroxine treatment for congenital hypothyroidism (Fig. 10-13).

Premature sutural fusion also may occur in Hurler syndrome, which is characterized by α-L-iduronidase deficiency. Craniosynostosis involves the sagittal and lambdoid sutures.

Craniosynostosis is observed in various etiologically distinct forms of rickets (Table 10-9). Premature sutural fusion was found in one-third of 59 rachitic children under 9 years of age in a study by Reilly and coworkers.[89] The severity of the rachitic process was not related to the type of rickets but rather to the extent of synostosis, and the more severe cases tended to have more severe degrees of craniosynostosis. The age at which rickets first occurred was also related to the extent of synostosis, the earlier diagnosed cases tending to be

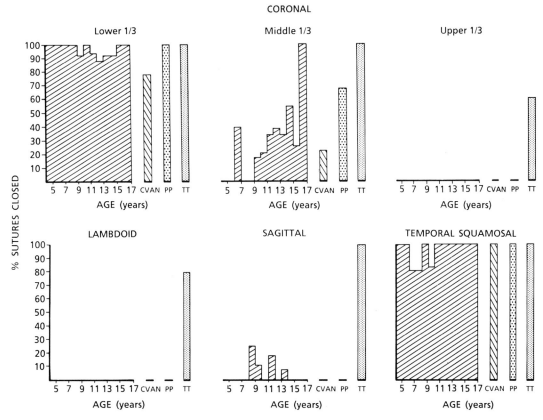

Figure 10-13. Percentage closure of each cranial suture. Control patients separated by age. TT, thyrotox-icosis patients; PP, precocious puberty patients; CVAN, congenital virilizing adrenal hyperplasia patients not separated by age. For control patients, n = 96; for TT patients, n = 10; for PP patients, n = 3; and for CVAN patients, n = 9. From Johnsonbaugh et al.[49]

more severe. Alkaline phosphatase, a reflection of the severity of the rachitic process (with the obvious exception of hypophosphatasia), was significantly re-lated, and higher values were associated with a correspondingly higher incidence of craniosynostosis. No demonstrable relationship was found between syn-ostosis and serum calcium levels or vitamin D intake.

Craniosynostosis may occur in various hematologic disorders. Hyperplasia of the marrow with compensatory bony overgrowth of the calvaria can *lock* the sutures. Conditions known to result in premature fusion of sutures include the thalassemias, sickle cell anemia, congenital hemolytic icterus, and polycythemia vera.[13]

Molecular Mutations

Some of the major craniosynostosis syndromes have been mapped to specific chromosomal locations, the genes identified, and the molecular mutations un-derlying a number of them identified (Table 10-10). To date, fibroblast growth factor receptor mutations have been responsible for most of them and the homeobox gene MSX2 for one of them. Two other syndromes have been mapped to the short arm of chromosome 7, but their genes have not been identified. The current state of knowledge has been reviewed by Cohen.[14,16,16a]

Table 10-9. Craniosynostosis and Rickets

Type of Rickets	Patients Studied	Craniosynostosis		Approximate Proportion Affected
		Present	Absent	
Vitamin D deficiency	16[a]	4	12	1/4
Vitamin D refractory				
Simple hypophosphatemic	14	6	8	1/3
Hypophosphatemic, hypocalcemic, amino-aciduric	5	1	4	1/5
Cystine storage disease	4	0	4	0
Hypophosphatemic, amino-aciduric, cirrhotic	2	1	1	1/2
Renal tubular acidosis	1	0	1	0
Azotemic osteodystrophy	4	1	3	1/4
Hepatic rickets	3	0	3	0
Hypophosphatasia	10	3(+3[b])	4	2/3
Total (all types of rickets)	59	16(+3[b])	40	1/3

From Reilly et al.[89]

[a]An additional 7-month-old male infant with severe vitamin D deficiency rickets had unilateral coronal synostosis that was probably present at birth. It is assumed that the occurrence was coincidental and the case was omitted from the study.

[b]Three very severely affected infants with almost completely uncalcified calvaria died in early infancy.

The field is advancing so rapidly that more mutations will be identified before this book is published.

Among the fibroblast growth factor receptors (FGFRs), mutations for various craniosynostosis syndromes are associated with FGFR1, FGFR2, and FGFR3, but mostly with FGFR2 (Table 10-10, Fig. 10-14). Heterogeneity has been demonstrated for craniosynostosis by genes on different chromosomes (8, 10, and 4 for FGFR1, FGFR2, and FGFR3, respectively; 5 and 7 for other cranio-synostosis syndromes).[8,41,46,56,83,91] There is also heterogeneity shown by mutations in different genes for the same syndrome (FGFR1 and FGFR2 for Pfeiffer syndrome)[67,97,100] and by different amino acid substitutions in the same gene for the same syndrome (e.g., Cys342Ser and Tyr328Cys from exon 9 and Cys278Phe and Gln289Pro from exon 7 in FGFR2, all resulting in Crouzon syndrome).[32,45,86,120] It is also clear that causal homogeneity may lead to phenotypic heterogeneity; a mutation such as Cys342Arg in exon 9 of FGFR2 can result in either Crouzon syndrome or Pfeiffer syndrome,[86,97,100] although both breed true within families.

Several generalizations emerge from the results shown in Table 10-10 and Figure 10-14. First, none of these genetic findings should surprise us. The same principles have been illustrated previously. Genes on different chromosomes have been mapped for tuberous sclerosis (9q33–q34 and 16p13).[50,78] Different amino acid substitutions in the RET proto-oncogene,* such as Cys635Arg in exon 11 and Cys619Ser in exon 10, can both result in MEN 2A.[117] Finally, the same mutation can result in different disorders as shown by the PRNP gene on chromosome 20; an Asp178Asn substitution can result either in one subtype of familial Creutzfeldt-Jakob disease or in familial fatal insomnia.[29]

Second, because Crouzon and Pfeiffer syndromes are etiologically hetero-

*Various mutations in the RET proto-oncogene are responsible for four different phenotypes: medullary thyroid carcinoma, MEN 2A, MEN 2B, and Hirschsprung disease.[117]

geneous, we can expect other mutations for these two syndromes in the future. Even Apert syndrome in which only two adjacent amino acids on FGFR2 (Ser252Trp and Pro253Arg) are involved in 75 of 76 reported cases[75,120] may have other rare mutations in the future.

Third, it can be deduced that Apert syndrome sites are more mutable than Crouzon syndrome sites. The birth prevalences of Apert and Crouzon syndromes are the same (~16/1,000,000),[22,23] but Apert syndrome sites are few in number and Crouzon syndrome sites are many (Table 10-10). Of the two Apert syndrome mutations, Ser252Trp is much more common than Pro253Arg. Of the many known Crouzon syndrome mutations Cys342Arg, Cy342Tyr, and Ala344Ala occur most frequently.

Fourth, most mutations for major craniosynostosis syndromes reported to date have been in the extracellular domain of FGFR2 including Apert syndrome, Crouzon syndrome, Pfeiffer syndrome, and Jackson-Weiss syndrome. Additionally, one mutation for Pfeiffer syndrome has been reported in the extracellular domain of FGFR1 (Table 10-10, Fig. 10-14).

However, the locations of several other mutations for disorders with craniosynostosis are noteworthy. When Crouzon syndrome occurs with acanthosis nigricans, an Ala391Glu substitution has been detected in the transmembrane domain of FGFR3, 11 amino acids away from the most common mutation for achondroplasia.[61b] Two cases of Beare-Stevenson cutis gyrata syndrome have been associated with a Tyr375Cys substitution in the transmembrane domain of FGFR2.[84a] In thanatophoric dysplasia, type II, a Lys560Glu substitution has been detected in the second kinase domain of FGFR3. On the other hand, thanatophoric dysplasia, type I, has been associated with several different mutations— some extracellular and some intracellular—on FGFR3[96a,110] (Table 10-10, Fig. 10-14).

Fifth, it is important to note that laboratory studies have failed to identify many specific mutations. For example, identification of Crouzon syndrome mutations (Table 10-10) has been successful in about 50% of the cases.[61a] At present, many exons of various FGFRs, particularly FGFR2, have yet to be extensively investigated.

Mutations have been identified in the linker region between IgII and IgIII on FGFR1, FGFR2, and FGFR3. The two amino acid substitutions on FGFR2 that result in Apert syndrome are both bulky mutations (Ser252Trp and Pro253Arg). Wilkie et al.[120] proposed that such substitutions may alter the relative orientation of IgII and IgIII, affecting the binding of FGF ligands or dimerization with other FGFRs. The analogous Pro252Arg change, resulting in some cases of Pfeiffer syndrome, is located in the same linker region on FGFR1.[67,100] Interestingly, thanatophoric dysplasia type I is associated with an Arg248Cys substitution in the linker region between IgII and IgIII on FGFR3.[110]

Mutations for Crouzon syndrome involve loss or gain of a cysteine residue in about 25% of cases. Such changes may alter the structure of the IgIII loop, which is maintained by a disulfide bond between two cysteine residues.[74] One common mutation, 1211G→A, does not result in an amino acid substitution (Ala344Ala). However, the mutation produces a cryptic donor splice site, causing a deletion of 17 amino acids and shortening the distance from the disulfide bond of IgIIIc to the transmembrane domain.[57]

Mutations on FGFR2 resulting in Pfeiffer syndrome cluster in one of two locations—the acceptor splice site for exon 9 or a cysteine residue essential for forming the disulfide-bonded loop of IgIII. Splice site mutations may disrupt the regular splicing mechanism of exon 9, and an absent cysteine from position

Table 10-10. Craniosynostosis Syndromes: Chromosome Localizations, Genes, and Molecular Mutations

Syndrome	Phenotype	Chromosome Localization	Gene	Exon/Domain[a]	Nucleotide Change[b]	Amino Acid Substitution
Apert syndrome[c]	Craniosynostosis, symmetric syndactyly of hands and feet, other anomalies	10q25.3-q26	FGFR2	7(U)/Linker:IgII-IgIII	934C→G	Ser252Trp
					937C→G	Pro253Arg
Crouzon syndrome[d]	Craniosynostosis, midface deficiency, ocular proptosis	10q25.3-q26	FGFR2	7(U)/IgIIIa	982insTGG	Thr268ThrGly
					978T→C	Ser267Pro
					1012G→T	Cys278Phe
					1038del	ΔHisIleGln
					CCACATCCA	287–289
					1045A→C	Gln289Pro
					1047T→G	Trp290Gly
					1047T→C	Trp290Arg
				9(B)/IgIIIc	1162A→G	Tyr328Cys
					1191G→C	Gly338Arg
					1197T→C	Tyr340His
					1203T→A	Cys342Ser
					1203T→C	Cys342Arg[e]
					1204G→A	Cys342Tyr[e]
					1204G→T	Cys342Phe
					1205C→G	Cys342Trp
					1210C→G	Ala344Gly[f]
					1211G→A	Ala344Ala[g]
					1219C→G	Ser347Cys
					1240C→G	Ser354Cys

Syndrome	Clinical features	Location	Gene	Exon/Domain	Nucleotide	Amino acid
Pfeiffer syndrome[b]	Craniosynostosis, broad thumbs, broad great toes, other anomalies	8p11.2-p12	FGFR1		755C→G	Pro252Arg
		10q25.3-q26	FGFR2	7(U)/IgIIIa 9(B)/IgIIIc	1012G→T	Cys278Phe[c]
					1141A→C	Asp321Ala
					1200A→C	Thr341Pro
					1203T→C	Cys342Arg[c]
					1203T→A	Cys342Ser[c]
					1204G→A	Cys342Tyr[c]
					1204G→C	Cys342Ser[c]
					1209G→C	Ala344Pro
					1254G→T	Val359Phe
					1263insTCAACA	ΔGly345-Pro361
					Acceptor splice site	
					T(−3)G	Intronic
					A(−2)G	Intronic
					G(+1)T, (1119G→T)	Ala314Ser
Jackson-Weiss syndrome[i]	Tarsal/metatarsal coalitions and, variably, craniosynostosis and broad great toes	10q25.3-q26	FGFR2	7(U)/IgIIIa 9(B)/IgIIIc	1045A→C	Gln289Pro[c]
					1203T→C	Cys342Arg[c]
					1211C→G	Ala344Gly[f]
Beare-Stevenson cutis gyrata syndrome[j]	Cloverleaf or Crouzonoid skull, cutis gyrata, furrowed palms and soles, cutaneous/mucosal tags, prominent umbilical stump	10q25.3-q26	FGFR2	10/IgIII-TM 10/TM	1294C→G	Ser372Cys
					1303A→G	Tyr375Cys

(continued)

Table 10-10. (Continued)

Syndrome	Phenotype	Chromosome Localization	Gene	Exon/Domain[a]	Nucleotide Change[b]	Amino Acid Substitution
Thanatophoric dysplasia[k]		4p16	FGFR3			
	Type I (curved humeri and femora; may have cloverleaf skull)			7/Linker:IgII-IgIII	742C→T	Arg248Cys
					746C→G	Ser249Cys
				9/IgIII-TM	1111A→T	Ser371Cys
				19/C-tail	2458T→G	Stop807Gly
					2458T→A	Stop807Arg
					2460A→T	Stop807Cys
	Type II (straight humeri and femora; cloverleaf skull more commonly found)			17/K2	1948A→G	Lys560Glu
Crouzon syndrome with acanthosis nigricans[l]	Craniofacial dysostosis, acanthosis nigricans	4p16	FGFR3	10/TM	1172C→A	Ala391Glu
Craniosynostosis, Boston type[m]	Fronto-orbital recession or frontal bossing or turribrachycephaly or cloverleaf skull	5qter	MSX2	2	64C→A	Pro7His
Craniosynostosis, Adelaide type[n]	Craniosynostosis, short stature, mental deficiency, hypoplastic middle and terminal phalanges in fingers	4p16	FGFR3? MSX1?			

| Saethre-Chotzen syndrome[o] | Craniosynostosis, characteristic facial appearance, brachydactyly other anomalies | 7p21 | |
| Greig cephalopoly-syndactyly[p] | Hypertelorism, polydactyly, craniosynostosis in 5% | 7p13 | GLI3[q] |

From Cohen.[16]

[a]FGFR2 exon numbers are based on Givol and Yayon[26] and exon letters in parentheses are based on Miki et al.[63] Linker:IgII-IgIII = linker region between IgII and IgIII. IgIIIa = first half of IgIII. IgIIIc = alternatively spliced second half of IgIII (most common form and transcripts highly expressed in mesenchyme). TM = transmembrane domain. K2 = second kinase domain. C-tail = carboxy-terminal tail.

[b]Numbering of nucleotides is based on FGFR2 cDNA sequence reported by Dionne et al. [1990] and used by Wilkie et al. [1995]. The original numbers are based on the sequence reported by Houssaint et al.[43] and used by Reardon et al.[86] and Rutland et al.[97]. To use the cDNA sequence numbers, add 167 to the original numbers.

[c]Wilkie et al.,[120] Park et al.[75]

[d]Preston et al.,[80] Li et al.,[56] Reardon et al.,[86] Jabs et al.,[45] Park et al.,[74] Malcolm and Reardon,[59] Gorry et al.,[32] Oldridge et al.,[72] Meyers et al.[61a]

[e]Cys342Arg has been found in Crouzon, Pfeiffer, and Jackson-Weiss syndromes. Cys278Phe, Cys342Tyr, and Cys342Ser have all been found in both Crouzon and Pfeiffer syndromes. Gln289Pro has been found in both Crouzon and Jackson-Weiss syndromes. However, families of Crouzon, Pfeiffer, and Jackson-Weiss syndromes each breed true for their respective phenotypes.

[f]Ala344Gly has been found in one Jackson-Weiss family [Jabs et al.[45]] and also in one Crouzon family [Gorry et al.[32]]. Ala344Gly in the Jackson-Weiss family [Jabs et al.[45]] has been misprinted as Arg344Gly and also as Ala342Gly [Jabs[44]]. The first of these misprints also appears as a misprint in Mulvihill.[69]

[g]Ala344 Ala obviously does not involve an amino acid change, but the G→A transition creates a donor splice site, causing a 17 amino acid deletion [Li et al.].[57]

[h]Robin et al.,[91] Muenke et al.,[67] Schell et al.,[100] Rutland et al.,[97] Lajeunie et al.,[53] Meyers et al.[61a]

[i]Jabs et al.,[45] Park et al.,[74] Meyers et al.[61a]

[j]Przylepa et al.,[84a]

[k]Tavormina et al.,[110] Rousseau et al.[96c]

[l]Meyers et al.[61b]

[m]Müller et al.,[68] Jabs et al.[46]

[n]Hollway et al.[47]

[o]Brueton et al.,[8] Reardon et al.,[85] Reid et al.,[88] Lewanda et al.,[55] van Herwerden et al.[116]

[p]Vortkamp et al.[119]

[q]Translocation breakpoints through GLI3.

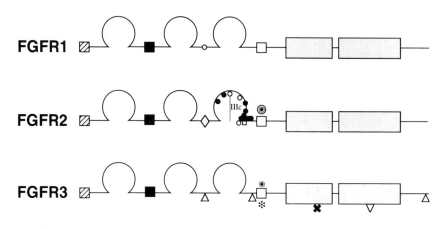

◊ Apert syndrome
○ Pfeiffer syndrome
● Crouzon syndrome
▫ Jackson-Weiss syndrome
◎ Beare-Stevenson cutis
   gyrata syndrome

△ Thanatophoric dysplasia, Type I
▽ Thanatophoric dysplasia, Type II
✳ Achondroplasia
✖ Hypochondroplasia
⊚ Crouzon syndrome with
   acanthosis nigricans

Figure 10-14. Most mutations for major craniosynostosis syndromes are on FGFR2 with only one known mutation on FGFR1. Note mutations for short limb skeletal dysplasias (achondroplasia, hypochondroplasia, thanatophoric dysplasia, type I, and thanatophoric dysplasia, type II) on FGFR3. Fibroblast growth factor receptors 1, 2, 3. Hatched squares, signal peptide; solid squares, acid box; open squares, transmembrane domain; dotted oblongs, kinase domains 1 and 2. Three loops from left to right are immunoglobulin-like domains (IgI, IgII, IgIII). IIIc is an alternatively spliced form of the second half of IgIII. From Cohen.[16]

342 may alter the IgIII loop. Both types of mutations may affect ligand binding or dimerization.[100]

    Stop codon FGFR3 mutations in thanatophoric dysplasia type I (Table 10-10) result in a receptor elongated by 141 amino acids, producing a hydrophobic domain in the C-tail. Such a hydrophobic region could act as a second transmembrane domain and affect either dimerization or kinase activity.[96a]

    It is clear from Table 10-10 and from Figure 10-14 that, particularly with respect to Crouzon and Pfeiffer syndromes, there are many more mutations than there are developmental pathways for craniosynostotic syndrome phenotypes. Thus, heterogeneous mutations for the same phenotype must be ca-

Table 10-11. WTP Family of Genes

WTP1	Christopher Robin
WTP2	Winnie-the-Pooh
WTP3	Piglet
WTP4	Eeyore
WTP5	Rabbit
WTP6	Kanga
WTP7	Baby Roo
WTP8	Owl
WTP9	Tigger

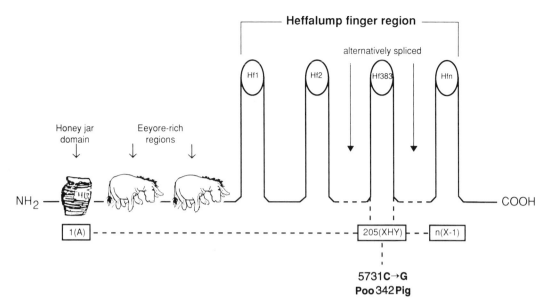

Figure 10-15. WTP4, the Eeyore gene; see Table 10-11. Note Poo342Pig, a Piglet substitution for a highly conserved Pooh resulting from a C→G transversion at nucleotide 5731. Note also alternatively spliced heffalump fingers. In this instance, the alternatively spliced form containing the mutation is exon 205, or XHY in the alternative nomenclature system. With alternative splicing there may be as few as 4 heffalump fingers or as many as 53; the last exon is n(X-1).

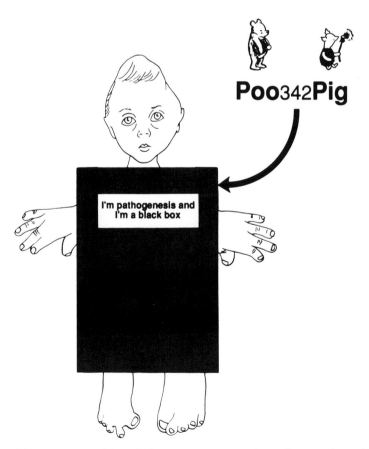

Figure 10-16. Although the mutation Poo342Pig is known, the pathogenesis of the syndrome is still a mystery.

nalized during development. An earlier concept of a single mutation resulting in a single disease is outmoded. On the other hand, the same mutation producing different phenotypes that breed true, such as Cys342Arg, which may result in either Crouzon syndrome or Pfeiffer syndrome, suggests the possibility of interaction with other gene products or of other alterations within the same gene.

Mutations identified on FGFRs may be located extracellularly, affecting ligand binding, or intracellularly, affecting activation of the signaling pathway. Almost all nucleotide changes are of the missense or splice-site type. Occasionally, insertions[61a] and deletions[72] are reported (Table 10-10).

FGFR mutations (Table 10-10) cannot be loss-of-function mutations because chromosomal deletions [del(8p), del(10q), del(4p)] that result in multiple anomalies do not include craniosynostosis.[8] Thus, such mutations are of the altered function or gain-of-function type. Study of the mutation for craniosynostosis of the Boston type in transgenic mice (Msx2Pro7His) suggests a gain-of-function mutation.[58a]

All human mutations on FGFRs known to date allow early human development to proceed normally but interfere with later development, particularly bone. When mesenchyme is converted to bone, the molecular cross-talk is highly complex and only partially understood. Much work remains to be done in unraveling the pathogenesis of these phenotypes. The idea that these molecular mutations might *explain* these craniosynostosis syndromes can best be understood by considering the WTP family of genes (Table 10-11) cloned in our laboratories. The primary structure of WTP4 is shown in Figure 10-15. It will be observed in Figure 10-16 that, even though the molecular mutation is known, the pathogenesis of the syndrome is still a mystery.

REFERENCES

1. Aleksic S, Budzilovich G, Greco MA, Epstein F, Feigin I, Pearson J: Encephalocele (cerebellocele) in the Goldenhar-Gorlin syndrome. *Eur J Pediatr* 140:137–138, 1983.
2. Aleksic S, Budzilovich G, Greco MA, Reuben J, Margolis S: Intracranial lipomas, hydrocephalus and other CNS anomalies in oculoauriculovertebral dysplasia (Goldenhar-Gorlin syndrome). *Childs Brain* 11:285–297, 1984.
3. Aleksic S, Budzilovich G, Reuben R, Lanuna J, McCarthy J, Converse JM, Feigin I: Unilateral arhinencephaly in Goldenhar-Gorlin syndrome. *Dev Med Child Neurol* 17:498–504, 1975.
4. Anderson FM, Geiger L: Craniosynostosis: A survey of 204 cases. *J Neurosurg* 22:229–240, 1965.
5. Arvystas M, Shprintzen RJ: Craniofacial morphology in the velo-cardio-facial syndrome. *J Craniofac Genet Dev Biol* 4:39–45, 1984.
6. Aurias A, Laurent C: Trisomie 11q. Individualisation d'un noveau syndrome. *Ann Génét* 18:189–191, 1975.
7. Bruce A, Winship I: Radial ray defect and Robin sequence: A new syndrome? *Clin Dysmorphol* 2:241–244, 1993.
8. Brueton LA, van Herwerden L, Chotai KA, Winter RM: The mapping of a gene for craniosynostosis: Evidence for linkage of the Saethre-Chotzen syndrome to distal chromosome 7p. *J Med Genet* 29:681–685, 1992.
9. Carey JC, Fineman RM, Ziter FA: The Robin sequence as a consequence of malformation, dysplasia and neuromuscular syndromes. *J Pediatr* 101:353–364, 1982.
10. Chisaka O, Capecchi MR: Regionally restricted developmental defects resulting from targeted disruption of the mouse homeobox gene hox-1.5. *Nature* 350:473–479, 1991.

11. Chitayat D, Meunier CM, Hodgkinson KA, Azouz ME: Robin sequence with facial and digital anomalies in two half-brothers by the same mother. *Am J Med Genet* 40:1167–1172, 1991.

12. Clarren SK, Salk DJ: Chromosome studies in hemifacial microsomia with radial ray defect. *Am J Med Genet* 15:169–170, 1983.

13. Cohen MM Jr: *Craniosynostosis: Diagnosis, Evaluation and Management.* New York: Raven Press, 1986.

14. Cohen MM Jr: Craniosynostoses: Phenotypic/molecular correlations. *Am J Med Genet* 56:334–339, 1995.

14a. Cohen MM Jr: Discussion: Need for velopharyngeal management following palatoplasty: An outcome analysis of syndromic and nonsyndromic patients with Robin sequence. *Plast Reconstr Surg,* in press.

15. Cohen MM Jr: Letter to the Editor: Will the real ophthalmologist please stand up? *Am J Med Genet* 56:425, 1995.

16. Cohen MM Jr: Molecular biology of craniosynostosis with special emphasis on fibroblast growth factor receptors. In Cohen MM Jr, Baum BJ (eds); *Studies in Stomatology and Craniofacial Biology.* IOS Press, Amsterdam 1996.

16a. Cohen MM Jr: Short-limb skeletal dysplasias and craniosynostosis: What do they have in common? *Pediatr Radiol* (in press).

17. Cohen MM Jr: Sutural biology and the correlates of craniosynostosis. *Am J Med Genet* 47:581–616, 1993.

18. Cohen MM Jr: Syndromology's message for craniofacial biology. *J Maxillofacial Surg* 7:89–109, 1979.

19. Cohen MM Jr: *The Child with Multiple Birth Defects.* New York: Raven Press, 1982.

20. Cohen MM Jr: The Robin anomalad—Its nonspecificity and associated syndromes. *J Oral Surg* 34:587–593, 1976.

21. Cohen MM Jr, Cole DEC: Origins of recognizable syndromes; Etiologic and pathogenetic mechanisms and the process of syndrome delineation. *J Pediatr* 115:161–164, 1989.

22. Cohen MM Jr, Kreiborg S: Birth prevalence studies of the Crouzon syndrome: Comparison of direct and indirect methods. *Clin Genet* 41:12–15, 1992.

23. Cohen MM Jr, Kreiborg S, Lammer EJ, Cordero JF, Mastroiacovo P, Erickson JD, Roeper P, Martínez-Frías ML: Birth prevalence study of the Apert syndrome. *Am J Med Genet* 42:655–659, 1992.

24. Cohen MM Jr, Rollnick BR, Kaye CI: Oculoauriculovertebral spectrum: An update critique. *Cleft Palate J* 26:276–286, 1989.

25. Dionne CA, Crumley G, Bellot F, Kaplow JM, Searfoss G, Ruta M, Burgess WH, Jaye M, Schlessinger J: Cloning and expression of two distinct high-affinity receptors cross-reacting with acidic and basic fibroblast growth factors. *EMBO J* 9:2685–2692, 1990.

26. Givol D, Yayon A: Complexity of FGF receptors: Genetic basis for structural diversity and functional specificity. *FASEB J* 6:3362–3369, 1992.

27. Glander K II, Cisneros GJ: Comparison of the craniofacial characteristics of two syndromes associated with the Pierre Robin sequence. *Cleft Palate-Craniofacial J* 29:210–219, 1992.

28. Glover TW: CATCHING a break on 22. *Nature Genet* 10:257–258, 1995.

29. Goldfarb LG, Peterson RB, Tabaton M, Brown P, LeBlanc AC, Montagna P, Cortelli P, Julien J, Vital C, Pendelbury WW, Haltia M, Wills PR, Hauw JJ, McKeever PE, Monari L, Schrank B, Swergold GD, Autilio-Gambetti L, Gajdusek DC, Lugaresi E, Gambetti P: Fatal familial insomnia and familial Creutzfeldt-Jakob disease: Disease phenotype determined by a DNA polymorphism. *Science* 258:806–808, 1992.

30. Goldfischer S, Collins J, Rapin I et al: Pseudo-Zellweger syndrome: Deficiencies in several peroxisomal oxidative activities. *J Pediatr* 108:25–32, 1986.

31. Gorlin RJ, Jue KL, Jacobson NP, Goldschmidt E: Oculoauriculovertebral dysplasia. *J Pediatr* 63:991–999, 1963.

32. Gorry MC, Preston RA, White GJ, Zhang Y, Singhal VK, Losken HW, Parker MG,

Nwokoro NA, Post JC, Ehrlich GD: Crouzon syndrome: Mutations in two spliceoforms of FGFR2 and a common point mutation shared with Jackson-Weiss syndrome. *Hum Mol Genet* 4:1387–1390, 1995.

33. Grabb WC: The first and second branchial arch syndrome. *Plast Reconstr Surg* 36:485–508, 1965.

34. Graham JM Jr, Hixon H, Bacino CA, Daack-Hirsch S, Stadler S, Murray JC: Autosomal dominant transmission of a Goldenhar-like syndrome: Description of a family and report of a sporadic case with a de novo 4;16; 8q24.11 translocation. David W. Smith Workshop on Malformations and Morphogenesis, Tampa, Florida, August 4–9, 1994.

35. Grix A Jr: Malformations in infants of diabetic mothers. *Am J Med Genet* 13:131–137, 1982.

36. Gustavson EE, Chen H: Goldenhar syndrome, anterior encephalocele and aqueductal stenosis following fetal primidone exposure. *Teratology* 32:13–17, 1985.

37. Hall BD: Syndromes and situations simulated by amniotic bands. Paper presented at the Birth Defects Conference, Chicago, Illinois, June 24–27, 1979.

38. Herrmann J, France TD, Spranger JW, Opitz JM, Wiffler C: The Stickler syndrome (hereditary arthroophthalmopathy). *Birth Defects* 11(2)76–103, 1975.

39. Herrmann J, Opitz JM: A dominantly inherited first arch syndrome. *Birth Defects* 5(2):110–112, 1969.

40. Herrmann J, Pallister PD, Opitz JM: Craniosynostosis and craniosynostosis syndromes. *Rocky Mt Med J* 66:45–56, 1959.

41. Hollway GE, Phillips HA, Adès LC, Haan EA, Mulley JC: Localisation of craniosynostosis Adelaide type to 4p16. *Hum Mol Genet* 4:681–683, 1995.

42. Holt SB: *The Genetics of Dermal Ridges.* Springfield, IL: Charles C Thomas, 1968.

43. Houssaint E, Blanquet PR, Champion-Arnaud P, Gesnel MC, Torriglia A, Courtois Y, Breathnach R: Related fibroblast growth factor receptor genes exist in the human genome. *Proc Natl Acad Sci USA* 87:8180–8184, 1990.

44. Jabs EW: Correction: Jackson-Weiss and Crouzon syndromes are allelic with mutations in fibroblast growth factor receptor 2. *Nature Genet* 9:451, 1995.

45. Jabs EW, Li X, Scott AF, Meyers G, Chen W, Eccles M, Mao J, Carnas LR, Jackson CE, Jaye M: Jackson-Weiss and Crouzon syndromes are allelic with mutations in fibroblast growth factor receptor 2. *Nature Genet* 8:275–279, 1994.

46. Jabs EW, Müller U, Li X, Ma L, Luo W, Haworth IS, Klisak I, Sparkes R, Warman ML, Mulliken JB, Snead ML, Maxson R: A mutation in the homeodomain of the human MSX2 gene in a family affected with autosomal dominant craniosynostosis. *Cell* 75:443–450, 1993.

47. Jackson CE, Weiss L, Reynolds WA, Forman TF, Peterson JA: Craniosynostosis, midfacial hypoplasia, and foot abnormalities: An autosomal dominant phenotype in a large Amish kindred. *J Pediatr* 88:963–968, 1976.

48. Johnson JP, Fineman RM: Branchial arch malformations in infants of diabetic mothers: Two case reports and a review. *Am J Med Genet* 13:125–130, 1982.

49. Johnsonbaugh RE, Bryan RN, Hierlwimmer UR, Georges LP: Premature craniosynostosis: A common complication of juvenile thyrotoxicosis. *J Pediatr* 93:181–191, 1978.

50. Kandt RS, Haines JL, Smith M, Northrup H, Gardner RJM, Short MP, Dumars K, Roach ES, Steingold S, Wall S, Blanton SH, Flodman P, Kwiatkowski DJ, Jewell A, Weber JL, Roses AD, Pericak-Vance MA: Linkage of a major gene locus for tuberous sclerosis to a chromosome 16 marker for polycystic kidney disease. *Am J Hum Genet* 51(Suppl):A4, 1992.

51. Kennedy LA, Persaud TVN: Pathogenesis of developmental defects induced in the rat by amniotic sac puncture. *Acta Anat* 97:23–35, 1977.

51a. Koskinen-Moffett L, Moffett BC: Sutures and intrauterine deformation. In Persing JA, Edgerton MT, Jane JA (eds): *Scientific Foundations and Surgical Treatment of Craniosynostosis.* Baltimore: Williams & Wilkins, pp 96–106.

52. Kurnit DM, Layton WM, Matthysee S: Genetics, chance, and morphogenesis. *Am J Hum Genet* 41:979–995, 1987.

53. Lajeunie E, Wei Ma H, Bonaventure J, Munnich A, Le Merrer M, Renier D: FGFR2 mutations in Pfeiffer syndrome. *Nature Genet* 9:108, 1995.

54. Lammer EJ, Chen DT, Hoar RM, Agnish ND, Benke PJ, Braun JT, Curry CJ, Fernhoff PM, Grix AW, Lott IT, Richard JM: Retinoic acid embryopathy. *N Eng J Med* 313:837–841, 1985.

55. Lewanda AF, Cohen MM Jr, Jackson CE, Taylor EW, Li X, Beloff M, Day D, Clarren SK, Ortiz R, Garcia C, Hauselman E, Figueroa A, Wulfsberg E, Wilson M, Warrman ML, Padwa BL, Whiteman DAH, Mulliken JB, Jabs EW: Genetic heterogeneity among craniosynostosis syndromes: Mapping the Saethre-Chotzen syndrome locus between D7S513 and D7S516 and exclusion of Jackson-Weiss and Crouzon loci form 7p. *Genomics* 19:115–119, 1994.

56. Li X, Lewanda AF, Eluma F, Jerald H, Choi H, Alozie I, Proukakis C, Talbot CC Jr, Kolk CV, Jones M, Cunningham M, Clarren SK, Pyeritz R, Weissenbach J, Jackson CE, Jabs EW: Two craniosynostotic syndrome loci, Crouzon and Jackson-Weiss, map to chromosome 10q23–q26. *Genomics* 22:418–424, 1994.

57. Li X, Park W-J, Pyeritz RE, Jabs EW: Effect on splicing of a silent FGFR2 mutation in Crouzon syndrome. *Nature Genet* 9:232–233, 1995.

58. Livingston G: Congenital ear abnormalities due to thalidomide. *Proc R Soc Med* 58:493–497, 1965.

58a. Liu Y-H, Kundu R, Wu L, Luo W, Ignelzi MA, Snead ML, Maxson RE Jr: Premature suture closure and ectopic cranial bone in mice expressing Msx2 transgenes in the developing skull. *Proc Natl Acad Sci USA* 92:6137–6141, 1995.

59. Malcolm S, Reardon W: Fibroblast growth factor receptor 2 and craniosynostosis: The molecular and clinical picture. International Genetic Workshop on Crouzon and Other Craniofacial Disorders, Pittsburgh, Pennsylvania, March 10–11, 1995.

60. McKusick VA: On lumpers and splitters, or the nosology of genetic disease. *Birth Defects* 5(1):23–30, 1969.

61. Melnick M, Myrianthopoulos NC: *External Ear Malformations: Epidemiology, Genetics and Natural History.* New York: Alan R Liss, p 21, 1979.

61a. Meyers GA, Day D, Goldberg R, Daentl DL, Przylepa KA, Abrams LJ, Graham JM Jr, Feingold M, Moeschler JB, Rawnsley E, Scott AF, Jabs EW: FGFR2 exon IIIa and IIIc mutations in Crouzon, Jackson-Weiss, and Pfeiffer syndromes: Evidence for missense changes, insertions, and a deletion due to alternative RNA splicing. *Am J Hum Genet* 58:491–498, 1996.

61b. Meyers GA, Orlow SJ, Munro IR, Przylepa KA, Jabs EW: Fibroblast growth factor receptor 3 (FGFR3) transmembrane mutation in Crouzon syndrome with acanthosis nigricans. *Nature Genet* 11:462–464, 1995.

62. Miehlke A, Partsch CJ: Ohrmissbildung, facialis-und abducenslähmung als syndrom der thalidomidschadigung. *Arch Ohrenheilkd* 181:154–174, 1963.

63. Miki T, Bottaro DP, Fleming TP, Smith CL, Burgess WH, Chan AM-L, Aaronson SA: Determination of ligand-binding specificity by alternative splicing: Two distinct growth factor receptors encoded by a single gene. *Biochemistry* 89:246–250, 1992.

64. Moeschler J, Clarren SK: Familial occurrence of hemifacial microsomia with radial limb defects. *Am J Med Genet* 12:371–375, 1982.

65. Moore CA, Wilroy RS, Tonkin I: Absence of the internal carotid in association with hemifacial defects and unilateral hydranencephaly. Paper presented at the Eighth Annual Workshop on Malformations and Morphogenesis, Greenville, SC, August 15–19, 1987.

66. Moss ML: The pathogenesis of premature cranial synostosis in man. *Acta Anat* 37:351–370, 1959.

67. Muenke M, Schell T, Hehr A, Robin NH, Losken HW, Schinzel A, Pulleyn LJ, Rutland P, Reardon W, Malcolm S, Winter RM: A common mutation in the fibroblast growth factor receptor 1 gene in Pfeiffer syndrome. *Nature Genet* 8:269–273, 1994.

68. Müller U, Warman ML, Mulliken JB, Weber JL: Assignment of a gene locus

involved in craniosynostosis to chromosome 5qter. *Hum Mol Genet* 2:119–122, 1993.

69. Mulvihill JJ: Craniofacial syndromes: No such thing as a single gene disease. *Nature Genet* 9:101–103, 1995.

70. Newman TB: Etiology for ventricular septal defects: An epidemiologic approach. *Pediatrics* 76:741–749, 1985.

71. Nishizuka Y: Protein kinase C and lipid signaling for sustained cellular responses. *FASEB J* 9:484–492, 1995.

72. Oldridge M, Wilkie AOM, Slaney SF, Poole MD, Pulleyn LJ, Rutland P, Hockley AD, Wake MJC, Goldin JH, Winter RM, Reardon W, Malcolm S: Mutations in the third immunoglobulin domain of the fibroblast growth factor receptor-2 gene in Crouzon syndrome. *Hum Mol Genet* 4:1077–1082, 1995.

73. Pagon R, Smith DW, Shepard TH: Urethral obstruction malformation complex: A cause of abdominal muscle deficiency and the "prune belly." *J Pediatr* 96:900–906, 1979.

74. Park W-J, Meyers GA, Li X, Theda C, Day D, Orlow SJ, Jones MC, Jabs EW: Novel FGFR2 mutations in Crouzon and Jackson-Weiss syndromes show allelic heterogeneity and phenotypic variability. *Hum Mol Genet* 4:1229–1233, 1995.

75. Park W-J, Theda C, Maestri NE, Meyers GA, Fryburg JS, Dufresne C, Cohen MM Jr, Jabs EW: Analysis of phenotypic features and FGFR2 mutations in Apert syndrome. *Am J Hum Genet* 57:321–328, 1995.

76. Pauli R, Jung JH, McPherson EW: Goldenhar association and cranial defects. *Am J Med Genet* 15:177–179, 1983.

77. Pawson T: Introduction: Protein kinases. *FASEB J* 8:1112–1113, 1994.

78. Pawson T: Protein modules and signalling networks. *Nature* 373:573–580, 1995.

79. Poll-The BT, Roels F, Ogier H et al: A new peroxisomal disorder with enlarged peroxisomes and a specific deficiency of acyl-CoA oxidase (pseudo-neonatal adrenoleukodystrophy). *Am J Hum Genet* 42:422–434, 1988.

80. Poswillo D: Observations of fetal posture and causal mechanisms of congenital deformity of palate, mandible, and limbs. *J Dent Res* 45:584–596, 1966.

81. Poswillo D: Otomandibular deformity: Pathogenesis as a guide to reconstruction. *J Maxillofac Surg* 2:64–72, 1974.

82. Poswillo D: The pathogenesis of the first and second branchial arch syndrome. *Oral Surg* 35:302–329, 1973.

83. Preston RA, Post JC, Keats BJB, Aston CE, Ferrell RE, Preist J, Nouri N, Losken HW, Morris CA, Hurtt MR, Mulvihill JJ, Ehrlich GD: A gene for Crouzon craniofacial dysostosis maps to the long arm of chromosome 10. *Nature Genet* 7:149–153, 1994.

84. Pruzansky S: Clinical investigation of the experiments of nature. *Oral Surg* 8:62–94, 1973.

84a. Przylepa KA, Paznekas W, Zhang M, Golabi M, Bias W, Bamshad MJ, Carey JC, Hall BD, Stevenson R, Orlow SJ, Cohen MM Jr, Jabs EW (1996): Fibroblast growth factor receptor 2 mutations in Beare-Stevenson cutis gyrata syndrome. *Nature Genet*, 73:492–494, 1996.

85. Reardon W, McManus SP, Summers D, Winter RM: Cytogenetic evidence that the Saethre-Chotzen gene maps to 7p21.2. *Am J Med Genet* 47:633–636, 1993.

86. Reardon W, Winter RM, Rutland P, Pulleyn LJ, Jones BM, Malcolm S: Mutations in the fibroblast growth factor receptor 2 gene cause Crouzon syndrome. *Nature Genet* 8:98–103, 1994.

87. Regenbogen L, Godel V, Goya V, Goodman RM: Further evidence for an autosomal dominant form of oculoauriculovertebral dysplasia. *Clin Genet* 21:161–167, 1982.

88. Reid CS, McMorrow LE, McDonald-McGinn DM, Grace KJ, Ramos FJ, Zackai EH, Cohen MM Jr, Jabs EW: Saethre-Chotzen syndrome with familial translocation at chromosome 7p22. *Am J Med Genet* 47:637–639, 1993.

89. Reilly BJ, Lemming JM, Fraser D: Craniosynostosis in the rachitic spectrum. *J Pediatr* 65:396–405, 1964.

90. Richieri-Costa A, Pereira SCS: Short-stature, Robin sequence, cleft mandible, pre/postaxial hand anomalies, and clubfoot: A new autosomal recessive syndrome. *Am J Med Genet* 42:681–687, 1992.

91. Robin NH, Feldman GJ, Mitchell HF, Lorenz P, Wilroy RS, Zackai EH, Allanson JE, Reich EW, Pfeiffer RA, Clarke LA, Warman ML, Mulliken JB, Brueton LA, Winter RM, Price RA, Gasser DL, Muenke M: Linkage of Pfeiffer syndrome to chromosome 8 centromere and evidence for genetic heterogeneity. *Human Mol Genet* 3:2153–2158, 1994.

92. Robinson LK, Hoyme HE, Edwards DK, Jones KL: The vascular pathogenesis of unilateral craniofacial defects. *J Pediatr* 111:236–239, 1987.

93. Rollnick BR, Kaye CI, Nagatoshi K, Hauck W, Martin AO: Oculoauriculovertebral dysplasia and variants: Phenotypic characteristics of 294 patients. *Am J Med Genet* 26:361–375, 1987.

94. Rollnick BR, Kaye CI: Hemifacial microsomia and variants: Pedigree data. *Am J Med Genet* 15:233–253, 1983.

95. Rollnick BR: Oculoauriculovertebral anomaly: Variability and causal heterogeneity. *Am J Med Genet*(Suppl 1):41–53, 1988.

96. Rosendal TH: Aplasia-hypoplasia of the otic labrynth after thalidomide. *Acta Radiol* 3:225–236, 1965.

96a. Rousseau F, Saugier P, Le Merrer M, Munnich A, Delezoide A-L, Maroteaux P, Bonaventure J, Narcy F, Sanak M: Stop codon FGFR3 mutations in thanatophoric dwarfism type 1. *Nature Genet* 10:11–12, 1995.

97. Rutland P, Pulleyn LJ, Reardon W, Baraitser M, Hayward R, Jones B, Malcolm S, Winter RM, Oldridge M, Slaney SF, Poole MD, Wilkie AOM: Identical mutations in the FGFR2 gene cause both Pfeiffer and Crouzon syndrome phenotypes. *Nature Genet* 9:173–176, 1995.

98. Sampson JR, Janssen LAJ, Sandkuijl LA, and the Tuberous Sclerosis Collaborative Group: Linkage investigation of three putative tuberous sclerosis determining loci on chromosomes 9q, 11q, and 12q. *J Med Genet* 29:861–866, 1992.

99. Sander LM: Fractal growth processes. *Nature* 322:789–793, 1986.

100. Schell U, Hehr A, Feldman GJ, Robin NH, Zackai EH, de Die-Smulders C, Viskochil DH, Stewart JM, Wolff G, Ohashi H, Price RA, Cohen MM Jr, Muenke M: Mutations in FGFR1 and FGFR2 cause familial and sporadic Pfeiffer syndrome. *Hum Mol Genet* 4:323–328, 1995.

101. Schimke RN, Collins DL, Hiebert JM: Congenital nonprogressive myopathy with Möbius and Robin sequence—The Carey-Fineman-Ziter syndrome: A confirmatory report. *Am J Med Genet* 46:721–723, 1993.

102. Schmickel RD: Contiguous gene syndromes. A component of recognizable syndromes. *J Pediatr* 109:231–241, 1986.

103. Setzer ES, Ruiz-Castaneda N, Severn C, Ryden S, Frias JL: Etiologic heterogeneity in the oculoauriculovertebral syndrome. *J Pediatr* 98:88–90, 1981.

104. Shprintzen RJ: Pierre Robin, micrognathia, and airway obstruction: The dependency of treatment on accurate diagnosis. *Angothesiol Clin* 26:64–71, 1988.

105. Soltan HC, Holmes LB: Familial occurrence of malformations possibly attributable to vascular abnormalities. *J Pediatr* 109:112–114, 1986.

106. Stoll C, Kleny J-R, Dott B, Alembik Y, Finck S: Ventricular extrasystoles with syncopal episodes, perodactyly, and Robin sequence in three generations: A new inherited MCA syndrome? *Am J Med Genet* 42:480–486, 1992.

107. Sulik KK, Johnston MC, Smiley SJ, Speight HS, Jarvis BE: Mandibulofacial dysostosis (Treacher Collins syndrome): A new proposal for its pathogenesis. *Am J Med Genet* 27:359–372, 1987.

108. Sulik KK, Smiley SJ, Turvey TA, Speight HS, Johnston MC: Pathogenesis of cleft palate in Treacher Collins, Nager, and Miller syndromes. *Cleft Palate J* 26:209–215, 1989.

109. Summitt R: Familial Goldenhar syndrome. *Birth Defects* 5(2):106–109, 1969.

110. Tavormina PL, Shiang R, Thompson LM, Zhu Y-Z, Wilkin DJ, Lachman RS, Wilcox WR, Rimoin DL, Cohn DH, Wasmuth JJ: Thanatophoric dysplasia

(types I and II) caused by distinct mutations in fibroblast growth factor receptor 3. *Nature Genet* 9:321–328, 1995.

111. Taysi K, Marsh JL, Wise DM: Familial hemifacial microsomia. *Cleft Palate J* 20:47–53, 1983.

112. Tenconi R, Hall BD: Hemifacial microsomia: Phenotypic classification, clinical implications and genetic aspects. In Harvold EP (ed): *Treatment of Hemifacial Microsomia*. New York: Alan R Liss, pp 39–49, 1983.

113. Thomas IT, Smith DW: Oligohydramnios, cause of the non-renal features of Potter's syndrome, including pulmonary hypoplasia. *J Pediatr* 84:811–814, 1974.

114. Thomas P: Goldenhar syndrome and hemifacial microsomia: Observations on three patients. *Eur J Pediatr* 133:287–292, 1980.

115. Ullrich A, Schlessinger J: Signal transduction by receptors with tyrosine kinase activity. *Cell* 61:203–212, 1990.

116. van Herwerden L, Rose CSP, Reardon W, Brueton LA, Weissenbach J, Malcolm S, Winter RM: Evidence for locus heterogeneity in acrocephalosyndactyly: A refined localization for the Saethre-Chotzen syndrome locus on distal chromosome 7p− and exclusion of Jackson-Weiss syndrome from craniosynostosis loci on 7p and 5q. *Am J Hum Genet* 84:669–674, 1994.

117. van Heyningen V: One gene—Four syndromes. *Nature* 367:319–320, 1994.

118. Verloes A, Soyeur-Broux M, Arrese-Estrada J, Piérand-Franchimont C, Dodinval P, Piérand GE: Poikiloderma, alopecia, retrognathia and cleft palate; the PARC syndrome. Is this an undescribed dominantly inherited syndrome? *Dermatologica* 181:142–144, 1990.

119. Vortkamp A, Gessler M, Grzeschik KH: GLI3 zinc finger interrupted by translocations in Greig syndrome families. *Nature* 352:539–540, 1991.

120. Wilkie AOM, Slaney SF, Oldridge M, Poole MD, Ashworth GJ, Hockley AD, Hayward RD, David DJ, Pulleyn LJ, Rutland P, Malcolm S, Winter RM, Reardon W: Apert syndrome results from localized mutations of FGFR2 and is allelic with Crouzon syndrome. *Nature Genet* 9:165–172, 1995.

121. Wilson GN, Barr M Jr: Trisomy 9 mosaicism: Another etiology for the manifestations of Goldenhar syndrome. *J Craniofac Genet Dev Biol* 3:313–315, 1983.

122. Wilson GN, Holmes RD, Hajra AK: Peroxisomal disorders; clinical commentary and future prospects. *Am J Med Genet* 30:771–792, 1988.

123. Wilson GN: Cranial defects in Goldenhar's syndrome. *Am J Med Genet* 14:435–443, 1983.

11

Approach to Syndrome Diagnosis

Because so many syndromes have been described, it is difficult to know or remember all of them except the more common ones. Obviously, the specialist in dysmorphology and medical genetics has the background and experience to know and diagnose many more. In dealing with the patient with multiple anomalies, it is important to avoid gathering useless or redundant information, particularly unnecessary laboratory tests. Economy of activity is the hallmark of a good syndromologist. Books that deal with the art of practicing dysmorphology are available (Table 11-1). A logical approach to any such patient is to narrow the possibilities systematically by first using the least expensive and invasive techniques and by consulting textbooks (Table 11-2) and database systems[4,6a,7a,16,17a,19,19b,31] (Table 11-3) devoted to the subject. If a syndrome can be identified in this way, a rational work-up of the patient can be planned from a description of the syndrome together with the clinical findings of the particular patient in question.

HISTORY

Obtaining a good history is important for all patients with multiple anomalies. The history should include pedigree analysis, maternal and paternal ages at the time of conception, presence or absence of parental consanguinity, number of abortions, and possible maternal exposure to environmental teratogens. A positive family history for the condition in question might indicate a monogenic, contiguous gene or possibly a chromosomal disorder. Advanced maternal age at the time of conception has been associated with trisomic conditions such as Down syndrome, trisomy 18 syndrome, and trisomy 13 syndrome. Advanced paternal age at the time of conception has been associated with new mutations

Table 11-1. Books About Approaches to Dysmorphology

Book	Author
Diagnostic Dysmorphology	Aase[1]
Smith's Recognizable Patterns of Human Deformation	Graham[9]
Smith's Recognizable Patterns of Human Malformation	Jones[10]

for some dominantly inherited conditions such as achondroplasia, Apert syndrome, and Marfan syndrome.[7,13] Parental consanguinity can be a factor in autosomal recessive disorders. A family history of abortion may be associated with X-linked dominant disorders and with chromosomal anomalies in which one parent is a balanced translocation carrier for the condition. Finally, a careful history for possible maternal exposure to environmental teratogens is important. Besides fetal alcohol syndrome, fetal hydantoin syndrome, valproate embryopathy, fetal trimethadione syndrome, warfarin embryopathy, retinoic acid

Table 11-2. Syndromology Textbooks

Authors/editors	Textbooks
Borgaonkar[2]	*Chromosomal Variation in Man: A Catalog of Chromosomal Variants and Anomalies.* Seventh Edition, New York: Wiley-Liss, 1994.
Buyse[3]	*Birth Defects Encyclopedia.* Birth Defects Information Services, Inc. Cambridge, MA: Blackwell Scientific, 1990.
Donnai and Winter[6b]	*Congenital Malformation Syndromes.* London: Chapman and Hall, 1995.
Gorlin, Cohen, and Levin[8]	*Syndromes of the Head and Neck.* Third Edition, New York: Oxford University Press, 1990.
Jones[10]	*Smith's Recognizable Patterns of Human Malformation.* Fifth Edition. Philadelphia: WB Saunders, 1996.
McKusick[15]	*Mendelian Inheritance in Man.* Eleventh Edition, Baltimore: Johns Hopkins University Press, 1994.
Schinzel[18]	*Catalog of Unbalanced Chromosome Aberrations in Man.* Berlin: de Gruyter, 1984.
Shepard[21]	*Catalog of Teratogenic Agents.* Eighth Edition, Baltimore: Johns Hopkins University Press, 1995.
Spranger, Langer, and Wiedemann[23]	*Bone Dysplasias: An Atlas of Constitutional Disorders of Skeletal Development.* Philadelphia: WB Saunders, 1974.
Stevenson, Hall, and Goodman[24]	*Human Malformations and Related Anomalies.* Vol. II. New York: Oxford University Press, 1993
Taybi and Lachman[25]	*Radiology of Syndromes, Metabolic Disorders, and Skeletal Dysplasias.* Fourth Edition. Chicago: Year Book Medical Publishers, 1996
Warkany[28]	*Congenital Malformations: Notes and Comments.* Chicago: Yearbook Medical Publishers, 1971
Wiedemann, Kunze, and Dibbern[29]	*An Atlas of Characteristic Syndromes.* Kent, UK: Wolfe Publishers, 1992
Winter, Knowles, Bieber, and Baraitser[32]	*The Malformed Fetus and Stillborn.* New York: John Wiley & Sons, 1988

Table 11-3. Computerized Database Systems

Systems[a]	Requirements for Use	References
BDIS (Birth Defects Information Services)	Coded anatomic description	Buyse[4]
LDDB (London Dysmorphology Database)	Coded anatomic description	Winter and Baraitser[30a]
POSSUM (Pictures of Standard Syndromes and Undiagnosed Malformations)	Coded anatomic description	Marquet[14a]
SYNDROC	Coded anatomic description	Schorderet[19a]
OMIM (On-Line Mendelian Inheritance in Man)	Key word searching	Schorderet[19]
Human Cytogenetic Database	Chromosomal abnormality or clinical features	Schinzel, Oxford Electronic Publishing[17b]

[a]To help assess possible teratogens, TERIS[26] and REPROTOX[20] are two computerized databases in which both human and animal studies are available.

embryopathy, and abnormalities associated with maternal hyperthermia during pregnancy, other teratogens have been reported such as toluene, misoprostol, and angiotensin-converting enzyme inhibitors (see Chapter 7).

CLINICAL ASSESSMENT

Physical examination should include careful assessment for both major and minor anomalies (see Chapter 3). In the interpretation of clinical findings, allowance should be made for variability in the expression of the condition, for changes in the phenotype with time, and for the ethnic background of the patient. Subjective judgments about clinical features that can be measured such as ocular hypertelorism should be avoided (see Chapter 5). The patient's features should be compared with those of siblings, parents, and other relatives when necessary. Because of the nonspecificity of individual anomalies, it is the *overall pattern of anomalies* that is significant for diagnosis, although an unusual abnormality, such as the pursed lips of the whistling face syndrome (see Fig. 1-4), may be helpful for rapid textbook diagnosis.

With the aid of the patient history and physical examination, the clinician should characterize the overall problem as being of either prenatal or postnatal onset (Fig. 11-1).[11,12] If the problem is of prenatal onset, it is important to decide whether the patient has a single anomaly or multiple anomalies. If the condition is interpreted as a single defect, it is important to decide whether it is a malformation, deformation, or disruption (see Chapter 2) because of differences in prognosis and recurrence rates. Deformations based on intrauterine constraint have a tendency to self-correct to some extent, depending on severity. Deformations tend to have even lower rates of recurrence than single malformations.* Disruptions tend to have negligible recurrence rates. If malfor-

*Although many single malformations can be monogenically inherited, the majority occur sporadically. Thus, the overall recurrence rate tends to be low. Some deformations such as congenital hip dislocation and clubfoot also have low multifactorial recurrence rates. Other types of deformations do not recur (see Chapter 2). Note also that with malformations, deformations, and disruptions we speak of *empiric recurrence rates*, which are commonly interpreted as *true risks*, when in fact they are not.

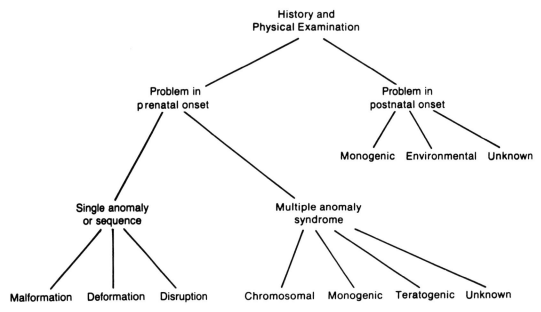

Figure 11-1. An approach to diagnosing patients with structural defects. See text. Modified from Jones and Higginbottom[11] and Jones and Jones.[12]

mations and deformations occur together, it is important to decide if the deformations can be explained as being secondary to the malformations.

If more than one malformation is present, it should be determined whether the anomalies can be reduced to a single malformation sequence or whether two or more embryonically *noncontiguous* malformations or sequences are present, representing a true multiple malformation syndrome. The distinction is important because a single malformation or malformation sequence is more likely to have a low recurrence rate, whereas an unknown multiple malformation syndrome is more likely to represent a discrete entity with a recurrence risk varying from negligible, as in a new mutation for an autosomal dominant disorder, to 25%, as in an autosomal recessive disorder.

If the overall problem is of postnatal onset, the majority of patients appear normal at birth and seem to have thrived *in utero*. Problems of postnatal onset commonly accompany dysmetabolic syndromes, dyshistogenetic syndromes, hamartoneoplastic syndromes, and some neurologic problems (Fig. 11-1). *Although many of these conditions are genetic and, therefore, prenatally determined, the most significant clinical manifestations usually evolve postnatally.* In some dysmetabolic syndromes, manifestations such as cataracts, sparse hair, coarse facial features, unusual skin pigmentation, and hepatosplenomegaly are frequently present. There are an increasing number of dysmorphic syndromes with demonstrable biochemical abnormalities.[*,5] Most involve the synthesis or degradation of macromolecules such as collagen, elastin, fibrillin, bone mineral, proteoglycans, glycoproteins, and triglycerides. Such defects may affect single or multiple enzymes in specific organelles, such as lysosomes or peroxisomes, or there may be a defect affecting hormonal control of synthesis and degradation. Disorders with dysmorphic features and biochemical abnormalities include,

*A reliable biochemical screening test is available for Down syndrome which measures α-fetoprotein, human chorionic gonadotropin, and estriol.[27]

among others, the osteogenesis imperfectas, the Ehlers-Danlos syndromes, Marfan syndrome, and the mucopolysaccharidoses. Investigations that may aid in diagnosing patients who develop coarse facial features are listed in Table 11-4. Investigations useful in delineating peroxisomal disorders are listed in Table 11-5. The Marfan syndrome (dyshistogenetic, 15q21, fibrillin-1 defect) with its evolving ectopia lentis and fusiform and dissecting aneurysms of the aorta, and neurofibromatosis (hamartoneoplastic, 17q11.2, neurofibromin defect) with its progressive tumor formation, evolve their most clinically relevant features during postnatal life, even though both conditions were initiated prenatally at the time of zygote formation. Finally, environmental factors such as trauma, infection, and hypoxia can result in structural defects of postnatal onset. Severe neurologic impairment may lead to progressive joint immobility, abnormal limb positioning, and paralysis.

Provisionally unique pattern syndromes and some of the less well-known recurrent pattern syndromes cannot be found in syndromology textbooks. Nevertheless, it is frequently possible to gain some insight into the nature of syndromes of unknown genesis. The clinician should strive to characterize the unknown condition as essentially dysmetabolic, dyshistogenetic, malformational, or deformational in type (Fig. 11-2). Classifying patients in this manner aids in doing a rational work-up. For example, if an unknown genesis syndrome is *malformational*, amino acid screening is not indicated, but a chromosomal study

Table 11-4. Investigations That May Aid In Diagnosing the Patient Who Develops Coarse Facial Features

Urine
  Glycosaminoglycans
  Oligosaccharides
  N-Aspartylglucosamine
  Sialic acid

Blood
  Thyroid function tests
  White cell histochemistry (vacuoles and metachromatic granules)
  I cell disease screen (e.g., plasma arylsulfatase A)
  White cell enzymes (as indicated by the above results)
    α-L-Iduronidase (Hurler, Scheie)
    Sulfoiduronate sulfatase (Hunter)
    Arylsulfatase B (Maroteaux-Lamy, Austin)
    Heparan N-sulfatase (Sanfilippo A)
    N-Acetyl-α-glucosaminidase (Sanfilippo B)
    Acetyl CoA: α-glucosaminide N-acetyltransferase (Sanfilippo C)
    N-Acetylglucosamine 6-sulfate sulfatase (Sanfilippo D)
    β-Glucuronidase (Sly)
    β-D-Galactosidase A (G_{M1} gangliosidosis, variant Morquio)
    α-Mannosidase (α mannosidosis)
    β-Mannosidase (β mannosidosis)
    α-L-Fucosidase (fucosidosis)
    1-Aspartamido-β-N-acetylglucosamine amidohydrolase
      (aspartylglycosaminuria)
    α-Neuraminidase (sialidosis)

Roentgenograms
  Skeletal survey for dysostosis multiplex

Modified after Clayton and Thompson.[5]

Table 11-5. Investigations Used to Delineate the Nature of a Peroxisomopathy

Demonstration of reduced numbers of peroxisomes
  Electron microscopy of liver biopsy
  Histochemistry of liver biopsy (staining for catalase activity)
  Fibroblast catalase latency test (release of catalase using digitonin)

Peroxisome morphology
  Electron microscopy of liver biopsy

Demonstration of impaired peroxisomal β-oxidation
  Plasma very long chain fatty acids (VLCFA)
  C27 bile acids in bile plasma or urine
  Fibroblast oxidation of ^{14}C-VLCFA

Localization of defect in peroxisomal β-oxidation
  Absence of peroxisomal β-oxidation protein in liver
    (immunoblotting)
  Fibroblast acyl-CoA oxidase activity
  C27 bile acid pattern

Demonstration of impaired plasmalogen synthesis
  Erythrocyte plasmalogens
  Fibroblast/platelet dihydroxyacetonephosphate acyltransferase
  Fibroblast de novo plasmalogen synthesis (hexadecanol
    incorporation into plasmalogens)

Demonstration of other biochemical abnormalities
  Plasma phytanic acid
  Oxidation of phytanic acid by fibroblasts
  Urinary pipecolic acid
  Hepatic D-amino acid oxidase activity
  Hepatic L-α-hydroxy acid oxidase activity
  Urinary organic acids

Modified after Clayton and Thompson.[5]

is.* If the patient has no malformations of the embryonic type, was normal at birth, and shows progressive deterioration with time for which no cause can be established, the patient most likely has a dysmetabolic syndrome.

If the overall condition can be characterized as dysmetabolic, dyshistogenetic, malformational, or deformational, then some cautious predictions can be made about the clinical course, growth, and recurrence risk. Figure 11-2 shows the triangular diagram of Chapter 8 modified to predict some features of unknown genesis syndromes. It has already been noted that malformational and deformational problems tend to be of prenatal onset, but that the most significant manifestations of dysmetabolic and dyshistogenetic syndromes tend to be of postnatal onset. The clinical course of most extrinsically caused deformations may improve with time once the fetus is out of the intrauterine constraining environment. Malformation syndromes tend to remain static, while dyshistogenetic and dysmetabolic syndromes tend to be progressive.

Many patients with multiple malformations may have growth deficiency of prenatal onset, in which case the infant is small for gestational age. If this type of growth deficiency is regarded as a malformation, that is, as hypoplasia of the whole individual, it is not surprising that other malformations, especially those of incomplete morphogenesis, frequently accompany the growth deficiency.

---

*In a study of 1,224 patients with severe mental retardation, Kaveggia et al.[14] found that 45% had single central nervous system malformations or malformation syndromes. Amino acid screening did not reveal a single biochemical abnormality in over 600 patients (see Chapter 13).

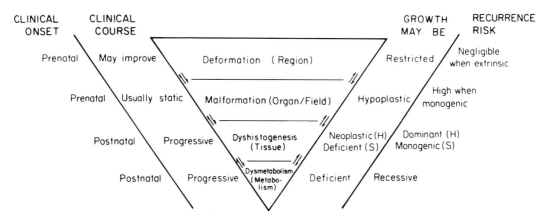

Figure 11-2. Triangular diagram modified to predict some features of unknown genesis syndromes. H, hamartoplastic type of dyshistogenetic syndrome; S, simple type of dyshistogenetic syndrome. See text. From Cohen.[6]

Organ formation and developmental placement are susceptible to malformation if hypoplasia occurs during the period of rapid differentiation and growth. Endocrine studies and various other tests for humorally mediated growth deficiency are generally contraindicated in pure malformation syndromes. Such growth deficiency usually persists into postnatal life.[22]

When growth deficiency accompanies one or more deformations, it is usually caused by intrauterine compression or uteroplacental insufficiency. Endocrine studies for humorally mediated growth deficiency are contraindicated. Catch-up growth is generally expected following birth once the fetus is no longer compressed within the uterus.[9]

Most deformations are extrinsically caused and have negligible recurrence risks.* The recurrence risk for an unknown malformation syndrome could be high if the condition is monogenic. After a chromosomal aberration is ruled out, a sporadically occurring, unrecognized malformation syndrome has a recurrence risk varying from negligible, based on a new mutation for an autosomal dominant disorder, to 25%, predicated on autosomal recessive inheritance.† Since most of the hamartoplastic syndromes are dominantly inherited, it is probable that an unrecognized hamartoplastic condition has a similar recurrence risk. Most known, simple dyshistogenetic syndromes are monogenic, but some occur only sporadically. The same is probably true for an unrecognized, simple dyshistogenetic syndrome. For an unrecognized, sporadically occurring dysmetabolic syndrome, the recurrence risk for future affected offspring should be 25%, since known dysmetabolic syndromes are recessive.

DIAGNOSIS: DEFINITIVE, PROBABLE, POSSIBLE, OR UNKNOWN

The best possible outcome of a dysmorphology examination is to establish a definitive diagnosis. In some instances, diagnosis may be probable, possible,

---

*A few intrinsically caused deformities such as some generalized types of arthrogryposis are monogenic.

†The risk could be as high as 50% if one parent has the same unrecognized syndrome, or a 25% risk with greater certainty if there are affected siblings.

deferred, or unknown. For probable or possible diagnoses several options may be available.

First, a number of formerly equivocal diagnoses now have established laboratory tests to rule in or rule out a particular disorder. A typical example is the Smith-Lemli-Opitz syndrome. Although diagnosis of a classic case presents no problem, many patients have abnormalities that *affect the same systems but do not have the classic phenotype.* Recently, the Smith-Lemli-Opitz syndrome was shown to have a defect in the conversion of 7-dehydrocholesterol to cholesterol. Diagnosis can be established by measuring elevated 7-dehydrocholesterol.[17]

Second, many syndromes have been mapped to specific chromosome locations by molecular techniques,[30] and, in a number of these, specific mutations are known. For example, hypochondroplasia can be difficult to diagnose in young children, but many instances can be confirmed at the molecular level (see Table 12-3).

Third, some phenotypes evolve with time, such as Proteus syndrome, and periodic reevaluation of a patient with a possible diagnosis may have a definitive diagnosis with time. Fourth, for a patient with a possible diagnosis or an unknown diagnosis with distinctive manifestations, consultation with other dysmorphologists by correspondence may be helpful.

Finally, in a number of instances, diagnosis has to be deferred because the syndrome is unknown and remains unknown even after consultation. Not having a specific diagnosis can be distressing to the family, but assigning an erroneous diagnosis can have negative prognostic and treatment implications. Also undoing a diagnosis or reassigning another diagnosis at a later time can be difficult for the family. It is much better to tell the family that no specific diagnosis can be made at present. Treatment, such as physical therapy and surgical repair, can be directed to specific problems even without an overall diagnosis.

SOME HYPOTHETICAL PROBLEMS IN SYNDROME DIAGNOSIS

Figure 11-3 diagrams various problems that arise in syndrome diagnosis. The rectangle, parallelogram, and trapezoid represent three different syndromes—specifically, the phenotypic spectra or boundaries of syndromes X, Y, and Z, respectively. The cross-hatched areas represent the phenotypic features of various patients.

In Figure 11-3A, the patient has enough features of syndrome X to make the diagnosis with certainty. For example, if a patient has nevoid basal cell carcinomas, jaw cysts, macrocephaly, ocular hypertelorism, bifid ribs, and shortened fourth metacarpals, a diagnosis of the nevoid basal cell carcinoma syndrome is assured. In Figure 11-3B, fewer features are present, but the diagnosis is still assured. For example, if a patient has all of the previously mentioned features except nevoid basal cell carcinomas, a diagnosis of the nevoid basal cell carcinoma syndrome can still be made with assurance. As shown in Figure 11-3C, if a patient has ocular hypertelorism and bifid ribs, a diagnosis of the nevoid basal cell carcinoma syndrome cannot be made with any assurance. Diagnosis could be made with more certainty if another family member were definitely known to be affected with syndrome X. For example, if one parent is known to have the nevoid basal cell carcinoma syndrome with certainty, diagnosis of the condition in an offspring who has only ocular hypertelorism and bifid ribs is much more

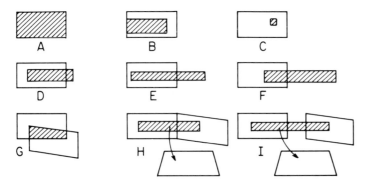

Figure 11-3. Diagram of various problems that arise in syndrome diagnosis. The rectangle, parellelogram, and trapezoid represent three different syndromes, specifically the phenotypic spectra or boundaries of syndromes X, Y, and Z respectively. Cross-hatched areas represent the phenotypic features of various patients. See text.

likely. It is highly probable that such a child will go on to develop other features of the syndrome such as jaw cysts, bridging of the sella turcica, and nevoid basal cell carcinomas.

In Figure 11-3D, most of the features of syndrome X are present, but an additional feature, not previously reported, is present. Suppose an infant has craniosynostosis, short clinodactylous fingers, preaxial polydactyly of the feet, ventricular septal defect, and cleft lip. This overall pattern of anomalies is diagnostic of Carpenter syndrome. All of the features have been reported previously as components of the syndrome except cleft lip, which may possibly represent a low frequency anomaly of the condition, or it might occur by chance.

In Figure 11-3E,F, only some features of syndrome X are present, but because several other features are at variance with the condition, a diagnosis of syndrome X cannot be made. If a patient has microcephaly, mental deficiency, downslanting palpebral fissures, beaked nose with the nasal septum extending below the alae, and short stature—all features compatible with the Rubinstein-Taybi syndrome—but, in addition, has webbed neck, omphalocele, radial aplasia, and lacks broad thumbs and broad great toes, the patient cannot be diagnosed as having the Rubinstein-Taybi syndrome.

In Figure 11-3G, several features are present that are shared by two different syndromes. A clear-cut diagnosis of either syndrome X or syndrome Y cannot be made. A patient with obesity, hypogenitalism, and postaxial polydactyly serves as an example. These features may be observed in both Bardet-Biedl syndrome and Biemond syndrome II. If the patient has retinitis pigmentosa in addition, a diagnosis of Bardet-Biedl syndrome can be made, but if the patient has iris colobomas and hypospadias in addition, a diagnosis of Biemond syndrome II can be made.[28]

In Figure 11-3H,I, the patient has some features of syndrome X and some features of syndrome Y. In Figure 11-3I, there are some additional features that are not found in either syndrome X or syndrome Y. Although both syndromes enter into the differential diagnosis, the patient cannot be said to have either syndrome. It is probably best to propose a new entity—provisionally unique pattern syndrome Z.

For example, if a patient has coronal synostosis, hypertelorism, cleft palate, fusion of C2–C3 and C5–C6, preaxial polydactyly of the fingers, radioulnar synostosis, and a ventricular septal defect, the differential diagnosis includes Greig cephalopolysyndactyly (hypertelorism and polysyndactyly) and Berant syndrome (craniosynostosis and radioulnar synostosis). However, most patients with Greig cephalopolysyndactyly have syndactyly of the feet, which the patient does not have. In the autosomal dominant Berant syndrome, synostosis involves the sagittal suture, resulting in scaphocephaly, which the patient does not have. Furthermore, since neither syndrome is associated with cleft palate, fusion of C2–C3 and C5–C6, and a ventricular septal defect, which the patient does have, it is best to postulate a newly recognized syndrome.

REFERENCES

1. Aase JM: *Diagnostic Dysmorphology*. New York: Plenum Medical, 1990.
2. Borgaonkar DS: *Chromosomal Variation in Man: A Catalog of Chromosomal Variants and Anomalies*. Seventh Edition, New York: Wiley-Liss, 1994.
3. Buyse ML: *Birth Defects Encyclopedia*. Center for Birth Defects Information Services, Inc. Cambridge, MA: Blackwell Scientific, 1990.
4. Buyse M: Center for Birth Defects Information Services. *Birth Defects* 16(5):83, 1980.
5. Clayton PT, Thompson E: Dysmorphic syndromes with demonstrable biochemical abnormalities. *J Med Genet* 25:463–472, 1988.
6. Cohen MM Jr: *The Child with Multiple Birth Defects*. New York: Raven Press, 1982.
6a. DiLiberti JH: Use of computers in dysmorphology. *J Med Genet* 25:445–453, 1989.
6b. Donnai D, Winter R: *Congenital Malformation Syndromes*. London: Chapman and Hall, 1995.
7. Erickson JD, Cohen MM Jr: A study of parental age effects on the occurrence of fresh mutations for the Apert syndrome. *Ann Hum Genet (Lond)*, 38:89–96, 1974.
7a. Evans CD: Computer systems in dysmorphology. *Clin Dysmorphol* 4:185–201, 1995.
8. Gorlin RJ, Cohen MM Jr, Levin S: *Syndromes of the Head and Neck*. Third Edition, New York: Oxford University Press, 1990.
9. Graham JM Jr: *Smith's Recognizable Patterns of Human Deformation*. Third Edition, Philadelphia: WB Saunders, 1996.
10. Jones KL: *Smith's Recognizable Patterns of Human Malformation*. Fifth Edition, Philadelphia: WB Saunders, 1996.
11. Jones KL, Higginbottom MC: Dysmorphology: An approach to diagnosing children with structural defects of the head and neck. *Head Neck Surg* 1:35–46, 1978.
12. Jones KL, Jones MC: A clinical approach to the dysmorphic child. In Emery AE, Rimoin DL (eds): *Principles and Practice of Medical Genetics*. Vol. 1. Edinburgh: Churchill Livingstone, pp 215–224, 1990.
13. Jones KL, Smith DW, Harvey MAS, Hall BD, Quan L: Older paternal age and fresh gene mutation: Data on additional disorders. *J Pediatr* 86:84–88, 1975.
14. Kaveggia EG, Durkin MV, Pendleton E, Opitz JM: Diagnostic/genetic studies on 1,224 patients with severe mental retardation. In *Proceedings of the Third Congress of the International Association for the Scientific Study of Mental Deficiency*. Warsaw: Polish Medical Publishers, pp 82–93, 1975.
14a. Marquet C: *P.O.S.S.U.M. User's Manual*. Fourth Edition, Melbourne: C.P. Expert Pty Ltd., 1991.
15. McKusick VA: *Mendelian Inheritance in Man*. Eleventh Edition. Baltimore: Johns Hopkins University Press, 1994.
16. Murdoch Institute: POSSUM Newsletter. September 1987.
17. Opitz JM: RSH ("Smith-Lemli-Opitz") syndrome as paradigmatic metabolic malformation syndrome. Fourth International Workshop on Fetal Genetic Pathology, Kruger National Park, South Africa, March 31–April 2, 1995.

17a. Pelz J, Arendt V, Kunze J: Computer assisted diagnosis of malformation syndromes: An evaluation of three databases (LDDB, POSSUM, and SYNDROC). *Am J Med Genet* 63:257–267, 1996.

17b. Schinzel A: Human Cytogenetic Database, Oxford University Press, Walton Street, Oxford, UK, OX2 6DP.

18. Schinzel A: *A Catalog of Unbalanced Chromosome Aberrations in Man.* Berlin: de Gruyter, 1984.

19. Schorderet DF: Using OMIM (On Line *Mendelian Inheritance in Man*) as an expert system in medical genetics. *Am J Med Genet* 39:278–284, 1991.

19a. Schorderet DF: *Diagnosing Human Malformation Patterns with SYNDROC. User's Manual,* Version 4.3, 1992.

19b. Schorderet D, Aebischer P: SYNDROC: Microcomputer based differential diagnosis of malformation patterns. *Arch Dis Child* 60:248–251, 1985.

20. Scialli AR: Data availability in reproductive and developmental toxicology. *Obstet Gynecol* 83:652–656, 1994.

21. Shepard TH: *Catalog of Teratogenic Agents.* Seventh Edition. Baltimore: Johns Hopkins University Press, 1992.

22. Smith DW: Growth deficiency: A new classification into primary cellular growth deficiency and secondary humoral growth deficiency. *South Med J* 64(Suppl):5–15, 1971.

23. Spranger JW, Langer LO, Wiedemann HR: *Bone Dysplasias.* Philadelphia: WB Saunders, 1974.

24. Stevenson RE, Hall JG, Goodman RM: *Human Malformations and Related Anomalies.* Vol II. New York: Oxford University Press, 1993.

25. Taybi R, Lachman RS: *Radiology of Syndromes, Metabolic Disorders, and Skeletal Dysplasias.* Fourth Edition. Chicago: Year Book Publishers, 1996.

26. TERIS (Teratogen Information System), c/o Dr. Janina E. Poliska, TERIS WJ-10, Department of Pediatrics, University of Washington, Seattle WA 98195.

27. Wald NJ, Kennaud A, Densem JW, Cuckle HS, Chard T, Butler L: Antenatal maternal screening for Down's syndrome: Results of a demonstration project. BMJ 305:391–394, 1992.

28. Warkany, J: *Congenital Malformations: Notes and Comments.* Chicago: Yearbook Medical Publishers, 1971.

29. Wiedemann H-R, Kunze J, Dibbern H: *An Atlas of Characteristic Syndromes.* Kent, UK: Wolfe Publishers, Inc., 1992.

30. Wilkie AOM, Amberger JS, McKusick VA: A gene map of congenital malformations. *J Med Genet* 31:507–517, 1994.

30a. Winter RM, Baraitser M: *London Dysmorphology Database.* Oxford: Oxford University Press, 1990.

31. Winter RM, Baraitser M, Douglas JM: A computerized data base for the diagnosis of rare dysmorphic syndromes. *J Med Genet* 21:121, 1984.

32. Winter RM, Knowles SAS, Bieber FR, Baraitser M: *The Malformed Fetus and Stillborn.* New York: John Wiley & Sons, 1988.

12

Dysmorphic Growth and Development

Many syndromes exhibit dysmorphic growth and development. The subject is considered in this chapter under the following headings: Growth deficiency; Overgrowth; Asymmetry; Radiologic Assessment in Dysmorphology; and Changes in Craniofacial Dysmorphism with Time.

GROWTH DEFICIENCY

Individuals with growth deficiency can be separated into three distinct categories: normal variants, prenatal-onset growth deficiency, and postnatal-onset growth deficiency. In prenatal-onset growth deficiency, the infant is small for gestational age. Such deficiency may be primary, as in some malformation syndromes and some chondrodysplasias, or secondary, as in deformational growth deficiency, prenatal infectious disease, and teratogenic growth deficiency.[65] A classification of short stature[57] is illustrated in Figure 12-1.

A major subtype is primary growth deficiency associated with both major and minor malformations. If prenatal-onset growth deficiency is regarded as a malformation—that is, as hypoplasia of the whole individual—it is not surprising that other malformations, especially those of incomplete morphogenesis, frequently accompany the growth deficiency.[65] Organ formation and developmental placement are susceptible to malformation if hypoplasia occurs during the period of rapid differentiation and growth. For example, trisomy 18 syndrome, characterized by growth deficiency of prenatal onset, also has many anomalies of organ formation, developmental placement, and insufficient growth such as microcephaly, short palpebral fissures, low-set hypoplastic ears, micrognathia, microstomia, short sternum, and ventricular septal defect. In

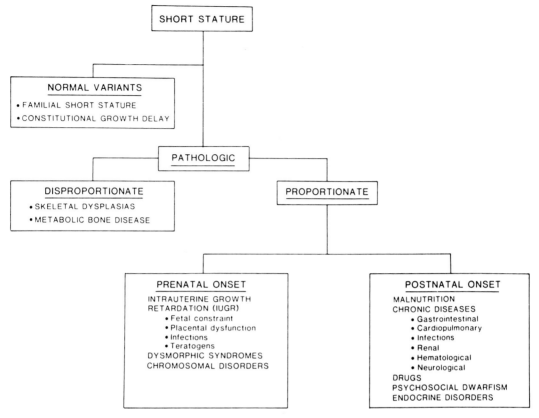

Figure 12-1. Classification of short stature. From Rimoin and Graham.[57]

Figure 12-2, growth deficiency is plotted for nine patients with de Lange syndrome (Figure 12-3), showing that in some malformation syndromes growth deficiency of prenatal onset tends to persist into postnatal life.

An expected consequence of a primary growth deficiency syndrome is that cell cultures from affected individuals should manifest the growth defect. Preliminary evidence for some disorders indicates that growth of cultured fibroblasts from trisomies 18 and 13 patients is slower than that from normal individuals (Table 12-1).[48]

GROWTH RESTRICTION

Deformational growth deficiency may be associated with deformities such as plagiocephaly and clubfoot. Since both growth deficiency and its associated deformities are caused by intrauterine constraint, catch-up growth is expected during postnatal growth once the fetus is out of the constraining intrauterine environment. Thus, *growth restriction* is a more appropriate term than growth deficiency.

OSTEOCHONDRODYSPLASIAS

The osteochondrodysplasias comprise a heterogeneous group of disorders involving abnormalities of bone or cartilage or both. Some, such as achondropla-

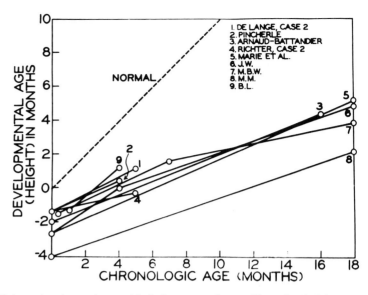

Figure 12-2. Primary growth deficiency in nine patients with de Lange syndrome. Plotted as height age. From Smith.[65]

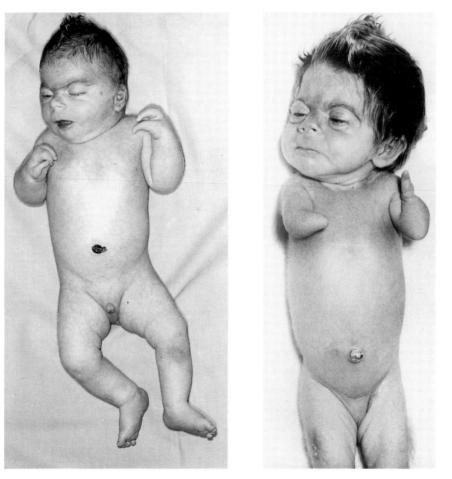

Figure 12-3. de Lange syndrome. Growth deficiency and hypoplastic limbs. Left, courtesy of M. Silverman, Atlanta, Georgia. Right, courtesy of R.W. Smithells, Leeds, England.

Table 12-1. Preliminary Study of *in vitro*
Fibroblast Doubling Time in Some Primary
Growth Deficiency Disorders

Condition	No. of Cases	Approximate Doubling Time
Trisomy 18 syndrome	3	40 h
Trisomy 13 syndrome	2	Slow
Rothmund-Thomson syndrome	1	41 h
Seckel syndrome	1	35 h
Normal controls	12	27 h

From Pious et al.[48]

Not all growth deficiency syndromes studied manifest slow fibroblast
growth. For example, cultures from del(4p) and Silver-Russell syndromes
did not differ significantly from normal growth.

sia and diastrophic dysplasia, are identifiable at birth. Others, such as hypochondroplasia, are not recognizable until childhood. Still others have an
impressive group of associated malformations. For example, in Majewski syndrome,[67] short limbs and narrow thorax occur together with polysyndactyly,
short flat nose, cleft lip or palate, low-set malformed ears, hypoplastic epiglottis,
transposition of the great vessels, renal cysts, and anomalies of the internal and
external genitalia.

Some Definitions

A distinction is usually made between chondrodysplasias and chondrodystrophies. A *chondrodysplasia* is a generalized disturbance of bone modeling, such as
in achondroplasia. A *chondrodystrophy* is a disturbance affecting various systems
including bone, such as in Hurler syndrome. A *dysostosis* is a malformation of
individual bones either singly or in combination. A good example is mandibulofacial dysostosis in which absence or hypoplasia of the zygomatic arches
occurs (see Fig. 4-12). A term frequently found in the literature, *cleidocranial
dysostosis*, is inappropriate because bone involvement is more generalized, affecting the clavicles, calvaria, pelvis, and phalanges. Thus, the term *cleidocranial
dysplasia* has been recommended.

Classification

The International Working Group on Constitutional Diseases of Bone based its
revised version[37] exclusively on radiodiagnostic criteria, grouping morphologi-
cally similar disorders (Table 12-2; Figs. 12-4 to 12-8). The mode of inheritance
is known for most of them. The histology of the growth plates has been studied
in a number of osteochondrodysplasias.[56] Many have been mapped to specific
chromosomal regions. In some, the gene and the defective protein have been
identified. Rapid advances in molecular biology (Table 12-3) will soon permit an
etiologic classification of the osteochondrodysplasias.

Disproportionate Short Stature

In disproportionate short stature, various discrepancies between limb length
and trunk length occur (Figs. 12-4 to 12-6).[56,57] In some conditions such as

Table 12-2. Abbreviated International Classification of Osteochondrodysplasias (1992)

Type of Osteochondrodysplasia	Example
Defects of tubular (and flat) bones and/or axial skeleton	
Achondroplasia group	Achondroplasia, hypochondroplasia, thanatophoric dysplasia (2 types)
Achondrogenesis	Several types
Spondylodysplastic group	Several types
Metatrophic dysplasia group	Metatropic dysplasia
Short rib dysplasia group	Short rib-polydactyly (type I Saldino-Noonan, type II Majewski), asphyxiating thoracic dysplasia, Ellis-van Creveld dysplasia
Atelosteogenesis/diastrophic dysplasia group	Atelosteogenesis (2 types), diastrophic dysplasia
Kniest-Stickler dysplasia group	Kniest dysplasia, Stickler dysplasia, dyssegmental dysplasia (2 types)
Spondyloepiphyseal dysplasia congenita group	Spondyloepiphyseal dysplasia congenita
Other spondylo epi-(meta)-physeal dysplasias	Pseudochondroplasia, Dyggve-Melchior-Clausen dysplasia
Dysostosis multiplex group	Mucopolysaccharidoses, mucolipidoses
Spondylometaphyseal dysplasias	Spondylometaphyseal dysplasia (Kozlowski type)
Epiphyseal dysplasias	Multiple epiphyseal dysplasia (Fairbanks/Ribbing)
Chondrodysplasia punctata (stippled epiphyses) group	Rhizomelic type, Conradi-Hünermann type
Metaphyseal dysplasias	Jansen type, Schmid type
Brachyrachia (short spine dysplasia)	Several types
Mesomelic dysplasias	Dyschondrosteosis, Robinow type
Acro/acromesomelic dysplasias	Geleophysic dysplasia, acrodysostosis, acromesomelic dysplasia
Dysplasias with significant (but not exclusive) membrane bone involvement	Cleidocranial dysplasia, Melnick-Needles osteodysplasty
Bent bone dysplasia group	Campomelic dysplasia, kyphomelic dysplasia
Multiple dislocations with dysplasias	Larsen syndrome
Osteodysplastic primordial dwarfism group	Several types
Dysplasias with decreased bone density	Osteogenesis imperfecta (several types, many mutations)
Dysplasias with defective mineralization	Hypophosphatasia, hypophosphatemic rickets
Dysplasias with increased bone density	Pycnodysostosis, craniometaphyseal dysplasia, craniodiaphyseal dysplasia, Lenz-Majewski dysplasia
Disorganized development of cartilaginous and fibrous components of skeleton	Multiple cartilaginous exostoses, osteoglophonic dysplasia
Idiopathic osteolyses	
Predominantly phalangeal	Hajdu-Cheney type
Predominantly carpal/tarsal	François syndrome
Multicentric	Mandibulo-acral dysplasia
Other	Familial expansile osteolysis

From International Classification of Osteochondrodysplasias.[37]

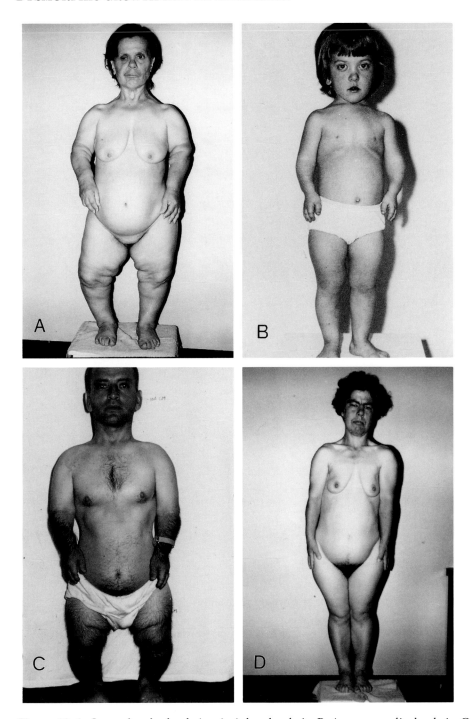

Figure 12-4. Some chondrodysplasias. A: Achondroplasia. B: Acromesomelic dysplasia. Courtesy of J.G. Hall, Vancouver, British Columbia. C: Pseudoachondroplasia (spondyloepiphyseal dysplasia of the pseudoachondroplastic type). D: Hypochondroplasia.

achondroplasia, limb length is shortened but trunk length is relatively normal. Depending on which segment is primarily shortened, a limb may be rhizomelic (short proximal segments, e.g., humerus and femur) as in achondroplasia, mesomelic (short middle segments, e.g., radius, ulna, tibia, and fibula) as in Ellis-van Creveld syndrome, or acromelic (short distal segments, e.g., metacarpals and

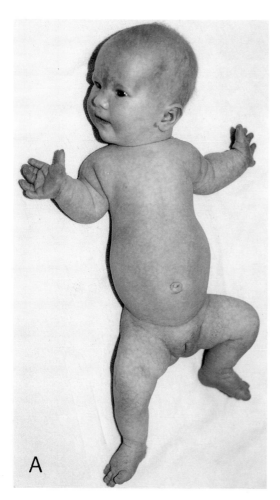
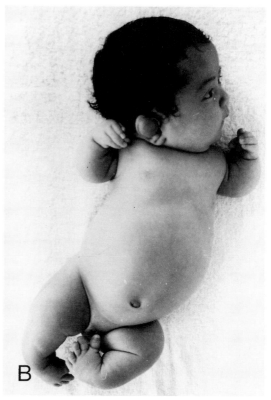

Figure 12-5. Some chondrodysplasias. A: Ellis-van Creveld syndrome. From Smith.[66] B: Diastrophic dysplasia. Courtesy of C. Gonzales, São Paulo, Brazil.

phalanges) as in peripheral dysostosis. Some chondrodysplasias have an impressive combination of alterations as in acromesomelic dysplasia[40] in which the forearms and hands are both short. In other conditions such as Morquio syndrome, trunk length is short and limb length is relatively normal.

Diagnosis

Clinical findings, radiographic findings, and family history are interpreted together (Table 12-4). Frequently, definitive diagnosis is radiographic and, increasingly, molecular. Prenatal diagnosis is possible in some of the osteochondrodysplasias and is radiographic and/or molecular.

OVERGROWTH

Normal newborns above 4,000 g whose mothers are not diabetic or prediabetic account for approximately 5% of all newborns. Features associated with new-

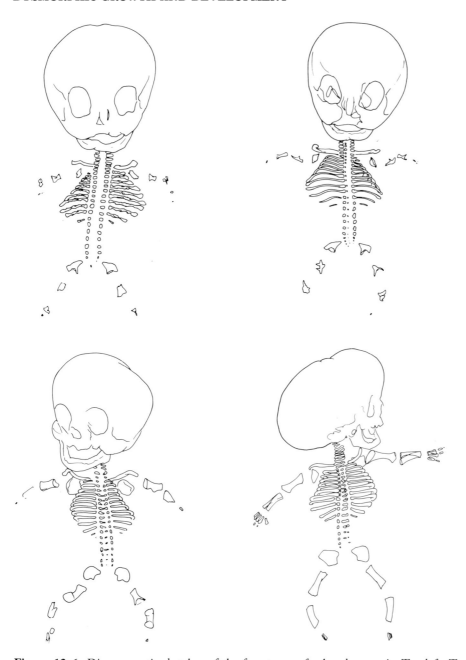

Figure 12-6. Diagrammatic sketches of the four types of achondrogenesis. Top left: Type 1 (Houston-Harris). Top right: Type II (Fraccaro). Bottom left: Type III (Langer-Saldino). Bottom right: Type IV (hypochondrogenesis). From Whitley and Gorlin.[76]

born macrosomia include genetic predisposition of the fetus, sex of the fetus, prepregnancy weight, weight gain during pregnancy, maternal age, population, and socioeconomic level.[7]

Overgrowth syndromes tend to have several characteristics in common. Although birth weight is often excessive, some infants may be of normal weight or even small for gestational age. In some instances, accelerated growth resulting in macrosomia occurs during the first year of life. Beckwith-Wiedemann syn-

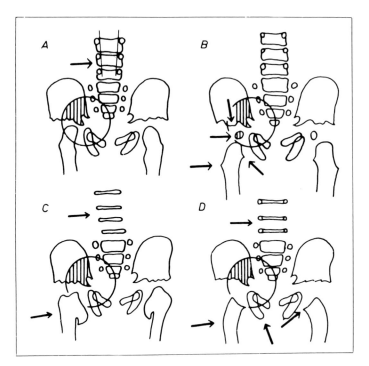

Figure 12-7. Schematic drawings of pelvic features of achondroplasia (A), Ellis-van Creveld syndrome (B), metatropic dysplasia (C), and thanatophoric dysplasia (D). Malformation of the acetabulum is nearly the same in the four conditions. In achondroplasia, interpediculate distances diminish downward. In Ellis-van Creveld syndrome, ossification centers of femur and spike-like exostoses at the trochanters are present. In metatropic dysplasia, reduced height of vertebral bodies, unusual form of the femur, and, occasionally, scoliosis are observed. In thanatophoric dysplasia, vertebral bodies are flat, and spike-like exostoses are present at the os pubis and the femur. The femur is also bowed. From Gefferth.[29]

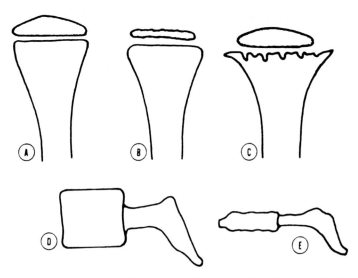

Figure 12-8. Classification of chondrodysplasias based on radiologic involvement of long bones (A,B,C) and vertebrae (D,E). A + D, normal; B + D, epiphyseal dysplasia; C + D, metaphyseal dysplasia; B + E, spondyloepiphyseal dysplasia; C + E, spondylometaphyseal dysplasia. From Rimoin and Horton.[57]

Table 12-3. Mutations of Short Limb Skeletal Dysplasias on Fibroblast Growth Factor Receptor 3

Phenotype	Nucleotide Change	Amino Acid Substitution	Comment
Achondroplasia[a]	1138G→A	Gly380Arg	Most common
	1138G→C	Gly380Arg	
	1125G→T	Gly375Cys	
	1037G→A	Gly346Glu	
Hypochondroplasia[b]	1620C→A	Asn540Lys	Two-thirds of cases
	1620C→G	Asn540Lys	One-third of cases
Thanatophoric dysplasia[c]			
Type I (curved humeri and femora, variably cloverleaf skull)	742C→T	Arg248Cys	Most common
	746C→G	Ser249Cys	
	1111A→T	Ser371Cys	
	2458T→G	Stop807Gly	
	2458T→A	Stop807Arg	
	2460A→T	Stop807Cys	
Type II (straight humeri and femora, cloverleaf skull)	1948A→G	Lys560Glu	All cases to date

From Cohen.[14]

[a]Bellus et al.,[3] Shiang et al.,[64] Superti-Furga et al.,[68] Prinos et al.[51]

[b]Bellus et al.[4] G. Bellus, personal communication, 1995.

[c]Tavormina et al.,[69] Rousseau et al.[60]

drome (Figs. 12-9 to 12-11), Proteus syndrome, and Sotos syndrome (Fig. 12-12) are examples. Anomalies and mental deficiency are frequently associated. Finally, some of these syndromes have a predilection for neoplasia (Fig. 12-11). Overgrowth syndromes have been extensively reviewed by Cohen[6,7,16] and Weksberg et al.,[74] and classifications have been proposed by Cohen[6] and Weaver.[73]

Overgrowth may result from (1) hyperplasia, (2) hypertrophy, (3) an increase in the interstitium (most commonly excessive fluid as in fetal hydrops), or (4) some combination of these.[6,7,16] In overgrowth syndromes, excessive cellular proliferation predominates and can be demonstrated or inferred to have occurred. An expected consequence of a primary overgrowth syndrome is that cell cultures from affected individuals should manifest the growth excess. Preliminary evidence from one disorder—Elejalde syndrome—indicates that cultured fibroblasts complete the whole cell cycle in 63% of the normal cell cycle time (Figs. 12-13, 12-14).[21]

Neoplasia and Overgrowth

That overgrowth syndromes are associated with neoplasia is not surprising, since rapidly dividing cells are a prerequisite for both processes. Mitotic activity, so pronounced during intrauterine life, becomes even more exaggerated in overgrowth syndromes. With respect to neoplasia, cells are most vulnerable to structural changes in DNA, disrupted transcription to RNA, and altered translation into protein–enzyme synthesis during mitotic activity.

The association of increased body size and neoplasia has been documented a number of times. Irving[38] reported that children who developed Wilms tumor tended to have higher birth weight. In an extensive study, Wertelecki and

Table 12-4. Key Clinical Features of Selected Osteochondrodysplasias

	Achondroplasia	Hypochondroplasia	Pseudoachondroplasia	Multiple Epiphyseal Dysplasia	Spondyloepiphyseal Dysplasia Tarda	Metaphyseal Dysplasias
Short at birth	Yes	Usually not	No	No	No	Usually not
Onset of decreased growth velocity	Infancy	Early childhood	Early childhood	Late childhood	Preadolescence	Early childhood
Short limbs	Yes; rhizomelic	Yes; rhizomelic	Yes; later in onset	Mild	No	Subtle to marked
Skin redundancy	Yes	Variable	No	No	No	No
Macrocephaly	Yes	Sometimes	No	No	No	No
Joint hypermobility	Yes; particularly hips and knees	Mild or absent	Yes; particularly wrists and hands	No	No	Variable
Upper:lower segment ratio	↑	↑	↑	Normal	→	Variable
Inheritance	Autosomal dominant	Autosomal dominant	Autosomal dominant (↑ gonadal mosaicism)	Autosomal dominant (usually)	X-linked recessive	Various

From Pauli.[45]

Table 12-5. Relationship of Overgrowth Syndromes to Neoplasia

Condition	Reported Neoplasms	Number Reported Patients	Infant Mortality
Diabetic macrosomia	No	Many	
Infant giants	No	Few	Increased
Beckwith-Wiedemann syndrome	Yes	Many	
Hemihyperplasia (hemihypertrophy)	Yes	Many	
Sotos syndrome	Yes	Many	
Nevo syndrome	No	Few	
Bannayan-Riley-Ruvalcaba syndrome	Yes	Some	
Weaver syndrome	Yes?[a]	Some	
Marshall-Smith syndrome	No	Few	50%
Elejalde syndrome	No	Few	All stillborn to date
Simpson-Golabi-Behmel syndrome	Yes	Many	
Proteus syndrome	Yes	Many	

From Cohen.[7]

[a]Two presumed cases possibly may be associated with neuroblastoma.

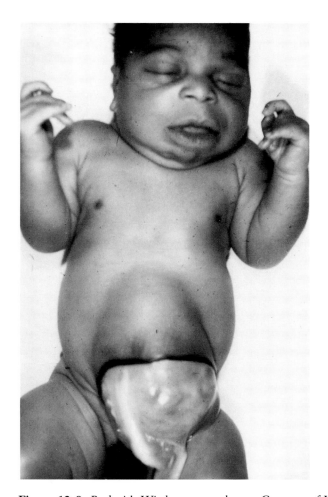

Figure 12-9. Beckwith-Wiedemann syndrome. Courtesy of J.B. Beckwith, Loma Linda, California.

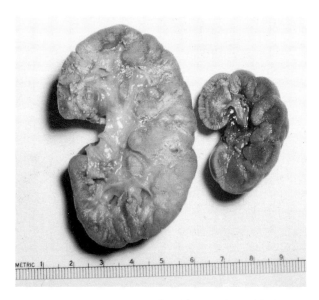

Figure 12-10. Enlarged kidney from Beckwith-Wiedemann case compared with normal-sized kidney at birth. Courtesy of J.B. Beckwith, Loma Linda, California.

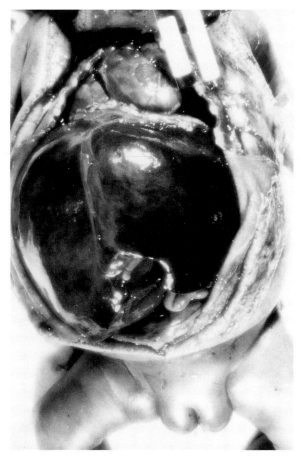

Figure 12-11. Beckwith-Wiedemann syndrome. Hepatoblastoma at autopsy.

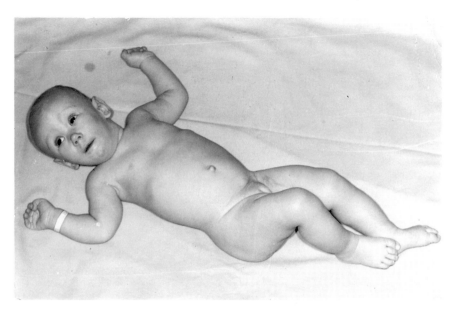

Figure 12-12. Sotos syndrome. Courtesy of R.J. Gorlin, Minneapolis, Minnesota.

Mantel[75] observed that leukemia was associated with increased birth weight. Fraumeni[23] showed that osteosarcoma tended to arise in bones that grew very rapidly, producing taller individuals. Tjalma[70] noted that larger breeds of dogs were more susceptible to osteosarcoma than were smaller breeds. Daling et al.[17] studied the birth certificates of 681 children with cancer who were linked with cancer registry data. These investigators found an increased proportion with birth weights in excess to 4,000 g. The relationship was strongest for children under age 2 years; about twice as many with neoplasia had high birth weights. Significant increases were observed for Wilms tumor, neuroblastoma, and leukemia. However, no relationship was observed for children with neoplasia diagnosed at age 4 years or older.

The relationship of overgrowth syndromes to neoplasia is summarized in Table 12-5. The first two data columns appear as simple qualitative terms; quantitation has been avoided because of problems of noncomparability of studies, ascertainment bias, and, in a number of instances, small sample size. Overgrowth syndromes of prenatal onset that are not known to be associated with neoplasia can be explained in several ways. First, with some overgrowth syndromes, too few cases have been reported thus far to establish or exclude relationships to neoplasia with certainty. Second, some syndromes with few reported cases also have high infant mortality rates, further limiting the possible expression of neoplasms during infancy. Third, an overgrowth disorder such as diabetic macrosomia is common and yet is not known to be associated with an increase in neoplasia. However, overgrowth is known to be humorally mediated.[6]

Fetal Hydrops

Fetal hydrops results from an increase in body fluid together with a relative increase in fluid in the interstitial space (Figs. 12-15, 12-16). When the latter is severe, free fluid may accumulate in the body cavities as well. Normal fluid

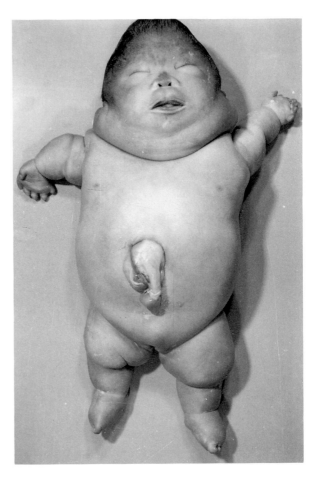

Figure 12-13. Elejalde syndrome. Female fetus weighing 4,300 g at 34 weeks gestation. Note excess subcutaneous connective tissue of trunk, neck, and limbs; short limbs with hexadactyly of hands; omphalocele; and facial dysmorphism. From Elejalde et al.[21]

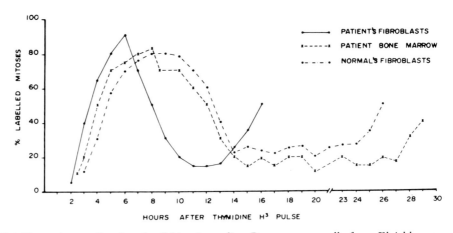

Figure 12-14. Elejalde syndrome. Results of cell kinetic studies. Bone marrow cells from Elejalde syndrome patient behave essentially like normal fibroblasts, taking approximately 37 hours to complete cell cycle. However, fibroblasts from Elejalde syndrome patient complete whole cycle in 16–18 hours (63% of normal time). From Elejalde et al.[21]

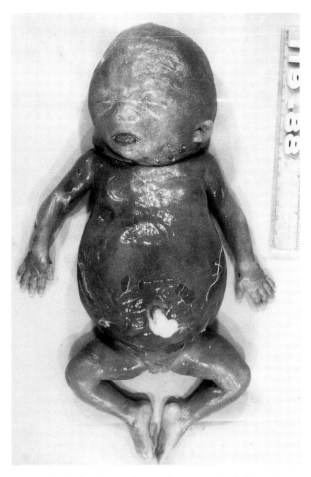

Figure 12-15. Fetal hydrops. Courtesy of M. Barr, Jr., Ann Arbor, Michigan.

distribution requires balanced osmotic and hydrostatic forces on either side of the cell membrane and an intact sodium pump. Initiating factors in hydrops include severe chronic anemia, hypoproteinemia, fetal heart failure, and obstruction of fetal circulation. Fetal hydrops has been extensively reviewed by Machin,[43] Boyd and Keeling,[5] and Van Maldergem et al.[71] Cardiovascular and chromosomal problems are identified most frequently (Table 12-6).

When fetal hydrops is recognized, amniocentesis should be considered to identify a chromosomal anomaly if present. Ultrasonography should be performed to study the rate, rhythm, and structure of the heart and to search for other structural anomalies as well. The family and obstetric history should be determined, and the mother should have an antibody screen, hemoglobin electrophoresis, and Kleihauer-Betke test for the presence of fetal blood.[19]

ASYMMETRY

Asymmetry has been discussed by many authors.[1,8–13,15,35]

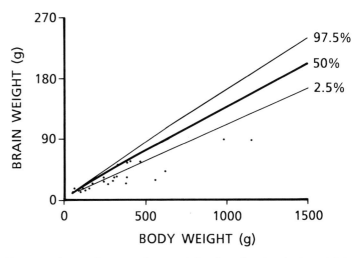

Figure 12-16. Hydrops cases caused by cervical cystic hygroma (brain weight plotted against body weight). Body weight too heavy for brain weight, i.e., 15 of 24 cases are <2.5%ile (brain weight is too light for body weight). Courtesy of M. Barr, Jr., Ann Arbor, Michigan.

Normal Variation

In humans, behavioral asymmetry is well illustrated by handedness. About 90% are right handed and 10% left handed. An exception occurs in major league baseball, in which the percentage of "south-paw" pitchers exceeds the percentage of "lefties" in the population as a whole.[2] Structural asymmetry is a normal state in human development. Human structural asymmetry is exemplified by many studies of the brain (Table 12-7, Fig. 12-17). Other paired structures known to be asymmetric include the humeri, radii, femorae, fibulae, clavicles, and ribs.[33,42,44,62] With respect to the normal face, subtle degrees of asymmetry become particularly evident when properly oriented frontal photographs are divided along the median plane and reprocessed, each side being paired with its mirror image, yielding two slightly different faces.[47]

Normal and Abnormal Laterality

Some developmental disturbances can augment the normal degree of asymmetry. Left–right tooth crown size asymmetry, evident by measurement but not by

Table 12-6. Some Causes of Nonimmune Fetal Hydrops[a]

Some Causes	Some Examples
Cardiovascular	Malformations with arrhythmias
Chromosomal	Turner syndrome, trisomy 21 syndrome
Thoracic	Chondrodysplasia, cystic adenomatoid malformation, diaphragmatic hernia
Twin transfusion	Hydropic donor, hydropic recipient
Anemia	α-Thalassemia
Infection	Cytomegalovirus, parvovirus B19
Urinary tract malformation	Urethral obstruction
Genetic metabolic disorder	Lysosomal storage disorders

[a]For complete coverage, see Machin,[43] Boyd and Keeling,[5] and Van Maldergem et al.[71]

Table 12-7. Left–Right Asymmetry of the Brain

Findings	References

Planum temporale
    Left side larger (65%)
    Right side larger (11%)
    Equal size (24%)
	Geschwind and Levitsky[30]

Temporoparietal cortex
    Larger volume left (88%)
    Larger volume right (12%)
	Galaburda et al.[25]

Medulla
    Decussation of left pyramid rostral
        to that of right pyramid (82%)
    Decussation of right pyramid rostral
        to that of left pyramid (18%)
	Kertesz and Geschwind[39]

Occipital lobe Wider on left side (more common)	LeMay[41]
Frontal lobe Wider on right side (more common)	LeMay[41]

From Cohen.[15]

visual inspection, is a normal state in the general population.[27] In trisomy 21 syndrome, left–right crown size asymmetry is definitely increased, although the asymmetry still cannot be appreciated visually.[26] Other developmental disturbances result in preferential laterality for various anomalies of paired structures, such as limb reduction defects. The predominantly involved side in such limb defects does not correspond to the preferred smaller side in normal development.[61] Preferential laterality for some anomalies is striking, as with left sidedness for cleft lip and postaxial polydactyly and with right sidedness for inguinal hernia and fibular aplasia (Table 12-8).[61] To date, no adequate hypotheses have been put forth to explain such phenomena. However, developmental interrelationships may account for similarities or differences in sidedness of at least a few defects such as right-sided inguinal hernia and cryptorchidism.

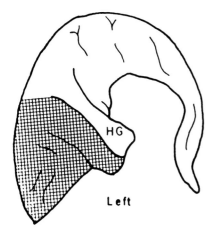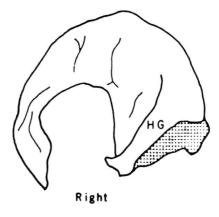

Figure 12-17. Diagram of superior temporal surface of brain showing planum temporale (hatched) caudal to Heschl's gyrus (HG). From Galaburda et al.[25]

Table 12-8. Sidedness of Unilateral Defects in Morphogenesis in Five Areas

Defect	No. of cases	Predominant Side	
		Left (%)	Right (%)
Craniofacial			
Cleft lip	2,403	68	
Agenesis of maxillary lateral incisor	298	55	
Hemifacial microsomia	200		62
Thoracoabdominal			
Renal agenesis	1,169	56	
Supernumerary nipples	13,530	55	
Poland anomaly	71		68
Pulmonary agenesis	71		57
Cryptorchidism	1,589		60
Inguinal hernia	1,310		67
Limb			
Postaxial polydactyly	242	77	
Congenital dislocated hip	827	62	
Clubfoot	1,401		55
Radial aplasia	168		58
Fibular aplasia	131		65
General			
"Hemihypertrophy"	251		62
Isolated limb asymmetry	22	73	
Limb asymmetry as a feature of Silver-Russell syndrome	30	70	
Neoplastic			
Neuroblastoma	520	55	
Wilms tumor	142	50	
Retinoblastoma	267		55

From Schnall and Smith.[61]

Establishing embryonic axes is essential in development, and normal left–right asymmetries are the last to appear. Although most parts of the human body are symmetric, organs such as the heart and great vessels, lungs, liver, gallbladder and biliary tract, gastrointestinal tract, and spleen are asymmetric. Mirror image reversal of normally asymmetric organs, known as *situs inversus*, may be partial or complete. When situs inversus is partial, the condition is frequently significant clinically. Total situs inversus is usually asymptomatic, however, although about 20% will have Kartagener syndrome and some 10% will have associated malformations.[1] A lethal malformation complex consisting of situs inversus, agnathia, and associated anomalies has been reported by Pauli et al.[46]

Work with experimental animals has been highly suggestive. A situs inversus mutation is known in the mouse and, recently, a recessive mutation was identified in a family of transgenic mice in 100% of the homozygotes tested.[78] A mutant disorganization (*Ds*) gene on chromosome 14 in the mouse results in a variety of developmental anomalies in structures derived from all three germ layers,[36] and asymmetric involvement is common. It has been suggested that some patients with unusual multiple anomalies and hamartomas, often asymmetric, may be the human homolog of the mouse disorganization gene.[18,20,59,72,77] In rat embryos, nitrous oxide results in altered laterality and increased mortality.[24] Asymmetric dysmorphogenesis of the limbs has been induced by various drugs and mutant genes.[63] Finally, Fantel et al.[22] have shown in rat embryos that left unilateral microphthalmia can be produced by *hyperoxia*, and right unilateral microphthalmia results from *hypoxia*.

Clinically Significant Asymmetry

Clinically significant asymmetry is etiologically and pathogenetically heterogeneous and may be localized or generalized. Causes may include trauma, infection, neurologic damage, chromosomal anomalies, and monogenic inheritance, among others.[15,35] There are a number of different ways to classify asymmetry. Some conditions with asymmetric dysmorphism are listed in Table 12-9. Distinctions among various types of asymmetry can be made, including hemihypertrophy, hemihyperplasia, hemihypoplasia, and hemiatrophy. The disorder

Table 12-9. Some Dysmorphic Conditions with Asymmetry

Categories	Examples	Comments
Malformation	Unilateral cleft lip	Assumes no *other* anomalies in a patient attributable to vascular disruption
	Plagiocephaly	Based on unilateral coronal synostosis
Disruption	Limb–body wall complex	
Deformation	Mandibular asymmetry	Assumes no intrinsic malformation of one side of mandible
	Plagiocephaly	Based on intrauterine constraint with normally patent sutures[a]
Hamartosis	Klippel-Trenaunay-Weber syndrome	Although some cases have vascular abnormalities such as hemangiomas and arteriovenous fistulas in the overgrown region, hypertrophy has occurred without the presence of vascular defects in some cases
	Proteus syndrome	
Hemihyperplasia	Beckwith-Wiedemann syndrome	Hemihyperplasia found in 13% of reported cases. Of Beckwith-Wiedemann patients with tumors, 30% have hemihyperplasia
Hemiatrophy	Romberg syndrome	Similar hemiatrophy of the face has been produced in experimental animals following cervical sympathectomy

[a] In some instances, *constraint itself* may result in unilateral coronal synostosis.

generally known as "hemihypertrophy" (Fig. 12-18) actually represents a hemi-hyperplastic process. It may be generalized, involving half the body, or it may occur on a more regional basis, as with a single affected limb or with unilateral facial involvement, or it may occur on a highly localized basis, as with macrodactyly.[6] "Hemihypertrophy" of a limb implies a discrepancy in both length and circumference of the affected limb compared with the normal limb. When considering a hemihyperplastic process, it is important to distinguish which tissues are involved. For example, in "hemihypertrophy" of the face, the abnormality involves both soft tissue and bone. In contrast, when facial asymmetry is caused by hyperplasia of the mandibular condyle, only bone is affected primarily, and this distinction has important surgical implications.[11]

RADIOLOGIC ASSESSMENT IN DYSMORPHOLOGY

Bone age determination is frequently abused in the assessment of growth, and an understanding of its uses and limitations is essential, especially in assessing dysmorphic syndromes. Radiologic assessment of bone maturation is commonly overrequested, underfilmed, and overread. Otherwise authoritative textbooks promote normal ranges that are much too narrow, being only one-half or even one-fourth as wide as the actual ranges.[32] Table 12-10 shows the normal ranges of the age-at-appearance of the principle ossification centers based on the excel-

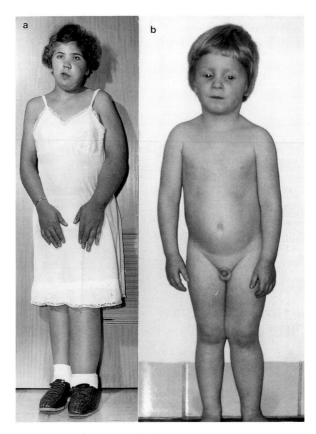

Figure 12-18. Hemihyperplasia (hemihypertrophy). a: Involvement of half the body. From Gorlin and Meskin.[31] b: Milder degree of involvement. From Cohen.[6]

Table 12-10. Normal Ranges of Age-at-Appearance of Principal Ossification Centers

	Age of Child	
Range	Male	Female
± 3–6 months	0–1 year	0–1 year
± 1–1.5 years	3–4 years	2–3 years
± 2 years	7–11 years	6–10 years
± 2 plus years	13–14 years	12–13 years

Table from Graham,[32] based on data from Garn et al.[28]

lent study of the Fels Research Institute.[28] It will be observed that the normal ranges are very broad. For example, a 3-year-old girl with a bone age between 1½ and 4½ years falls within the normal range. Because the estimation of osseous maturation from hand–wrist films alone is often misleading, while the routine study of all the hemiskeletal ossification centers is usually superfluous, a sampling method based on the usual age-at-appearance ranges of the most important ossification centers has been recommended (Fig. 12-19).[32]

Dysharmonic Maturation

In syndromic dysmorphism, unusual radiographic features may be observed such as bizarre ossification sequences, delay or advance of specific ossification

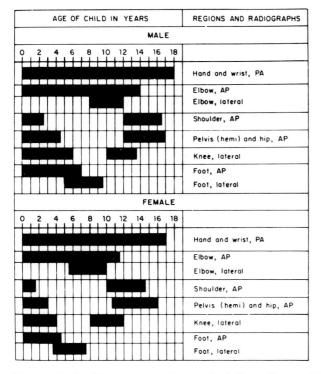

Figure 12-19. Bone age sampling method. From Graham.[32]

centers, side-to-side asymmetry, abnormal configuration of various bones, and patterned dimensional alterations of various bones.[49,50] Figure 12-20 shows a hand–wrist film of a 42-month-old female with trisomy 18. The finding of absent carpal centers of ossification with most of the epiphyses present represents an unusual ossification sequence not found in the general population. The hand–wrist film of a 6-year-old female with Hurler syndrome is shown in Figure 12-21. With such markedly abnormal bone configuration, accurate estimation of skeletal age becomes virtually impossible. The hand–wrist films of two patients with the hand-foot-uterus syndrome are shown in Figure 12-22. Although relative shortening of various bones can be appreciated to some extent in the radiographs, the patterned dimensional alterations in these x-rays, known as *metacarpophalangeal profile patterns* (Fig. 12-23), provide information far beyond the capabilities of the most experienced radiographic observer.

In metacarpophalangeal profile pattern analysis, the relationship between the lengths of various tubular bones in the hand can be illustrated graphically. The lengths of the tubular bones in the condition to be studied are plotted in terms of standard deviation units derived from normal tubular bone lengths. Because profiles are plotted against standards for age and sex, they allow comparison between various individuals. For example, in the hand-foot-uterus syndrome graphed in Figure 12-23, it will be observed that an affected adult female profile pattern, an affected 12-year-old male profile pattern, and a mean profile pattern for eight affected individuals all bear strong similarity to one another.

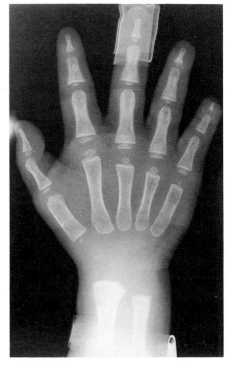

Figure 12-20. Trisomy 18. Forty-two-month-old female showing differential carpal delay. No carpal ossification centers are apparent, while most of the epiphyses are present. This unusual ossification sequence is not found in the general population. From Poznanski et al.[49]

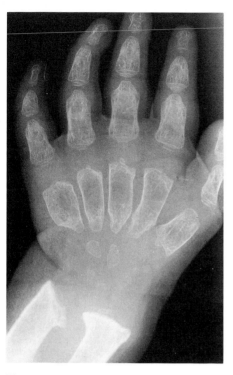

Figure 12-21. Hurler syndrome. Six-year-old female with markedly abnormal configuration of metacarpals and phalanges. There is marked retardation of the capitate and hamate with irregularity of their margins. The epiphyses are also irregular and retarded. When marked abnormality of configuration is present, accurate bone age estimation is virtually impossible. From Poznanski et al.[49]

Limitations and Cautions

Caution is indicated when interpreting the relevance of bone age for syndromes with either growth deficiency or overgrowth of prenatal onset. In syndromes with prenatal onset growth deficiency, a lag in the appearance of various ossification centers does not necessarily mean that such findings are secondary to an abnormality in the maturation rate. Similarly, the precocious bone development in some prenatal onset overgrowth syndromes does not necessarily indicate accelerated maturation; it may indicate a mesenchymal defect that has resulted in early mineralization of ossification centers. With chondrodysplasias, the bones commonly used to assess maturation are part of the disorder, thus rendering bone age determination meaningless. However, complete radiologic assessment of the abnormal configuration of various bones can be extremely helpful in diagnosing the particular chondrodysplasia.[15]

Growth predictions for various syndromes must be based on knowledge of the particular condition in question. For example, stature and final height attainment in achondroplasia can be predicted only from standard curves constructed for that particular disorder (Fig. 12-24). The same principle holds for other aspects of dysmorphic growth and development. For example, in normal human development, growth of the maxilla is essentially complete by age 14 years. In Apert syndrome, midfacial growth is arrested because of faciostenosis, and it would be erroneous to conclude that maxillary growth in this condition

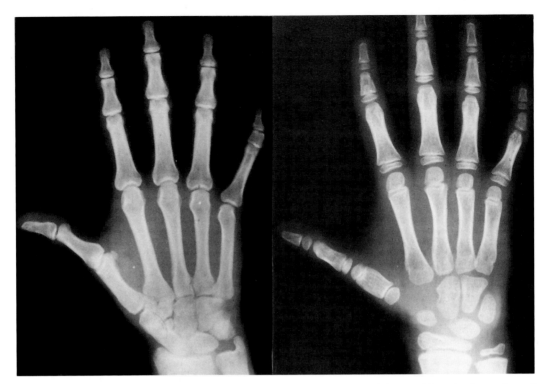

Figure 12-22. Radiographs of two patients with hand-foot-uterus syndrome. Although shortening of various tubular bones is evident on radiographs, metacarpophalangeal profile patterns (illustrated in Fig. 12-23) are more sensitive indices for detecting similarity of hand radiographs than simple inspection of the radiographs. From Poznanski et al.[50]

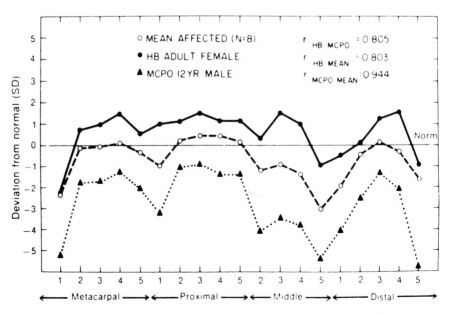

Figure 12-23. Hand-foot-uterus syndrome. Metacarpophalangeal profile patterns showing relative shortening of the first metacarpal, first proximal phalanx, second middle phalanx, fifth middle phalanx, and fifth distal phalanx. Since profile patterns are plotted against appropriate standards for age and sex, an affected adult female, an affected 12-year-old male, and a mean profile pattern for eight affected individuals can be compared. All bear strong similarity to one another. From Poznanski et al.[50]

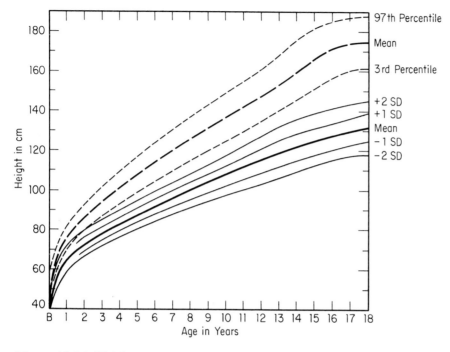

Figure 12-24. Height (mean and SD) for males with achondroplasia, shown by solid lines (N = 189), compared with normal male standard height curve (3rd, 50th, and 97th percentile), shown by dashed lines. From Horton et al.[34]

continues until 14 years of age; it is arrested much earlier than that. This fact has obvious surgical implications.[15]

Changes in Craniofacial Dysmorphism With Time

Craniofacial dysmorphism may become more severe, may remain the same, or may improve with time, depending on the nature of the particular syndrome. In mandibulofacial dysostosis, the osseous abnormalities remain essentially unchanged throughout the entire postnatal growth period (see Fig. 10-6). The curvature of the lower border of the mandible has been shown to be syndrome specific and can be defined by a computer-generated polynomial equation. Deformational Robin sequence improves with time. Catch-up growth occurs once the fetus has been released from the intrauterine constraining environment (see Fig. 10-3). Finally, studies of the major craniosynostosis syndromes have demonstrated an increased severity over time in both Apert and Crouzon syndromes. Increasing severity is caused by disproportionate growth of the craniofacial structures, which results in displacement, compression, and dysfunction.[52-55]

REFERENCES

1. Aylsworth AS: The spleen. In Stevenson RE, Hall JG, Goodman RW (eds): *Human Malformations and Related Anomalies.* Vol II, New York: Oxford University Press, 1993, pp 307–315.
2. Babcock LE: The right and the sinister. *Natural History* 102:32–39, 1993.

3. Bellus GA, Hefferon TW, Ortiz de Luna RI, Hecht JT, Horton WA, Machado M, Kaitila I, McIntosh I, Francomano CA: Achondroplasia is defined by recurrent G380R mutations of FGFR3. *Am J Hum Genet* 56:368–373, 1995.

4. Bellus GA, McIntosh I, Smith EA, Aylsworth AS, Kaitila I, Horton WA, Greenhaw GA, Hecht JT, Francomano CA: A recurrent mutation in the tyrosine kinase domain of fibroblast growth factor receptor 3 causes hypochondroplasia. *Nature Genet* 10:357–359, 1995.

5. Boyd PA, Keeling JW: Fetal hydrops. *J Med Genet* 29:91–97, 1992.

6. Cohen MM Jr: A comprehensive and critical assessment of overgrowth and overgrowth syndromes. In Harris H, Hirschhorn K (eds): *Advances in Human Genetics.* Vol 18. New York: Plenum Press, 1989, pp 181–303.

7. Cohen MM Jr: Overgrowth syndromes. In El Shafie M, Klippel CH (eds): *Associated Congenital Anomalies.* Baltimore, Williams & Wilkins, 1981, pp 71–104.

8. Cohen MM Jr: Perspectives on craniofacial asymmetry. I. The biology of asymmetry. *Int J Oral Maxillofac Surg* 24:2–7, 1995.

9. Cohen MM Jr: Perspectives on craniofacial asymmetry. II. Asymmetric embryopathies. *Int J Oral Maxillofac Surg* 24:8–12, 1995.

10. Cohen MM Jr: Perspectives on craniofacial asymmetry. III. Common and/or well-known causes of asymmetry. *Int J Oral Maxillofac Surg* 24:127–133, 1995.

11. Cohen MM Jr: Perspectives on craniofacial asymmetry. IV. Hemiasymmetries. *Int J Oral Maxillofac Surg* 24:134–141, 1995.

12. Cohen MM Jr: Perspectives on craniofacial asymmetry. V. The craniosynostoses. *Int J Oral Maxillofac Surg* 24:191–194, 1995.

13. Cohen MM Jr: Perspectives on craniofacial asymmetry. VI. The hamartoses. *Int J Oral Maxillofac Surg* 24:195–200, 1995.

14. Cohen MM Jr: Short-limb skeletal dysplasias and craniosynostosis: What do they have in common? *Pediatr Radiol* (in press).

15. Cohen MM Jr: *The Child with Multiple Birth Defects.* New York: Raven Press, 1982.

16. Cohen MM Jr: The large-for-gestational age (LGA) infant in dysmorphic perspective. In Willey AM, Carter TM, Kelly S, Porter IH (eds): *Clinical Genetics: Problems in Diagnosis and Counseling.* New York: Academic Press, 1982, pp 153–169.

17. Daling JR, Starzyk P, Plshan AF, Weiss NS: Birth weight and the incidence of childhood cancer. *J Natl Cancer Inst* 72:1039–1041, 1984.

18. De Michelena MI, Stachurska A: Multiple anomalies possibly caused by a human homologue to the mouse disorganization (*Ds*) gene. *Clin Dysmorphol* 2:131–134, 1983.

19. Donnai D: Fetal hydrops: Mechanisms and syndromes. *Proc Greenwood Genet Center* 8:108–110, 1989.

20. Donnai D, Winter RM: Disorganization: A model for "early amnion rupture." *J Med Genet* 25:241–245, 1989.

21. Elejalde BR, Giraldo C, Jimenez R, Gilbert EF: Acrocephalopolydactylous dysplasia. *Birth Defects* 13(B):53–67, 1977.

22. Fantel AG, Person RE, Burought-Gleim C, Shepard TH, Juchau MR, Mackler B: Asymmetric development of mitochondrial activity in rat embryos as a determinant of the defect patterns induced by exposure to hypoxia, hyperoxia, and redox cyclers *in vitro*. *Teratology* 44:355–362, 1991.

23. Fraumeni JF Jr: Stature and malignant tumors of bone in childhood and adolescence. *Cancer* 20:967–973, 1967.

24. Fujinaga M, Baden JM, Shepard TH, Mazze RI: Nitrous oxide alters body laterality in rats. *Teratology* 41:131–135, 1990.

25. Galaburda AM, LeMay M, Kemper TL, Geschwind N: Right–left asymmetries in the brain. *Science* 199:852, 1978.

26. Garn SM, Cohen MM Jr, Geciauskas MA: Increased crown-size asymmetry in trisomy G. *J Dent Res* 49:465, 1970.

27. Garn SM, Lewis AB, Kerewsky RS: The meaning of bilateral asymmetry in the permanent dentition. *Angle Orthod* 36:55–62, 1966.

28. Garn SM, Rohmann CG, Silverman FN: Radiographic standards for postnatal ossification and tooth calcification. *Med Radiogr Photogr* 43:45–66, 1967.
29. Gefferth K: Metatropic dwarfism. *Prog Pediatr Radiol* 4:137–151, 1973.
30. Geschwind N, Levitsky W: Human brain: Left right asymmetries in temporal speech region. *Science* 161:186–187, 1968.
31. Gorlin RJ, Meskin LG: Congenital hemihypertrophy. *J Pediatr* 61:870–879, 1962.
32. Graham CB: Assessment of bone maturation—Methods and pitfalls. *Radiol Clin North Am* 10:185–202, 1972.
33. Halperin G: Normal asymmetry and unilateral hypertrophy. *Arch Intern Med* 49:676–682, 1931.
34. Horton WA, Rotter JI, Rimoin DL, Scott CI Jr, Hall JG: Standard growth curves for achondroplasia. *J Pediatr* 93:435–438, 1978.
35. Hoyme HE: Asymmetry and hemihypertrophy. In Stevenson RE, Hall JG, Goodman RW (eds): *Human Malformations and Related Anomalies.* Vol II. New York: Oxford University Press, 1993, pp 1031–1045.
36. Hummel KP: The inheritance and expression of disorganization, an unusual mutation in the mouse. *J Exp Zool* 137:389–432, 1958.
37. International Working Group on Constitutional Diseases of Bone: International Classification of Osteochondrodysplasias. *Am J Med Genet* 44:223–229, 1992.
38. Irving I: The EMG syndrome (exomphalos, macroglossia, gigantism). In Rickham RP, Hacker WC, Prevolt J (eds): *Progress in Pediatrics.* Vol 1. Munich: Urban and Schwarzenberg, 1970, pp 1–61.
39. Kertesz A, Geschwind N: Patterns of pyramidal decussation and their relationship to handedness. *Arch Neurol* 24:326–332, 1971.
40. Langer LO Jr, Beals RK, Solomon IL, Bard PA, Bard LA, Rissman EM, Rogers JG, Dorst JP, Hall JG, Sparkes RS, Franken EA Jr: Acromesomelic dwarfism: Manifestations in childhood. *Am J Med Genet* 1:87–100, 1977.
41. LeMay M: Origins and evolution of language and speech. *NY Acad Sci,* 349, 1976.
42. LeMay M, Clebras A: Human brain: morphologic differences in the hemispheres demonstrable by carotid arteriography. *N Engl J Med* 287:168–171, 1972.
43. Machin GA: Hydrops revisited: Literature review of 1,414 cases published in the 1980s. *Am J Med Genet* 34:366–390, 1989.
44. Meredith HV: Length of upper extremities in *Homo sapiens* from birth through adolescence. *Growth* 11:1–50, 1947.
45. Pauli RM: Osteochondrodysplasias with mild clinical manifestations: A guide for endocrinologists and others. *Growth Genet Hormones* 11:1–5, 1995.
46. Pauli RM, Graham JM Jr, Barr M Jr: Agnathia, situs inversus and associated malformations. *Teratology* 23:85–93, 1981.
47. Peck H, Peck S: A concept of facial esthetics. *Angle Orthod* 40:284–318, 1970.
48. Pious D, Millis AJT, Sabo K: *In vitro* growth rates in primary cellular growth deficiency syndromes. *Pediatr Res* 9:279, 1975.
49. Poznanski AK, Garn SM, Kuhns LR, Sandusky ST: Dysharmonic maturation of the hand in the congenital malformation syndromes. *Am J Phys Anthropol* 35:417–432, 1971.
50. Poznanski AK, Garn SM, Nagy JM, Gall JC Jr: Metacarpophalangeal pattern profiles in the evaluation of skeletal malformations. *Radiology* 104:1–11, 1972.
51. Prinos P, Kilpatrick MW, Tsipouras P: A novel G345E FGFR3 mutation in achondroplasia. *Pediatr Res* 37:151A, 1995.
52. Pruzansky S: Clinical investigation for the experiments of nature. *ASHA Rep* 8:62–94, 1973.
53. Pruzansky S: Not all dwarfed mandibles are alike. *Birth Defects* 5(2):120–129, 1969.
54. Pruzansky S: Radiocephalometric studies of the basicranium in craniofacial malformations. In Bosma JF (ed): *Development of the Basicranium.* Bethesda, MD: U.S. DHEW, Pub. No. (NIH) 76-989, 1976, pp 278–300.
55. Pruzansky S: Time: The fourth dimension in syndrome analysis applied to craniofacial malformations. *Birth Defects* 13(3C):3–28, 1977.

56. Rimoin DL: The chondrodystrophies. In Harris H, Hirschhorn K (eds): *Advances in Human Genetics.* New York: Plenum Press, 1975, pp 1–118.

57. Rimoin DL, Graham JM Jr: Short stature. In Emery AEH, Rimoin DL, eds. *Principles and Practice of Medical Genetics.* Vol. I. 2nd Ed. Edinburgh: Churchill Livingstone, 1990, pp 225–234.

58. Rimoin DL, Horton WA: Short stature. Part II. *J Pediatr* 92:679–704, 1978.

59. Robin NH, Adewale OO, McDonald-McGinn D, Nadeau JA: Human malformations similar to those in the mouse mutation disorganization (*Ds*). *Hum Genet* 92:461–464, 1993.

60. Rousseau F, Saugier P, Le Merrer M, Munnich A, Delezoide A-L, Maroteaux P, Bonaventure J, Narcy F, Sanak M: Stop codon FGFR3 mutations in thanatophoric dwarfism type 1. *Nature Genet* 10:110–112, 1995.

61. Schnall BS, Smith DW: Nonrandom laterality of malformations in paired structures. *J Pediatr* 85:509–511, 1974.

62. Schultz AH: Proportions, variability and asymmetries of the long bones of the limbs and the clavicles in man and apes. *Hum Biol* 9:281–328, 1937.

63. Scott WJ: Asymmetric limb malformations induced by drugs and mutant genes. *Prog Clin Biol Res* 163C:111–113, 1985.

64. Shiang R, Thompson LM, Zhu Y-Z, Church DM, Fielder TJ, Bocian M, Winokur ST, Wasmuth JJ: Mutations in the transmembrane domain of FGFR3 cause the most common genetic form of dwarfism, achondroplasia. *Cell* 78:335–342, 1994.

65. Smith DW: Growth deficiency: A new classification into primary cellular growth deficiency and secondary humoral growth deficiency. *S Med J* 64(Suppl):5–15, 1971.

66. Smith DW: *Recognizable Patterns of Human Malformation.* Second Edition, Philadelphia: WB Saunders, 1976.

67. Spranger J, Langer LO Jr, Wiedemann H-R: *Bone Dysplasia: An Atlas of Constitutional Disorders of Skeletal Development.* Philadelphia: WB Saunders, 1974.

68. Superti-Furga A, Eich G, Bucher HU, Wisser J, Giedion A, Gizelmann R, Steinmann B: A glycine 375-to-cysteine substitution in the transmembrane domain of the fibroblast growth factor receptor-3 in a newborn with achondroplasia. *Eur J Pediatr* 154:215–219, 1995.

69. Tavormina PL, Shiang R, Thompson LM, Zhu Y-Z, Wilkin DJ, Lachman RS, Wilcox WR, Rimoin DL, Cohn DH, Wasmuth JJ: Thanatophoric dysplasia (types I and II) caused by distinct mutations in fibroblast growth factor receptor 3. *Nature Genet* 9:321–328, 1995.

70. Tjalma RA: Canine bone sarcoma: Estimation of relative risk as a function of body size. *J Natl Cancer Found* 36:1137–1150, 1966.

71. Van Maldergem L, Jauniaux E, Fourneau C, Gillerot Y: Genetic causes of hydrops fetalis. *Pediatrics* 89:81–86, 1992.

72. Wainwright H, Viljoen D: Developmental anomalies in monozygous twins resembling the human homologue of the mouse mutant disorganization. *Clin Dysmorphol* 2:135–139, 1993.

73. Weaver DD: Overgrowth syndromes and disorders: Definition, classification and discussion. *Growth Genet Hormones* 10:1–4, 1994.

74. Weksberg R, Terespolsky D, Squire J, Cohen MM Jr: Overgrowth syndromes and cancer. In D. Malkin (Ed) *Inherited Tumors.* London: Springer-Verlag, 1996.

75. Wertelecki W, Mantel N: Increased birth weight in leukemia. *Pediatr Res* 7:132–138, 1973.

76. Whitley CB, Gorlin RJ: Achondrogenesis: New nosology with evidence of genetic heterogeneity. *Radiology* 148:693–698, 1983.

77. Winter RM, Donnai D: A possible human homologue for the mouse mutant disorganization. *J Med Genet* 26:417–420, 1989.

78. Yokoyama T, Copeland NG, Jenkins NA, Montogomery CA, Elder FFB, Overbeek PA: Reversal of left–right asymmetry: A situs inversus mutation. *Science* 260:679–682, 1993.

13

Mental Deficiency

Mental deficiency is both etiologically and pathogenetically heterogeneous. Many surveys of mentally retarded populations have been carried out using various types of ascertainment, various classifications, and different terminologies. These have been reviewed elsewhere.[10] *In the aggregate, such studies indicate that in severe mental deficiency prenatal factors must be sought in approximately two-thirds of the cases; perinatal and postnatal factors are implicated in no more than 15% of the cases; dysmetabolic syndromes are only responsible for approximately 5% of the cases; and causes cannot be found for a high percentage of cases.*

Complex interrelationships exist between mental retardation and patients with multiple anomalies.[10] Some congenital malformations, both major and minor as well as both single and multiple, may serve as indicators of mental retardation. Malformations of prenatal onset may imply structural defects of the brain that also date back to early periods of development. Trisomy 13 syndrome, the Meckel syndrome, and the fetal alcohol syndrome serve as examples of discrete disorders of chromosomal, monogenic, and teratogenic origins, respectively, in which structural defects of the central nervous system arise during intrauterine life. Crome,[1] in examining the brains at necropsy of 282 individuals with mental deficiency, found that over 70% of clinically defined cases and 95% of idiopathic cases had abnormalities of the brain. Malamud,[4] in analyzing 1,410 consecutive necropsies from three hospitals for mentally retarded patients, found that 61% had structural defects of the central nervous system. Of these, 19% were grossly visible anomalies and 81% were less conspicuous anomalies. Smith and Bostian[7] noted that 42% of patients with idiopathic mental retardation had three or more anomalies of which 80% were externally visible minor anomalies detectable on clinical examination. Thus, minor anomalies may indicate that an infant's developmental progress should be carefully monitored.

The association between mental deficiency and patients with multiple anomalies must be considered cautiously. First, because infants with anomalies of prenatal onset frequently have difficult deliveries and problems in perinatal adaptation, these complications may be held responsible retrospectively for the patient's mental retardation. Such erroneous interpretations should be avoided. Second, it is important to know the limitations of prognosticating mental deficiency when anomalies are present. Many malformations, either singly or in combination, are compatible with normal mental development. Furthermore, mental retardation is a variable feature of many discrete disorders such as Apert syndrome. Finally, although an association between minor congenital anomalies and behavioral problems has been suggested in several studies,[5,6,9] the assessment of minor anomalies in early life has not been found to be a practical screening device for predicting later, aberrant behavior.[3] Thus, caution should be exercised in making assumptions about psychomotor development, cognitive development, and behavioral characteristics on the basis of minor congenital anomalies observed in infancy. To some extent, faulty predictions can become self-fulfilling prophesies.

In general, a specific overall diagnosis can be made more frequently in cases of severe mental deficiency (IQ <50) than in cases of mild retardation (IQ = 50 to 70). The latter group is primarily composed of individuals from mentally dull or socioeconomically deprived families. Polygenic and environmental factors play the major role in most of these cases. However, this group also contains a few individuals with X-aneuploidy states (especially Klinefelter syndrome), malformation syndromes, milder defects of central nervous system development, dysmetabolic disorders, and residual central nervous system insults.[8]

A classification of severe mental deficiency based on a large study is presented in Table 13-1. Of all such patients, 45% had either a single central nervous system malformation or a malformation syndrome in which a defect in brain morphogenesis also occurred or was thought to occur by inference. The total malformation group (45%) stood in marked contrast to the dysmetabolic syndromes (5.8%).[2] These two groups were mutually exclusive with respect to (1) major and minor anomalies, occurring in the former but not in the latter; and (2) biochemical abnormalities, occurring in the latter but not in the former. Amino acid screening did not reveal a single biochemical abnormality in over 600 patients with either a major central nervous system malformation or a malformation syndrome.

Table 13-1. Study of a Severely Retarded Population Consisting of 1,224 Patients

Type of Disorder		Frequency (%)
Malformation syndromes	45 {	29
Primary central nervous system malformations		15.7
Dysmetabolic disorders		5.8
Hypothyroidism		0.7
Cerebral palsy, seizures, or hypotonia		31.4
Environmental damage		12.4
Pure mental deficiency		4.1
Psychosis and mental deficiency		1.2
		100

From Kaveggia et al.[2]

Patients with mental deficiency can be divided into four categories based on the age of onset of central nervous system dysfunction: prenatal onset, perinatal onset, postnatal onset, and unknown time of onset.[8] In the first and largest category are patients with a defect in prenatal morphogenesis of the brain. Included are patients (discussed above) who have either a single central nervous system malformation or a malformation syndrome. In the second category are patients who have sustained an insult to the brain perinatally. Included in this group are patients with severe hypoglycemia, kernicterus, cerebral hemorrhage, perinatal hypoxia, and meningitis. Although problems in perinatal adaptation also occur in patients in the first category, such problems are secondary and not the cause of the mental deficiency. The third category consists of patients with a problem in brain function of postnatal onset. Included in this group are patients with central nervous system insults such as trauma, meningitis, encephalitis, hypernatremia, and lead encephalopathy, in addition to patients with enzymatic defects in amino acid, carbohydrate, uric acid, mucopolysaccharide, and lipid metabolism. Although dysmetabolic disorders are of prenatal onset, the clinical manifestations are usually of postnatal onset. Patients for whom the time of onset of brain dysfunction cannot be established belong to the fourth category, which is second in size only to the group of patients with central nervous system malformations and malformation syndromes. In this fourth group, developmental progress is slow, and spasticity, hypotonia, seizures, or aberrant behavior may accompany the developmental delay. Finally, some disorders, such as rubella, toxoplasmosis, and hypothyroidism may present clinically in several of the four categories.[8]

REFERENCES

1. Crome L: The brain and mental retardation. *BMJ* 1:897–904, 1960.
2. Kaveggia EG, Durkin MV, Pendleton E, Opitz JM: Diagnostic/genetic studies on 1,224 patients with severe mental retardation. In *Proceedings of the Third Congress of the International Association for the Scientific Study of Mental Deficiency.* Warsaw: Polish Medical Publishers, 1975, pp 82–93.
3. LaVeck B, Hammond MA, LaVeck GD: Minor congenital anomalies and behavior in different home environments. *J Pediatr* 96:940–943, 1980.
4. Malamud N: Neuropathology. In Stevens HA, Heber R (eds): *Mental Retardation. A Review of Research.* Chicago: University of Chicago Press, 1974.
5. Quinn PQ, Rapoport JL: Minor physical anomalies and neurologic status in hyperactive boys. *Pediatrics* 53:742–746, 1974.
6. Rosenberg JB, Weller GM: Minor physical anomalies and academic performance in young school-age children. *Dev Med Child Neurol* 15:131–135, 1973.
7. Smith DW, Bostian KE: Congenital anomalies associated with idiopathic mental retardation. *J Pediatr* 65:189–196, 1964.
8. Smith DW, Simons ER: Rational diagnostic evaluation of the child with mental deficiency. *Am J Dis Child* 129:1285–1290, 1975.
9. Waldrop MF, Bell RQ, McLaughlin B, Halverson CF: Newborn minor physical anomalies predict short attention span, peer aggression, and impulsivity at age 3. *Science* 199:563–565, 1978.
10. Warkany J, Lemire RJ, Cohen MM Jr: *Mental Retardation and Congenital Malformations of the Central Nervous System.* Chicago: Year Book Publishers, 1981.

14

Psychosocial Considerations

Dear Miss Lonelyhearts:

I am sixteen years old now and I don't know what to do and would appreciate it if you could tell me what to do. When I was a little girl it was not so bad because I got used to the kids on the block making fun of me, but now I would like to have boy friends like the other girls and go out on Saturday nights, but no boy will take me because I was born without a nose—although I am a good dancer and have a nice shape and my father buys me pretty clothes.

I sit and look at myself all day and cry. I have a big hole in the middle of my face that scares people even myself so I can't blame the boys for not wanting to take me out. My mother loves me, but she cries terrible when she looks at me.

What did I do to deserve such a terrible fate? Even if I did do some bad things I didn't do any before I was a year old and I was born this way. I asked my Papa and he says he doesn't know, but that maybe I did something in the other world before I was born or that maybe I was being punished for his sins. I don't believe that because he is a very nice man. Ought I commit suicide?

Sincerely yours,

Desperate

From *Miss Lonelyhearts*, by Nathaniel West[86]

This chapter is organized under the following headings: Parents of Malformed Children; Malformed Children; General Problems of Adaptation; Specific Problems of Adaptation (Short Stature, Mental Deficiency, Cancer, Craniofacial Anomalies, and Genital Malformations); Studies of Specific Syndromes; and Critique of Psychosocial Studies.

PARENTS OF MALFORMED CHILDREN

In sociocultural perspective, responses to infants with congenital malformations have been remarkably variable, ranging from protection to exclusion, and, at the extremes, from adoration to extermination, and sometimes both. The birth of a malformed infant often precipitates a major family crisis that disrupts the usual pathways to parent–infant bonding. One of the early tasks of the parents is to resolve the discrepancy between their idealized image of the infant and the infant's actual appearance. Parental reaction, parent–infant bonding, and parental adjustment depend on many factors, such as the cultural background, social factors, personalities, attitudes, and coping patterns of the parents.

The reactions of parents to their malformed infant and the degree to which parent–infant bonding is disrupted also depend on the properties of the defect. Is the anomaly visible, especially involving the craniofacial area, or is it invisible? The reaction of mothers toward infants who have cleft lip tends to be much stronger than the reaction of mothers with infants who have cleft palate.[69] Is the anomaly correctable or uncorrectable? Is the condition life threatening, or will it affect the future development of the child? Parents must mourn the loss of the dreamed-of or planned-for infant before they can become fully attached to their defective infant. In contrast to the situation in which the malformed infant dies, the mourning process is less effective when the child survives. Because parents may be confronted constantly with their child's problems, such as mental retardation, it is unreasonable to expect serene acceptance; residues of distress and grief may remain.[20] Are features such as short stature or genital malformations part of the picture? Does the condition involve a single malformation, or are multiple anomalies present? Do other members of the family have the condition? Will there be a need for repeated hospitalizations, outpatient visits (Fig. 14-1), or visits to various agencies?[36,68]

Generally, parents with malformed infants go through an identifiable sequence of complex emotional reactions (Fig. 14-2), although the amount of time required to work through the problems of each stage varies. The initial period is usually one of overwhelming shock. Some parents do not react with shock, but tend to intellectualize the problem and focus on the facts related to their infant's condition. A second stage of disbelief follows in which most parents practice denial, the intensity of which varies considerably. Feelings of sadness and anger follow the stage of disbelief. A gradual lessening of sadness, anger, and anxiety gives way to a stage of equilibrium in which the parents become increasingly comfortable with their situation and develop confidence in their ability to care for their infant. Equilibrium takes a variable amount of time to reach; some parents remain in a state of chronic sorrow long after the birth of a malformed child. During the fifth stage, the period of reorganization, parents deal with the responsibility for their child's problems and achieve an adequate adaptation.[17]

Parental adjustments are quite variable and influence the manner in which the child handles feelings about his or her problems. The following reactions are commonly found to some degree in most parents and are not necessarily mutually exclusive. Anger and disappointment may cause some parents to withdraw emotionally from their malformed child. Some parents may continue to practice denial. An element of guilt is found in most parental reactions. For some, guilt feelings may be overwhelming, such as in a mother who devotes herself entirely to the welfare of her malformed child while excluding her other children and her

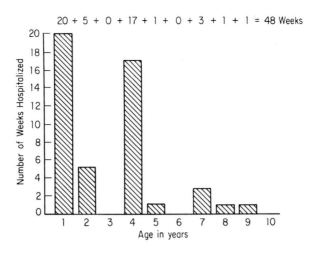

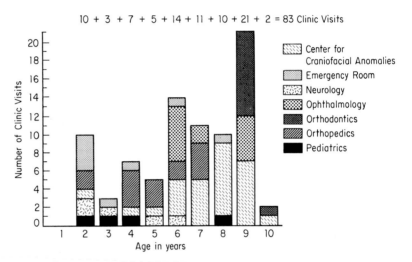

Figure 14-1. Number of weeks of hospitalization and number of outpatient clinic visits for one patient with Apert syndrome over a 10-year-period. Courtesy of S. Pruzansky, Chicago, Illinois.

husband. Parents may regard the problem as something that makes their child special. They may also acknowledge the problem while focusing on the positive qualities of the child. Some parents may become preoccupied with social reactions to their child. Parental responses also may include chronic sorrow, social withdrawal, alcoholism, psychosis, divorce, and child abuse.[4,6,36,38,79]

Responding to the birth of a malformed child in the best possible way is exceedingly difficult because of the ambiguities involved. For example, what is the difference between the special needs of such a child and overprotectiveness? What constitutes optimal adaptation? If sorrow, depression, and anger are the natural responses evoked in parents of malformed infants, what is the right balance between mourning and acceptance? To expect that such feelings must be *completely resolved* only forces parents to deny their real feelings to professionals who wish to help them.[36]

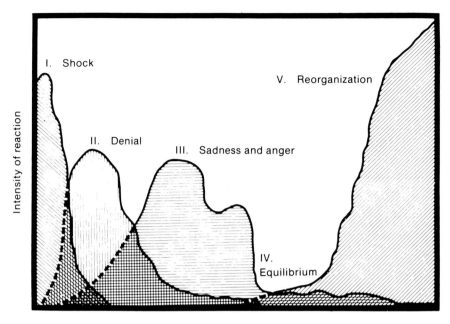

Figure 14-2. Hypothetical model showing sequence of parental reactions to birth of a malformed infant. From Drotar et al.[17]

MALFORMED CHILDREN

Belfer and his colleagues[4,47] have presented a model of body image development in the malformed child based on their experience with complex craniofacial anomalies such as hemifacial microsomia and Apert syndrome. Normal and distorted body image are contrasted in Figure 14-3. The malformed infant is more likely to experience disrupted parental bonding during the neonatal period, to develop a sense of incompetence during infancy, to become isolated from peers during school age, to experience an uncertain sense of identity and have diminished career goals during adolescence, and to have feelings of seclusion, incompleteness, failure, conflict, and hostility together with diminished achievement during adulthood. A distorted developmental pathway diverges from the normal, becoming more constricted with each milestone. Surgical intervention for a craniofacial anomaly tends to shift the malformed patient's development toward normal pathways. In contrast, a craniofacial defect resulting from trauma or a neoplasm in a normal individual tends to shift development toward distorted pathways.

Because society attaches a stigma to those who are different, the victim of any malformation may receive negative feedback, resulting in self-devaluation. When the physical appearance exceeds the variability of normative expectations, others commonly respond with emotional arousal, anxiety, and fear. Based on various studies of initial social encounters between physically disabled and nondisabled persons, Richardson[57] developed two sets of generalizations, one dealing with reactions of those who are not physically disabled, the other dealing with reactions of those who are, as given below:

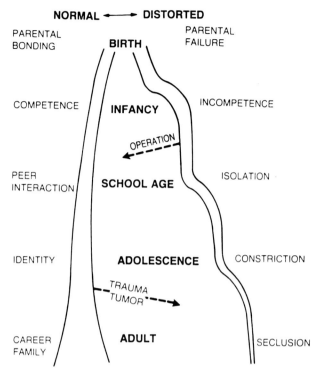

Figure 14-3. Contrasting pathways of body image development. Divergence between normal and distorted pathways with each milestone. Note progressive constriction leading to isolation and seclusion in the malformed person. From Murray et al.[47]

Reactions of Those Who Are Not Physically Disabled:

1. Initial reactions toward those who are physically disabled are less favorable than toward those who are not disabled.
2. There is considerable agreement among subcultures as to which physical disabilities are more or less preferred.
3. Emotional arousal and anxiety occur in varying degrees in an initial encounter with a disabled person.
4. Reactions described in 1–3 above are present early in childhood.
5. The physical disability initially dominates the attention of the nondisabled person. The salience of the disability leads to inattention to the other attributes of the disabled person—attributes that normally would be included in initial interpersonal evaluation and used in guiding the initial stages of the interpersonal relationship.
6. The initial interaction frequently includes a feeling of ambivalence on the part of the nondisabled person. For fear of revealing the negative aspect of the ambivalence, the nondisabled person is more formal and controlled in the behavior he or she exhibits.
7. Depending on the experience in the initial social encounter, the ambivalence felt may later be expressed as denigration of the disabled or as giving overly favorable impressions.
8. There is inhibition of nonverbal behavior, such as gesture, and a tendency to come less close physically.

9. The nondisabled exhibit less variability in their behavior, and they distort their opinions in the directions they feel are more acceptable to the disabled person.

Consequences of Reactions for Those Who Are Physically Disabled:

1. In a social gathering where individuals have not previously met, the disabled person is likely to be the recipient of fewer social contacts. Negative and ambivalent feelings in the nondisabled may lead them to avoid social encounters with the disabled, especially when there are other nondisabled people in the group from which to choose and when the nondisabled have greater mobility than the disabled.
2. The disabled person is at a disadvantage if his or her impairment initially becomes a focus of attention. It is difficult for him or her to present other attributes of himself or herself which may gain attention and form the basis of developing a social relationship.
3. The combination of anxiety, ambivalence, and formalization of behavior in the nondisabled person results in the disabled person not experiencing as wide a range of behavior as the nondisabled.
4. The distortion of information given the disabled person by the nondisabled person, because he or she does not wish to offend or hurt the disabled person, will result in the disabled person not obtaining honest feedback when he or she behaves inappropriately. This reduces the likelihood of learning the appropriateness and inappropriateness of certain forms of social competence.
5. The negative values toward physical disability are learned in childhood by the disabled, who accept and incorporate these values. This results in loss of self-esteem.

Several coping mechanisms are employed by individuals with malformations to protect their self-esteem.[23] One is to deny that the problem matters very much, rationalizing that he or she has many other positive attributes. The individual may dismiss those who are critical of his or her appearance as being shallow, ignorant, or cruel. The stigmatized person may use the disability for secondary gain, as with the attempt to get sympathy or special consideration or to explain failure that may be due to some other personal flaw. Another mechanism is to deprecate others who are not disabled. Some malformed individuals come to view their misfortune as an enriching experience. Others may make a special effort to overcome the disability, as in the case of a lame individual who learns to swim or a facially malformed person who seeks to correct the defect through plastic surgery.

GENERAL PROBLEMS OF ADAPTATION

Although the shock of having a malformed infant is overwhelming, attachment can be facilitated by showing the parents their newborn as soon as possible. Some parents may wish to delay seeing their baby at first because of the need to temper the intensity of their experience. Unnecessary delay in showing the parents their baby or in giving some perspective on the problem, however, should be avoided, because it heightens parental anxiety. Parents attach great importance to the approach and general attitude of the medical and nursing staff. They may be so distressed that whereas the specific details of the initial counseling session may not be recalled, the kindness and sympathy of the staff make a deep and lasting impression.[36] This cannot be overemphasized, because studies have shown that parents of malformed infants and professionals are usually both at a loss as to how to behave.[57] The medical staff, nursing staff, and social worker should not interpret parental grief for the parents as being caused by the loss of the anticipated normal child; such intellectualization may rob the parents of the full strength and depth of their grief.[36]

Parental mourning of the malformed stillborn is problematic; although a sense of loss occurs, death without seeing a body seems unreal and is intensified because there are not experiences with the baby to remember. Therefore, bereaved parents should be offered the opportunity to look at and touch or hold their dead infant. They should be encouraged to take an active role in naming the baby and arranging a funeral. This facilitates the mourning process and, ultimately, the family is likely to adjust better to bereavement.[39]

Depending on the nature of the condition and the wishes of the parents, management may vary from no medical intervention when limited survival is anticipated to full medical intervention when survival and functional adaptation can be anticipated. In conditions such an anencephaly, trisomy 13 syndrome, and trisomy 18 syndrome, parents may be given the option of no medical intervention. Central nervous system anomalies can be explained from a developmental perspective, and the situation is interpreted as a late miscarriage. The mother may be told that she is well suited for carrying children to full term because in most instances such malformed babies do not survive early fetal life and are miscarried. With malformations such as cleft lip, polydactyly, and pyloric stenosis, the anomaly can be explained from a developmental perspective, its management discussed, and its impact on the child explained. Acceptance of the whole child as being normal* becomes the key to the approach, the malformation problem being defined in realistic terms. For the chronically handicapped child, the approach is usually an individualized one—depending on the nature and severity of the condition—aimed at helping the parents accept the child with the attendant problem. The usual range of functional limitations for the disorder in question should be explained and the parents told what can be done to help their child adapt.[67]

Parents need an opportunity to discuss their own ideas about the cause of their malformed infant and the meaning that they attach to the medical terms and labels employed. Counseling about the nature of the condition and its cause, when known, can clear up a number of misconceptions the parents may have. The clinician should answer any questions the parents may ask, recognize that parental anger may be directed toward him or her initially, accede to parental wishes for another opinion gracefully and indicate willingness to continue working with them thereafter, be available for further information and discussion, and be prepared to repeat the information several times until it is absorbed. The parents should know that they are not alone, that support services, agencies, clinics, schools, and counseling services are available. For many conditions, it is appropriate to bring the family into contact with groups who have the same problem, such as Little People of America, Support Organization for Trisomy 18/13, the Prader-Willi Syndrome Association, and many others. The clinician should be prepared to monitor parental adaptation to the malformed child over time, hoping to avoid the extremes of rejection and overprotection.

---

*With normal strengths and weaknesses like any other child.

SPECIFIC PROBLEMS OF ADAPTATION

Short Stature

Short stature is discussed in Chapter 12. The reactions of others to short stature can range from derogatory comments to protective overtures to mild inquisitiveness. Most dwarfed children do not become intensely sensitive about their height until they are subjected to comparisons, ridicule, and verbal abuse by their peers at school (Fig. 14-4). Dwarfed children react to teasing in various ways, such as passive resignation and withdrawal, assuming the role of mascot and laughing at one's self with the crowd, fighting back physically, becoming friendly with a larger child who helps ward off offenders, and using humor in the form of sharp verbal retorts. Ironically, in the process of socialization, the dwarfed child incorporates negative attitudes and schemas while simultaneously being victimized by them. Because the dwarfed child usually has no contact with other dwarfed individuals in society with whom to identify, he or she learns a negative response to others with the same problem. Dwarfed children are subjected to the silhouette effect, in which they are treated according to their size rather than their chronologic age. It is not uncommon for a 5-year-old dwarf to be cuddled as if he or she were only 2 years old. Although the dwarfed child may have difficulty in manipulating the environment through gross motor activities,

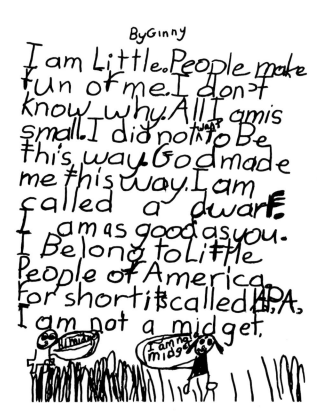

Figure 14-4. Letter written by an achondroplastic child for circulation in her elementary school. Note difference in size of child's name and sentences in body of letter. Members of Little People of America use the terms *midget* and *dwarf* purposely to distinguish between proportionately and disproportionately short-statured individuals. From Scott.[61]

the child easily manipulates adults in the environment. The silhouette effect facilitates such manipulation, because adults tend to have lower expectations for the dwarfed child. As the child becomes older, dwarfed stature confers instant recognition in school and in the community at large. He or she becomes widely known without any effort at all and must face undue social attention at some times and social isolation at other times.[16,23,61,85]

Families with individuals of short stature need to know what problems they will face during the course of the child's development and propitious courses of action to follow in order to mitigate such problems. Various articles such as the ones by Drash,[16] Scott,[61] and Weinberg[85] can be recommended, and contact with other families who have the same problem may be especially helpful. The most important advice that can be given to parents of a dwarfed child is to make every effort to treat the child according to chronologic age, not size. The greater the degree of overprotection, the more immature and insecure the child tends to be. Often this leads to social withdrawal, in which the dwarfed child retreats to the more rewarding and less demanding sphere of adults and younger children. Mascotism is a much healthier response, and many short-statured children become adept at playing such a role with their peer group.[16,61]

Little People of America provides organizational remedies for its short-statured members. Functions of the organization include socializing, dating, finding spouses, overcoming employment difficulties, dealing with clothing problems, purchasing brake and accelerator extensions for driving, and increasing medical knowledge about dwarfism. The organization expands the field of eligible partners to an extraordinary degree, providing many adults with their first date, dance, or party with adult peers. Since the dating–engagement–marriage sequence tends to start at a much later time for organization members than for people of normal stature, the sequence of events is usually accelerated. The sharing of common problems such as short stature and loneliness tends to override the usual role of similarity of values in the process of mate selection.[61,85]

Short-statured individuals do not typically seek out other dwarfed individuals, as this tends to focus attention on themselves when they are often unwilling to accept their condition. The initial encounter with another dwarfed individual may be a shock, for in such encounters the dwarfed individual is forced to recognize and acknowledge his or her own condition. When a member of the Little People of America approaches another dwarfed individual to discuss the organization, the nonmember often becomes embarrassed and attempts to avoid the encounter. Both the threat of acknowledging one's condition and the threat of acknowledgment by others produce fear. The same response may be found among relatives of the dwarfed individual. When members of the Little People of America attempt to visit the home of a nonmember, they are often refused admittance by the parents. The discredit of the stigmatized individual, shared in part by the relatives, may help to explain such actions by these parents.[23,61,85]

Mental Deficiency

Mental deficiency is discussed in Chapter 13. Unless a syndrome is invariably associated with mental retardation, especially of severe degree, the spectrum of possible outcomes should be kept clearly in mind. It is best to handle each situation on an individual basis when providing some perspective for the family. Some parents associate mental retardation with a vegetative state of developmental arrest. They need to know that many retarded children grow, develop, and learn, although at a slower rate. Some parents may not know that developmental and psychological tests become more predictive with advancing age or that the functioning of many retarded individuals depends more on socialization than on intelligence quotient. Some parents do better when they have hope that the child will "grow out of it," even though this is unrealistic. Although professionals tend to regard such denial as an ominous sign, it is not necessarily so, because such parents sometimes resist the pejorative label of retardation but actually understand their child's capabilities very well.[20]

For a particular syndrome in which mental deficiency may or may not be a feature and, if present, is known to vary widely in degree, the possibility of retardation in the infant should not be discussed with the parents unless there is almost absolute certainty that their baby is damaged. Faulty prediction can alter the parental expectations for the child and hence the parent–child relationship, perhaps masking potential abilities. In this connection, a high-risk nursery study has shown that neonatologists and neurologists made correct predictions of normality and abnormality in complicated high-risk infants only 50% of the time. Because of the appropriateness of uncertainty in some cases, the developmental level of the child can be indicated—perhaps reinforcing parental observations—without giving a firm prognosis.[20,36]

Cancer

When cancer is diagnosed, universal concerns surface, including fear of death, morbidity associated with treatment, fear of recurrence, fear of abandonment, and loss of functional ability, social values, self-esteem, economic competence, and familiar role behavior. These concerns may be augmented or diminished by the particular type of neoplasm and its location, the stage of the life cycle during which the tumor arises, a history of previous tumors, and the presence or absence of a family history of cancer. In counseling cancer-prone families that should be monitored for possible development of neoplasia, the clinician should exercise caution to avoid engendering either a cancer phobia or hypochondriasis that may give rise to feelings of fatalism, denial, or crippling apprehension.[40,84]

Craniofacial Anomalies

Among the body parts, the face serves as a major source of communication, reflecting the emotions, character, and personality of an individual. Self-concept is formed, in part, by one's own, and other's, reactions to facial features and facial expression. A person with a craniofacial malformation may receive negative social messages, resulting in lowered self-esteem. The closer a defect is to an individual's communication channels, such as the eyes or the mouth, the smaller the defect needs to be to throw a participant in the exchange off balance.[22] The severity of facial disfigurement is not necessarily proportional to the degree of psychic stress it engenders in affected individuals or to the kinds of adjustments they make; factors such as parental attitudes, the individual's own personality, and the social setting play a stronger role.[41] A particularly comprehensive and sensitive review of psychological studies of the effects of craniofacial anomalies and reconstructive surgery is that of Pertschuk.[51] In children with craniofacial anomalies, the Draw-A-Person test may reveal a distorted body image (Fig. 14-5). Excessive denial is frequently used as a coping mechanism, especially among severely malformed children.[4,47] In the study of Lefebvre and Munro,[38] patients with craniofacial anomalies usually rated themselves as being *less* malformed than did either their parents or members of the craniofacial team.

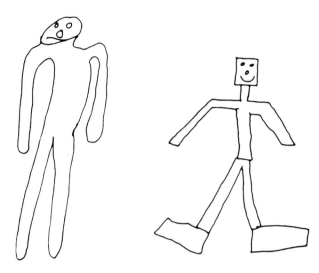

Figure 14-5. Left: *Draw-A-Person* test by an 11-year-old boy with hemifacial microsomia. Right: *Draw-A-Person* test repeated 6 weeks later following surgery to correct facial asymmetry. Note striking change in body image. From Murray et al.[47]

Belfer and his coworkers[4,47] have hypothesized four stages in the modification of body image in malformed children undergoing reconstructive surgery for complex craniofacial anomalies such as mandibulofacial dysostosis and Crouzon syndrome. The first stage, the decision to undergo surgery, represents the beginning of the dissolution of what, for many children, has been pathologic denial. The timing of the complex decision to undergo surgery is based on self-recognition, emotional state, parental and peer group pressure, social awareness, and the surgeon's assessment of reconstructive potential. During the second stage, the operative experience, the reality of physical intervention is acknowledged by the child. The third stage, the immediate postoperative period, is characterized by pain and swelling with *increased* distortion of the face. The period constitutes a psychological crisis in which the decision to undergo surgery and the hoped-for changes are reassessed. Previous psychological defenses are disrupted, leading to introspection and acknowledgment of the previously existing malformation. During the final stage, the reintegration period, the psychological defenses are reorganized, resulting in increased intellectual freedom, reordering of social priorities, and an upsurge in interpersonal relationships.

Denial as a coping mechanism can be abandoned after body image change.[4] The change in body image does not necessarily correlate with the degree of anatomic improvement.[47] In the study of Lefebvre and Munro,[38] patients rated themselves as being more attractive postoperatively than did either their parents or members of the craniofacial team. In general, a high degree of satisfaction has been reported with the results of craniofacial surgery by patients, surgeons, and psychiatrists.[38,47] Contraindications for reconstructive surgery include patients whose request for surgery is vague, patients whose request is obviously in response to parental pressure, and patients who are clearly irrational.[38]

Genital Anomalies

For the infant with genital ambiguity, it is important to establish proper diagnosis and the sex of rearing as soon as possible after birth. However, sex assignment must be delayed until all necessary tests have been completed. In the 11-and 21-hydroxylase–deficient forms of congenital adrenal hyperplasia, fertility is of decisive importance. Such infants should be reared as females regardless of the degree of masculinization of the external genitalia. In such patients the internal genitalia and gonads are those of a normal female, and, with the proper reconstructive surgery, patients can attain the total function of the female, including reproduction. Male sex assignment is obvious in isolated hypospadias, isolated cryptorchidism, and males with hernia uteri inguinale. All other conditions with genital ambiguity are associated with sterility,* and the sex of rearing should be based on assessment of whether the phallus ultimately can result in a penis that is adequate for coitus. Assigned sex need not necessarily agree with chromosomal or gonadal sex, but should agree with the morphology of the surgically corrected external genitalia. Hormonal sex should be properly regulated at puberty.[12,65,77]

For the infant with genital ambiguity, a team approach is essential. Members of the team should include a gynecologist, urologist, pediatrician, endocrinologist, geneticist, and psychiatrist. The facts should not be hidden from the new parents. Explanations should be geared to their intellectual and emotional capacities to understand. It is often useful to equate ambiguous genitalia with being *sexually unfinished*, using embryonic diagrams to show the development of the genital tubercle and labioscrotal swellings. The parents should be counseled that their child can expect normal psychosocial development regardless of the sex of rearing chosen. Birth announcements should be deferred and, if legally possible, the first name should be withheld from the birth certificate until sex assignment can be made. Alternately, names suitable for either a boy or a girl, such as Chris, Leslie, or Pat, might be considered. Once sex has been assigned, the parents should be convinced that the decision for their baby was the only possible one. Gender role should be reinforced by whatever psychological measures are necessary. Residual uncertainty in their minds may have an adverse influence on the child. Openness about the problem within the immediate family should be encouraged and seems preferable to living with the fear that one day the family skeleton will be let out of the closet. The affected child will eventually need an explanation to rationalize the need for medical check-ups, later hormonal therapy, possible further surgery, and even later counseling about parenthood, adoption, and the like.[12,46,65,77]

In sex assignment or reassignment of newborns or young infants, there is some latitude in choice because psychosexual identity is still undifferentiated. Reassigning sex in a child who is already differentiated psychosexually is hazardous and should be undertaken only with preliminary psychiatric preparation and follow-up. An older child with a peniform clitoris raised as a boy serves as an example; since surgical repair to produce a functional penis is not possible, it is sometimes worth the psychological risk involved to reassign the child's sex as a girl. The resultant psychosexual adjustment may be questionable, but will not be any worse than adjustment as a male and is likely to be much better. Reassigning the sex of a hermaphroditic child is much easier in those instances in which the child's psychosexual identity itself is ambiguous or incongruous with current sex assignment.[46]

For the male infant with a micropenis, a short course of early testosterone therapy may enlarge the penis to normal size for his age. The likelihood of

---

*With the possible exception of 5α-reductase deficiency and some cases of true hermaphroditism.[16]

success is high when the micropenis is caused by primary testicular insufficiency, as in XXY Klinefelter syndrome, or secondary testosterone deficiency, as in Prader-Willi syndrome. Enlarging the penis to normal size during infancy may facilitate acceptance of the child by the parents, not only in cases of isolated micropenis, but also in syndromes with micropenis in which mental deficiency is part of the picture.[27,66]

Delay in the onset of puberty and continued persistence of sexual infantilism can be associated with psychopathology. The more obvious the defect, the more likely the personality adaptations are to be distorted.[32] In individuals with XXY Klinefelter syndrome, the presence of a small phallus, small testes, and gynecomastia may have profoundly disturbing effects on body image and ability to function as a male both sexually and socially.[37]

STUDIES OF SPECIFIC SYNDROMES

Four general types of psychosocial studies are found in the literature: (1) the effects of cultural differences in perception[18,29,80]; (2) the effects of dysmorphic conditions on patients and their families, e.g., osteogenesis imperfecta[62]; (3) the effects of craniofacial anomalies and their surgical correction[1,4,8,35,38,41–43,47,51–53] (discussed previously); and (4) behavioral characteristics of specific syndromes, which are considered in this section.

Behavioral phenotypes are patterns of behavior in many or most patients with specific syndromes.[82] Turk and Hill[82] have recommended several categories for describing each condition: intellectual functioning, speech and language, attention deficits, social impairments, and other behavioral disturbances (e.g., lip biting in Lesch-Nyhan syndrome). To date, the most extensive research of a behavioral phenotype has been carried out on patients with fragile X syndrome.[2,28,31,45,81] Studies of the behavioral characteristics of various dysmorphic syndromes are listed in Table 14-1. Sometimes certain features may be present in only a minority of patients with a given syndrome that cannot properly be considered a behavioral phenotype. Nevertheless, such features need to be described and explained. A good example is tuberous sclerosis in which autism and hyperactivity occur more frequently and more severely than in the general population.[32a]

CRITIQUE OF PSYCHOSOCIAL STUDIES

More systematic psychosocial research is needed in the future. Sophisticated social science methodologies are available, and many genetics services have large patient pools from which to draw subjects.

A great deal of research in the field to date has been anecdotal in nature. Furthermore, some papers suggest approaches based on *good common sense* that, with further repetition in various authoritative sources, become *truth* when, in fact, well-controlled studies for proper evaluation are needed. Finally, some studies suffer from problems such as small sample size, biased sampling that does not permit generalization, inappropriate sampling that lumps too many different disorders together, generalization from one condition to others thought to be similar when they may not be, and stereotyped or typologic conclusions about disorders with characteristics that are variable and spectral in nature.

Table 14-1. Behavioral Characteristics of Some Dysmorphic Syndromes

Syndromes	References
Turner syndrome	Downey et al.[15]
	Silbert et al.[64]
Klinefelter syndrome	Bolton and Holland[7a]
	Mandoki et al.[44]
	Ratcliffe et al.[55]
	Ratcliffe et al.[56]
	Stewart et al.[71]
XYY	Ratcliffe et al.[56]
	Schiavi et al.[60]
	Witkin et al.[88]
Fragile X syndrome	Bailey et al.[2]
	Hagerman and Silverman[28]
	Hodapp et al.[31]
	Mazzocco et al.[45]
	Turk[81]
Down syndrome	Blackwood et al.[7]
	Oliver and Holland[48]
	Pueschel et al.[54]
	Whalley[87]
Prader-Willi syndrome	Cassidy[9]
	Donaldson et al.[14]
	Greenswag[26]
Angelman syndrome	Clayton-Smith[10]
	Jolleff and Ryan[34]
	Penner et al.[50]
	Robb et al.[58]
Velocardiofacial syndrome	Golding-Kushner et al.[24]
Smith-Magenis syndrome	Colley et al.[11]
de Lange syndrome	Barr et al.[3]
	Fraser and Campbell[19]
	Gadoth et al.[21]
	Hawley et al.[30]
	Johnson et al.[33]
	Shear et al.[63]
Rubinstein-Taybi syndrome	Stevens et al.[70]
Williams syndrome	Bellugi et al.[5]
	Dilts et al.[13]
	Gosch and Pankau[25]
	Gosch and Pankau[25a]
	Udwin and Yule[83]
	Tew[78]
Sotos syndrome	Rutter and Cole[59]
Fetal alcohol syndrome	Streissguth[73]
	Streissguth et al.[76]
	Streissguth[75]
	Streissguth[74]
Tuberous sclerosis	Hunt and Dennis[32a]
Dubowitz syndrome	Parrish and Wilroy[49]
Oculocerebrorenal syndrome of Lowe	Kenworthy and Charnas[35a]
Straussberg partial alopecia syndrome	Straussberg et al.[72]

Long-term studies should be carried out for many specific syndromes with emphasis on the problems of adaptation and with specific suggestions about the ways in which affected individuals and their families may best cope. Longitudinal studies are also needed to evaluate medical or surgical intervention in various disorders with emphasis on treatment timing and on changes observed in the personalities of affected individuals. Finally, the effects of syndrome labeling on families should be studied, especially in provisionally unique pattern syndromes in which specific labels cannot be applied and in conditions in which patients have been mislabeled, necessitating a change of labels.

REFERENCES

1. Andreasen NC, Bardach J: Dysmorphophobia: Symptom or disease? *Am J Psychiatry* 134:673–676, 1977.
2. Bailey A, Bolton P, Butler L, LeCouteur A, Murphy M, Scott S, Webb T, Rutter M: Prevalence of the fragile X anomaly amongst autistic twins and singletons. *J Child Psychol Psychiatry* 34:673–688, 1993.
3. Barr AN, Grabow JD, Matthews CG, Grosse FR, Motl ML, Opitz JM: Neurologic and psychometric findings in the Brachmann-de Lange syndrome. *Neuropädiatrie* 3:46–66, 1971.
4. Belfer MD, Harrison AM, Murray JE: Body image and the process of reconstructive surgery. *Am J Dis Child* 133:532–535, 1979.
5. Bellugi U, Bihrle A, Jernigan T, Trauner D, Doherty S: Neuropsychological, neurological, and neuroanatomical profile of Williams syndrome. *Am J Med Genet Suppl* 6:115–125, 1990.
6. Bentovim A: The impact of malformation on the emotional development of the child and his family. In Berry CL, Poswillo DE, (eds): *Teratology—Trends and Applications*. Berlin: Springer-Verlag, 1975, pp 223–233.
7. Blackwood DHR, St Clair DM, Muir WJ, Oliver CJ, Dickens P: The development of Alzheimer's disease in Down's syndrome assessed by auditory event-related potentials. *J Ment Defic Res* 32:439–453, 1988.
7a. Bolton P, Holland A: Chromosomal abnormalities. In Rutter M, Taylor E, Hersov L (eds): *Child and Adolescent Psychiatry: Modern Approaches*. Oxford: Blackwell Scientific, 1994.
8. Campis LB, DeMaso DR, Twente AW: The role of maternal factors in the adaptation of children with craniofacial disfigurement. *Cleft Palate Craniofacial J* 32:55–61, 1995.
9. Cassidy SB: Prader-Willi syndrome. *Curr Probl Pediatr* 14:1–55, 1984.
10. Clayton-Smith J: Clinical research on Angelman syndrome in the United Kingdom: Observations on 82 affected individuals. *Am J Med Genet* 46:12–15, 1993.
11. Colley AF, Leversha MA, Voullaire LA, Rogers JG: Five cases demonstrating the distinctive behavioural features of chromosome deletion 17(p11.2) (Smith-Magenis syndrome). *J Pediatr Child Health* 26:17–21, 1990.
12. Conte F, Grumbach MM: Pathogenesis, classification, diagnosis, and treatment of anomalies of sex. In DeGroot LJ (ed): Endocrinology. Vol 3. New York: Grune & Stratton, 1979, pp 1317–1351.
13. Dilts CV, Morris CA, Leonard CO: Hypothesis for development of a behavioral phenotype in Williams syndrome. *Am J Med Genet Suppl* 6:126–131, 1990.
14. Donaldson MDC, Chu CE, Cooke A, Wilson A, Greene SA, Stephenson JBP: The Prader-Willi syndrome. *Arch Dis Child* 70:58–63, 1994.
15. Downey J, Ehrhardt AA, Gruen R, Bell JJ, Morishima A: Psychopathology and social functioning in women with Turner syndrome. *J Nervous Ment Disord* 177:191–201, 1989.
16. Drash PW: Psychologic counseling: Dwarfism. In Gardner LI (ed): *Endocrine and Genetic Diseases of Childhood*. Philadelphia: WB Saunders, 1969, pp 1015–1022.

17. Drotar D, Baskiewicz A, Irvin N, Kennell J, Klaus M: The adaptation of parents to the birth of an infant with a congenital malformation. A hypothetical model. *Pediatrics* 56:710–717, 1975.

18. Fisher NL: Ethnocultural approaches to genetics. *Pediatr Clin North Am* 39:55–64, 1992.

19. Fraser WI, Campbell BM: A study of six cases of the de Lange Amsterdam dwarf syndrome, with special attention to voice, speech and language characteristics. *Dev Med Child Neurol* 20:189–198, 1978.

20. Freeman RD: Psychological management of the retarded child and the family. *Pediatr Ann* 2:53–58, 1973.

21. Gadoth N, Lerman M, Garty B-Z, Shmuelewitz O: Normal intelligence in the Cornelia de Lange syndrome. *Johns Hopkins Med J* 150:70–72, 1982.

22. Goffman E: *Encounters: Two Studies in the Sociology of Interaction.* Indianapolis: Bobbs-Merrill, 1963.

23. Goffman E: *Stigma: Notes on the Management of Spoiled Identity.* Englewood Cliffs, NJ: Prentice-Hall, 1963.

24. Golding-Kushner KJ, Weller G, Shprintzen RJ: Velo-cardio-facial syndrome: Language and psychological profiles. *J Craniofac Genet Dev Biol* 5:259–266, 1985.

25. Gosch A, Pankau R: Letter to the Editor: "Autistic" behavior in two children with Williams-Beuren syndrome. *Am J Med Genet* 53:83–84, 1994.

25a. Gosch A, Pankau R: Longitudinal study of the cognitive development in children with Williams-Beuren syndrome. *Am J Med Genet* 61:26–29, 1996.

26. Greenswag LR: Adults with Prader-Willi syndrome: A survey of 232 cases. *Dev Med Child Neurol* 29:145–152, 1987.

27. Guthrie RD, Smith DW, Graham CB: Testosterone treatment for micropenis during early childhood. *J Pediatr* 83:247–252, 1973.

28. Hagerman RJ, Silverman AC: *Fragile X Syndrome: Diagnosis, Research and Treatment.* Baltimore: Johns Hopkins University Press, 1991.

29. Harper DC: Children's attitudes to physical differences among youth from western and non-western cultures. *Cleft Palate Craniofacial J* 32:14–119, 1995.

30. Hawley PP, Jackson LG, Kurnit DM: Sixty-four patients with Brachmann-de Lange syndrome: A survey. *Am J Med Genet* 20:453–459, 1985.

31. Hodapp RM, Dykens EM, Ort SI, Selinsky DG, Leckman JG: Changing patterns of intellectual strengths and weaknesses in males with fragile X syndrome. *J Autism Dev Disord* 21:503–516, 1991.

32. Huffer V, Scott WH, Connor TB, Lovice H: Psychological studies of adult male patients with sexual infantilism before and after androgen therapy. *Ann Intern Med* 61:255–268, 1964.

32a. Hunt A, Dennis J: Psychiatric disorder among children with tuberous sclerosis. *Dev Med Child Neurol* 29:190–198, 1987.

33. Johnson HG, Ekman P, Friesen W, Nyhan W, Shear C: A behavioral phenotype in the de Lange syndrome. *Pediatr Res* 10:843–850, 1976.

34. Jolleff N, Ryan MM: Communication development in Angelman's syndrome. *Arch Dis Child* 69:148–150, 1993.

35. Kapp-Simon KA, Simon DJ, Kristovich S: Self-perception, social skills, adjustment, and inhibition in young adolescents with craniofacial anomalies. *Cleft Palate Craniofacial J* 29:352–356, 1992.

35a. Kenworthy L, Charnas L: Evidence for a discrete behavioral phenotype in the oculocerebrorenal syndrome of Lowe. *Am J Med Genet* 59:283–290, 1995.

36. Klaus MH, Kennell HH: *Maternal–Infant Bonding.* St. Louis: CV Mosby, 1976.

37. Kvale JN, Fishman JR: The psychosocial aspects of Klinefelter's syndrome. *J Am Med Assoc* 193:97–102, 1965.

38. Lefebvre A, Munro I: The role of psychiatry in a craniofacial team. *Plast Reconstr Surg* 61:564–569, 1978.

39. Lewis E: The management of stillbirth: coping with an unreality. *Lancet* 2:619–620, 1976.

40. Lynch HT, Harris RE, Organ CH, Guirgis HA, Lynch PM, Lynch JF, Nelson EJ:

The surgeon, genetics, and cancer control: The cancer family syndrome. *Ann Surg* 1985:435–440, 1977.

41. MacGregor FC: Some psycho-social problems associated with facial deformities. *Am Soc Rev* 16:629–638, 1951.

42. MacGregor FC: Social and psychological implications of dentofacial disfigurement. *Angle Orthod* 40:231–233, 1970.

43. MacGregor FC: *After Plastic Surgery*. New York: Prager, 1979.

44. Mandoki MW, Summer OS, Hoffman RP, Riconda DL: A review of Klinefelter's syndrome in children and adolescents. *J Am Acad Child Adolescent Psychiatry* 30:167–172, 1991.

45. Mazzocco MM, Hagerman RJ, Cronister-Silverman A, Pennington BF: Specific frontal lobe deficits among women with the fragile X gene. *J Am Acad Child Adolescent Psychiatry* 31:1141–1148, 1992.

46. Money J: Psychologic counseling: Hermaphroditism. In Gardner LI (ed): *Endocrine and Genetic Diseases of Childhood*. Philadelphia: WB Saunders, 1969, pp 539–544.

47. Murray JE, Mulliken JB, Kaban LB, Belfer M: Twenty years experience in maxillo-craniofacial surgery: An evaluation of early surgery on growth, function and body image. *Ann Surg* 190:320–331, 1979.

48. Oliver C, Holland AJ: Down's syndrome and Alzheimer's disease: A review. *Psychol Med* 16:307–322, 1986.

49. Parrish JM, Wilroy RS Jr: The Dubowitz syndrome: The psychological status of ten cases at follow-up. *Am J Med Genet* 6:3–8, 1980.

50. Penner KA, Johnston J, Faircloth BH, Irish P, Williams CA: Communication, cognition, and social interaction in the Angelman syndrome. *Am J Med Genet* 46:34–39, 1993.

51. Pertschuk MJ: Reconstructive surgery: Objective change of objective deformity. In Cash TF, Pruzinsky T: *Body Images: Development, Deviance, and Change*. New York: Guilford Press, 1990, pp 237–252.

52. Pertschuk MJ, Whitaker LA: Psychosocial adjustment and craniofacial malformations in childhood. *Plast Reconstr Surg* 75:177–182, 1985.

53. Pertschuk MJ, Whitaker LA: Psychosocial outcome of craniofacial surgery in children. *Plast Reconstr Surg* 82:741–744, 1988.

54. Pueschel SM, Bernier JC, Pezzullo JC: Behavioural observations in children with Down's syndrome. *J Ment Defic Res* 35:502–511, 1991.

55. Ratcliffe SG, Bancroft J, Axworthy D, McLaren W: Klinefelter's syndrome in adolescence. *Arch Dis Child* 57:13–17, 1982.

56. Ratcliffe SG, Butler GE, Jones M: Edinburgh study of growth and development of children with sex chromosome abnormalities. *Birth Defects* 26(4):1–44, 1991.

57. Richardson SA: Attitudes and behavior toward the physically handicapped. *Birth Defects* 12(4):15–34, 1976.

58. Robb SA, Pohl KRE, Baraitser M, Wilson J, Brett EM: The "happy puppet" syndrome of Angelman: Review of the clinical features. *Arch Dis Child* 64:83–86, 1989.

59. Rutter SC, Cole TRP: Psychological characteristics of Sotos syndrome. *Dev Med Child Neurol* 33:898–902, 1991.

60. Schiavi RC, Theilgaard A, Owen DR, White D: Sex chromosome anomalies, hormones and aggressivity. *Arch Gen Psychiatry* 41:93–99, 1984.

61. Scott CI: Medical and social adaptation in dwarfing conditions. *Birth Defects* 13(3C):29–43, 1977.

62. Shea-Landry GL, Cole DEC: Psychosocial aspects of osteogenesis imperfecta. *Can Med Assoc J* 135:977–991, 1986.

63. Shear CS, Nyhan WL, Kirman BH, Stern J: Self-mutilative behavior as a feature of the de Lange syndrome. *J Pediatr* 78:506–507, 1971.

64. Silbert A, Wolff PH, Lilienthal J: Spatial and temporal processing in patients with Turner's syndrome. *Behav Genet* 7:11–21, 1977.

65. Simpson JL: Diagnosis and management of the infant with genital ambiguity. *Am J Obstet Gynecol* 128:137–145, 1977.

66. Smith DW: Male genital defects in patterns of malformation. *Birth Defects* 14(6C):57–67, 1978.

67. Smith DW: *Recognizable Patterns of Human Malformation.* Second Edition. Philadelphia: WB Saunders, 1976.

68. Solnit AJ, Stark NH: Mourning and the birth of a defective child. *Psychoanal Study Child* 16:523–537, 1961.

69. Spriestersbach DC: *Psychosocial Aspects of the "Cleft Palate Problem."* Iowa City: University of Iowa Press, 1973.

70. Stevens CA, Carey JC, Blackburn BL: Rubinstein-Taybi syndrome: A natural history study. *Am J Med Genet Suppl* 6:30–37, 1990.

71. Stewart DA, Bailey JD, Netley CT, Park E: Growth, development, and behavioural outcome from mid-adolescence to adulthood in subjects with chromosomal aneuploidy: The Toronto study. *Birth Defects* 26:131–188, 1991.

72. Straussberg R, Regenbogen L, Goodman RM: A newly recognized partial alopecia syndrome associated with distinct personality traits. *J Craniofac Genet Dev Biol* 11:3–6, 1991.

73. Streissguth AP: Attention, distraction and reaction time at age 7 years and prenatal alcohol exposure. *Neurobehav Toxicol Teratol* 8:717–725, 1986.

74. Streissguth AP: Psychological handicaps in children with fetal alcohol syndrome. *Ann NY Acad Sci* 273:140–145, 1976.

75. Streissguth AP: The behavioral teratology of alcohol: Performance behavioral, and intellectual deficits in prenatally exposed children. In West J (ed): *Alcohol and Brain Development.* New York: Oxford University Press, 1986, pp 3–44.

76. Streissguth AP, Herman CS, Smith DW: Intelligence, behavior, and dysmorphogenesis in the fetal alcohol syndrome: A report on 20 patients. *J Pediatr* 92:363–367, 1978.

77. Summitt RL: Differential diagnosis of genital ambiguity in the newborn. *Clin Obstet Gynecol* 15:112–140, 1972.

78. Tew BJ: The "cocktail party syndrome" in children with hydrocephalus and spina bifida. *Br J Disord Commun* 14:89–101, 1979.

79. Tew BJ, Laurence KM, Payne H, Rawnsley K: Marital stability following the birth of a child with spina bifida. *Br J Psychiatry* 131:79–82, 1977.

80. Toliver-Weddington G: Cultural considerations in the treatment of craniofacial malformations in African Americans. *Cleft Palate Craniofacial J* 27:289–293, 1990.

81. Turk J: The fragile X syndrome: On the way to a behavioural phenotype. *Br J Psychiatry* 160:24–35, 1992.

82. Turk J, Hill P: Behavioural phenotypes in dysmorphic syndromes. *Clin Dysmorphol* 4:105–115, 1995.

83. Udwin O, Yule W: Expressive language of children with Williams syndrome. *Am J Med Genet Suppl* 6:108–114, 1990.

84. Vaeth JM, Blomberg RC, Adler L: *Frontiers of Radiation Therapy and Oncology.* Vol 14. Basel: S Karger, 1979.

85. Weinberg MS: The problems of midgets and dwarfs and organizational remedies: A study of the Little People of America. *J Health Soc Behav* 9:65–71, 1968.

86. West Nathaniel: *Miss Lonelyhearts.* New York: Avon, 1959.

87. Whalley LJ: The dementia of Down's syndrome and its relevance to aetiological studies of Alzheimer's disease. *Ann NY Acad Sci* 396:39–53, 1982.

88. Witkin HA, Mednick SA, Schulsinger F, Bakkestrom E, Christiansen KO, Goodenough DR, Hirschhorn K, Lundsteen C, Owen DR, Philip J, Rubin DB, Stocking M: XYY and XXY men: Criminality and aggression. *Science* 193:547–555, 1976.

Index

Page references with the suffix 't' refer to tables.
Page references in italics refer to illustrations.